NEURODEVELOPMENTAL DISEASES - LABORATORY AND CLINICAL RESEARCH

DYSLEXIA

PERSPECTIVES, CHALLENGES AND TREATMENT OPTIONS

NEURODEVELOPMENTAL DISEASES - LABORATORY AND CLINICAL RESEARCH

Additional books in this series can be found on Nova's website under the Series tab.

Additional e-books in this series can be found on Nova's website under the e-book tab.

NEURODEVELOPMENTAL DISEASES - LABORATORY AND CLINICAL RESEARCH

DYSLEXIA

PERSPECTIVES, CHALLENGES AND TREATMENT OPTIONS

MARILYN FRAZIER
EDITOR

NOVA BIOMEDICAL
New York

Library of Congress Cataloging-in-Publication Data

ISBN: 978-1-63485-328-6
Library of Congress Control Number: 2016939453

Published by Nova Science Publishers, Inc. † New York

Contents

PREFACE

Dyslexia is a reading disability in which speed and accuracy in word decoding is impaired. It is usually accompanied by spelling and/or arithmetic difficulties. This book discusses the perspectives, challenges and treatment options available for dyslexia. Chapter One reviews dyslexia from its definition and neurobiological basis to the neurophysiology and central auditory processes. Chapter Two examines how dyslexia affects perception of academic performance in elementary school pupils and how it affects their sociometric position in the classroom. Chapter Three reviews dyslexia from an educological perspective. Chapter Four investigates the views of parents of pupils with dyslexia concerning their collaboration with teachers. Chapter Five describes and compares the response of parents and teachers of Brazilian and Italian Dyslexic's students about learning skills. Chapter Six outlines the key findings from the Dyslexia and Multilingualism project (Mortimore et al, 2012) focusing on the challenges and lessons learnt from a research project on a literacy intervention for vulnerable learners with English as an additional language in English primary schools. It also focuses on issues relating to screening processes and assessments used for identifying SpLD/dyslexia within complex multilingual schools. Chapter Seven investigates whether Brazilian students with developmental dyslexia could be classified according with subtypes. Chapter Eight discusses new assessment trends and challenges for the future of dyslexia. Chapter Nine examines complexities and challenges of selecting participants for dyslexia studies. Chapter Ten discusses the use of children's literature as a resource tool to help such children address their psychosocial-emotional needs. Chapter Eleven discusses diagnostic interventions by operationalizing the definition of dyslexia. Chapter Twelve describes the development of the neuropsychological rehabilitation program in executive functions for students with dyslexia. Chapter Thirteen examines the integration of proprioceptive signals, postural control and dyslexia. Chapter Fourteen provides a few remarks on magnocellular responses and brief stimuli. The final chapter provides a synthesis of research concerning the socio-emotional dimension of Dyslexia in adulthood.

In: Dyslexia: Perspectives, Challenges and Treatment Options ISBN: 978-1-63485-328-6
Editor: Marilyn Frazier

Chapter 1

DYSLEXIA: FROM DEFINITION AND NEUROBIOLOGICAL BASIS TO NEUROPHYSIOLOGY AND CENTRAL AUDITORY PROCESSES

Yolanda Peñaloza-López, Paulina C. Murphy-Ruiz and Adrián Poblano
Laboratory of Central Auditory Processes Alterations,
National Institute of Rehabilitation, Mexico City, Mexico

ABSTRACT

In this chapter we analyzed at deep the current definition of developmental Dyslexia, because we propose, following other researchers, that the disorder is the result from alteration of the wide distributed cortical neural network, mainly located near at the area of Broca at the left hemisphere frontal lobe that alters the phonological decoding of language. We presented a discussion of some paper from our work group team and other that supports our hypothesis, and the role of the right hemisphere in the disorder, and some examples of many types of neurophysiological studies that supports our hypothesis.

INTRODUCTION

In last decades, interest to change definition of developmental Dyslexia has prevailing (see Table 1). Reports of some authors defined Dyslexia in children as: a severe, persistent, and unexpected disability for reading and spelling during development [1, 2]. The prevailing definition was published in the fourth version of the Diagnostic and statistical manual of mental disorders (DSM-IV), of the American Psychiatric Association, and was expressed in terms of the exclusion criteria, it means, developmental Dyslexia is an unexpected reading disability in children with no sensory alteration, no cognitive, neither educational, and others difficulties (American Psychiatric Association, DSM-IV) [3]. In the new published version of the Diagnostic and statistical manual of mental disorders (American Psychiatric Association, DSM-5) [4], definition of developmental Dyslexia was included in the Learning disorders section, in the same group with dysgraphia, and dyscalculia, but far from Language alterations, who was in other section.

Table 1. Central auditory processes alterations and developmental Dyslexia

Author/year	Publication	Dyslexia definition or key issues	Statement applies/author	Author proposal
Lyon 1995	DSM-IV APA 1994	"Reading accuracy or comprehension is substantially below that expected given persons chronological age measured intelligence and age-appropriate education. Significant interferes with academic achievement. If sensory deficit is present, reading deficit are in excess".	"There is a critical need to have a valid and operational definition of dyslexia"	"Guidelines for definition: 1-Must be theory driven.2- Supported by substantial body of convergent research and clinical information 3- Based on studies of well described samples of subjects 4- Based on constructs that are relevant to the theory, measured objectively, internally valid. 5- Externally valid and useful".
Ramus F 2004		"Developmental dyslexia is a mild hereditary neurological disorder that manifest as a persistent difficulty in learning to read in children with otherwise normal intellectual functioning and educational opportunities"	"Researchers attempt to characterize dyslexia at genetic, neurobiological and cognitive levels of description and to uncover causal pathways between the different levels"	"The future belongs to longitudinal studies that will be able to trace causal pathways throughout development, across genetic, neurological and cognitive measures, and within each individual subject"
Dawes P Bishop D 2010	TallalP, 2004	"It has been suggested that APD is not a separate disorder but rather is a reflection of an attention deficit, a learning disability or a language disorder"	"The auditory processing problems may co-occur with specific learning disabilities, and some have suggested that they may be causally related"	"Around half of the children diagnosed as having APD would fit a diagnosis of dyslexia or SLI or both. Difference between APD/Dyslexia is quantitative rather that qualitative. APD diagnosed children tending to have more severe problems, including autism"
Snowling, Hulme 2012	DSM-5	Learning Disorders list (3), and Communication Disorders (7)	"The relationships between reading speech and language impairments are not transparent".	"A more inclusive classification of Learning Disorders is required"
Peterson, Pennington 2012	Lyon, Shaywitz, Shaywitz, 2003 Nation, et al. 2010. Rodgers 1983, Shaywitz 1992	"Individual have difficulties with accurate and /or fluent word recognition and spelling despite adequate instruction and intelligence and intact sensory abilities". "Poor comprehenders show adequate decoding but poor understanding for what is read".	"Difficulties with decoding while comprehension is typically relatively intact". "There are other forms of learning disability that impact reading". "Dyslexia represents the lower end of a normal distribution of word reading ability".	"This research underscores the complexity of the development reading difficulties. We need to learn more about the nature of phonological deficit and how this problem interacts k with other linguistic and non-linguistic risk factors, the developmental course of neural abnormalities and how this predict treatment response"

Author/year	Publication	Dyslexia definition or key issues	Statement applies/author	Author proposal
Boets 2014	Ramus 2008 Boetz 2013	"Is a hereditary neurological disorder characterized by severe and persistent reading or spelling impairments despite normal intelligence and adequate schooling"	"Analogous to the adult findings, in dyslexic children the phonological deficit, occurs in short term memory, conscious attention and time constraint, they will not appear in the more basic speech processing measures. A functional connectivity study did reveal reduced communication between Broca's area and left and right superior gyrus temporal in cases with Dyslexia".	"It is required to conduct research with longitudinal design among cases of children with dyslexia continue into adulthood. Meta-analysis of dyslexia studies covering basic speech perception Vs higher order phonological processing".
Finn E et al. 2014	Lyon, Schaywitz, Schaywitz 2003	"Developmental dyslexia or specific reading disability is an unexpected difficulty in accuracy or fluency of reading for the age, intelligence, level of education or professional status of an individual"	"There had been some functional connectivity studies of dyslexia, all of these have examined connections between specific regions chosen a priori. These regions follow the literature of task-based results and represent only a small fraction of the brain".	"Previous studies, potentially fail in provide a complete picture of the connectivity profiles of dyslexic/ non-impaired readers. From 20 000 connections investigated in each dataset, results suggest that dyslexia is not simply attributable to dysfunction in a few specific language nodes".
Bishop 2015	Hallgren 1950	"Development Dyslexia: Some highly intelligent people struggle to learn to read and even if they master basic literacy, they continue as adults to find reading a slow and ponderous process. The popular view of dyslexia is that it is a clear cut-disorder, distinct from normal development, and with specific organic basis. It runs in families".	"Common medical condition run in families but family pedigrees do not usually show a Mendelian pattern of inheritance. Genetic association studies do not find common mutations that cause these illnesses. Instead there appear to be many genetic variants that individually have a small influence on likelihood of developing the condition, but which in combination can create a high risk for disorder".	"We do have much simpler behavioural, familial and environmental measures that do a pretty good job of identifying young children at risk for reading difficulties. It would only be worth developing a genetic screening test if we could demonstrate that it improved sensitivity and specificity when combined, with behavioural measures".
Goswami 2015	Psicología Educativa U Goswami 2015	"Reading acquisition by children is predicted across languages by individual differences in children's awareness of the phonological (sound based) structures of speech"	"Across languages, the core perceptual unit reflecting these sound structures is now thought to be the syllable rather that the phoneme".	"To examine whether early pedagogical practices based on language play or combining motor movements with language or singing to music modulate the activity of the Theta oscillatory networks".

APA American Psychiatric Association 1994.

TOWARD A NEW DEFINITION

From the scope of some researchers, and clinicians, it was observed the wish to change that definition of developmental Dyslexia, because it no manifest the real magnitude of the problem [5, 6, 7]. It is important to remember that Satz and Sparrow, since 1970 [8], called the attention that cases of Dyslexia during development not only presented reading disability, instead, children with Dyslexia presented also no-consolidated right-left handedness, incapability to identify and recognize digits sequences, dyscalculia, verbal and intelligence limitations, visual and auditory perceptual disorders, alterations in motor coordination, among other symptoms. However, these authors hypothesized that alteration is due to a maturation delay, which our group of research attributes to a Central nervous system (CNS) damage restructuring in phonological decoding neural network, and plasticity from rehabilitation therapeutics.

PHONOLOGICAL BASIS OF DYSLEXIA

It is interesting that some authors chose a specific definition of developmental Dyslexia, for example Peterson and Pennington (2012), and other researchers postulated definitions in base to a phonological etiology [6, 7, 9, 10]. In other cases, the neurobiological pathophysiology of Dyslexia, is related to a dysfunction of cerebral connectivity [11, 12], or to a genetic basis of the alteration [1, 9, 13].

Despite that point of view of some researches, search for the etiology of developmental Dyslexia represent a significant advance, but the investigation lines are not concluded at all. In this way, the need to looking for interaction among etiological factors is seen, such as the relationship between phonological basis and cortical connectivity [11, 12].

Boets et al. (2013) evaluated 23 adult subjects with Dyslexia and 22 normal readers by means of functional Magnetic resonance images (fMRI) with a multi-voxel pattern analysis; they searched whether phonological alterations presented by dyslexics could be detected in the cortical phonological network [11]. Authors concluded that adults with developmental Dyslexia had an intact cortical phonological representation, but alterations in these subjects, results from difficulties in access to phonological decoding network.

Pars opercularis, of the area of Broca in the left frontal lobe, are engaged with phonological processing from its connections with primary and association auditory cortex of left temporal lobe by the *arcuate fasiculus* [11]. Boets et al. (2013) found that connection among both auditory areas and left frontal inferior gyrus were deficient in subjects with developmental Dyslexia; moreover, they found a significant relationship of alterations with words reading, non-words reading, spelling, phonological awareness, verbal short memory, and lexical access [11].

Analysis of alterations in neural networks in developmental Dyslexia was studied by fRMI by Finn et al. (2014). They compared groups of normal readers of 8-9, and 19-20 years of age and groups of dyslexics in the same age range, searching for neural networks supporting the complex cognitive task of reading. Authors found: 1. functional decrease of connectivity among the visual pathway and prefrontal regions; 2. reduction of language left hemispheric lateralization; 3. increased connectivity among both limbic regions; 4. reduced connectivity of the visual area engaged with words reading; and 5. persistent of aberrant connectivity with left hemisphere language region. These results confirm the complex interaction of anatomic distant areas of reading, such as frontal and occipital areas [12].

Relationships between language alterations processing and developmental Dyslexia had been the objective of several studies. Bishop (2014) criticized definition and the meaning of developmental language delay, who proposed that the current theory is weak [14]. From his point of view, the denomination problem leads to a lack of understanding among educators and physicians, and highlights the interest in no harm children labeling with the words "specific language disorder" because "specific" is imprecise. An alternative scope to Bishop proposed, that is more harmful no labeling children with specific language disorders for a correct identification and therapeutics, while other views had searched for phonological alterations.

GENETICS OF DYSLEXIA

There are several studies in search for the genetic transmission mechanisms of Dyslexia. There is an agreement that Dyslexia has a family transmission [1]. However, the heritage pattern has not a Mendelian fashion of expression. Instead, it has been proposed that combination of several altered genes, and many environmental factors exposure may results in developmental Dyslexia. Bishop (2015) suggested observe among genotype and phenotype relationships to search in this complex alteration [1]. A separated issue is the study of the participation of co-morbidities with Dyslexia, such as: Developmental language delay, Attention deficit-hyperactivity disorder, or alterations in the Central auditory processes [7]. Taking into account that there is not agreement in Intelligence quotient (IQ), there is not consensus whether heritage alterations in developmental Dyslexia results in high or low IQ [15]. Genetics studies in developmental Dyslexia merits more research in the future with genomic and proteomics techniques.

RIGHT HEMISPHERE ROLE IN DYSLEXIA

The brain processes the information with a double integrated system, in which each hemisphere specializes in some functions, playing a complementary part with the intervention of the inter-hemispheric communication [16]. The left hemisphere specializes in the analysis of verbal auditory stimuli, while the right hemisphere in the non verbal stimuli [17].

The right hemisphere has a predominant function in the analysis of the prosodic information, acknowledge of voices and pitch, natural sounds, melody and auditory patterns [18]. In patients with dyslexia there are some reports of disorder of the central auditory processing, which could be the result of the dysfunctions listed in the theories than try to explain the physiopathology. The Dyslexia has a complex genetic and ambient background, some theories have been described in order to explain the findings, such as the phonological, in rapid auditory processing, the visual, cerebellar and magnocelular theory. There are some reports of cortical and subcortical anatomic malformations, and cellular migration errors. There are findings of different hemispheric activation pattern in the imaging studies.

In a trial with children that have Dyslexia, compared to controls, it was reported a minor achievement in all tests of auditory processing involving right hemisphere functions (frequency and duration patterns, ambient sounds and music) in all children with dyslexia [19]. Shaywitz and Shaywitz (2005) had mentioned that the dyslexia represents a disorder of the language neural system, precisely of the phonologic processing sub-component, so it might be considered that the errors found are not exclusive of the left hemisphere but that are consequence of alterations in the homologue areas of the right hemisphere, that would produce the non verbal stimuli processing to fail [20]. It could be considered that this errors are consequence of the failure in the fast processing of the auditory stimuli, analysis of the temporal processing and of the supra-segmental information [21].

NEUROPHYSIOLOGICAL STUDIES

There are many neurophysiological studies that can be used in the research of children with Dyslexia. The most frequently employed have been: Event-related potentials (ERP), Magnetoencephalography (MEG), and Electro-oculography (EOG). Thus we present here, some examples of contemporary studies carried-out in children with Dyslexia searching for alterations in central auditory processing.

Event Related Potentials (ERP)

Event-related potentials (ERP) are evoked to several kind of stimuli, such as memory recalling, paying attention to different quality of stimuli, identify mismatch, or discriminate to some special features of a stimuli. ERP potentials are recorder at scalp, mainly in frontal locations.

It is widely accepted that Dyslexia is associated with difficulties in phonological awareness and that rhyme awareness in young children can predict later reading success. However, little is known regarding the underlying phonological mechanisms of rhyme awareness in Dyslexia, as rhyme awareness is typically assessed using explicit behavioural measures that represent only the endpoint of processing and often lack phonological distracters. ERP in response to auditory word pairs that differed in phonological overlap during a rhyme judgement task, were given to 6-year-old beginning readers who were at high-risk for Dyslexia (n = 30) and typical-reading age-matched controls (n = 29). ERP were recorded in response to word pairs with various types of phonological overlap, including rhyming (e.g., wall-ball), non-rhyming overlapping (e.g., bell-ball) and non-rhyming unrelated (e.g., sock-ball) word pairs. Both groups of participants exhibited N400 responses for basic rhyme judgements vs. unrelated targets. In the typical-reading controls, the neural responses also differed between the rhyming targets and the non-rhyming overlapping targets, whereas neural responses to these targets were similar in the group of children at high-risk for Dyslexia, indicating difficulties in their ability to process similar-sounding, non-rhyming targets. These findings suggest that typical-reading children solve the rhyme judgement task using a more analytical approach, whereas children who are at high-risk for Dyslexia base their judgments on a comparison of overall sound similarity [22].

It has been suggested that Dyslexia is linked to a core cognitive deficit in phonological awareness tasks and/or in the processing of auditory stimuli. ERP are a valid, objective measure of the accuracy of central auditory processing in humans. For example, Maciejewska et al., assessed Auditory evoked potentials (AEP) in children with Dyslexia. Sixty-six children participated in the study. A set of hearing tests and the recording of complex event-related potentials (ERP) were performed. Mismatch negativity (MMN) and P300 waves were significantly more frequent in the control healthy children than in children with dyslexia, complex ERP were recorded only in 33% of the time, and latencies of complex ERP in children with Dyslexia were greater than latencies in controls. A wide range of MMN and P300 responses was observed across children with Dyslexia. Thus, complex ERP may be useful in determining the condition of audiological functions; however, on their own they are not sufficient to recognize Dyslexia because of the heterogeneity of nonspecific changes [23].

Both ERP studies are in line with our hypothesis, showing the possibility of alteration of the central auditory processing as the core of disturbs in children with a high-risk for Dyslexia, and in children with Dyslexia.

Magnetoencephalography (MEG)

Recording the magnetic fields and currents of the brain suggest that in fluent reading, visual processing occurs around 100 milliseconds after seeing a word, in the postero-medial extrastriate cortex bilaterally. Afterward the first reading-specific signal is detected about 150 msec after word onset in the left inferior occipital and temporal cortex. After 200 msec, the left superior temporal cortex is engaged in semantic processing, and is disrupted in dyslexics around 200 msec after seeing a word [24].

Poor readers perform worse than their normal reading peers on a variety of speech perception tasks, which may be linked to their phonological-processing abilities. Wehner et al., compared the brain activation patterns of normal and impaired readers on speech perception to better understand the phonological basis in reading disability. Whole-head magnetoencephalography (MEG) was recorded as good and poor readers, of 7-13 years of age, performed an auditory word discrimination task. They used an auditory oddball paradigm in which the 'deviant' stimuli (/bat/, /kat/, /rat/) differed in the degree of phonological contrast (one versus three features) from a repeated standard word (/pat/). Both good and poor readers responded more slowly to deviants that were phonologically similar compared to deviants that were phonologically dissimilar to the standard word. Source analysis of the MEG data using minimum norm estimation (MNE) showed that compared to good readers, poor readers had reduced left-hemisphere activation to the most demanding phonological condition, reflecting their difficulties with phonological processing. Unlike good readers, poor readers did not show differences in activation as a function of the degree of phonological contrast. These results were consistent with a phonological account of reading disability [25].

Dyslexia seems to be related to a lack of *Planum temporale* (PT) asymmetry that is accompanied by functional differences to control subjects in both left and right hemispheric temporal regions during language tasks. PT asymmetry has been found to correlate with phonological and verbal skills. In accordance, reduced asymmetry of the magnetic auditory N100m sources in dyslexic adults and in P100m sources in dyslexic children has been reported. These results might also be related to an atypical PT symmetry or the recruitment of other structures than the PT for speech processing in Dyslexia. Paul et al., tried to replicate and extend previous findings by examining a sample of 64 dyslexic and 22 control children with MEG. They measured cortical activity during a passive auditory oddball-paradigm and localized Event related field (ERF) sources evoked by a /ba/. Reduced hemispheric asymmetry in the localization of the auditory N260m was revealed. While control children displayed a typical asymmetrical pattern with more anterior sources in the right hemisphere, this asymmetry was not present for the children with Dyslexia. Further, a correlation between N260m asymmetry and spelling test performance was found. Results suggested that localization of ERF components is indeed an applicative tool for investigating cortical deviances in Dyslexia. A lack of source localization asymmetry in Dyslexia appears to be a robust finding across different samples children and adults with Dyslexia. It appears that cortical auditory language processing is organized differently in subjects with Dyslexia than in controls. This might be the consequence of a more symmetrical PT organization, which in turn might be the result of maturational delay [26].

Electro-Oculography (EOG)

Eye movements can be recorded by means of electrodes in external angles of eyes. It provides information about strategies of lecture. Several authors held that difficulty in learning to read is associated with abnormal eye movements. Great effort has been devoted to the analysis of eye movements in reading. Differences with respect to this typically exhibited by expert readers has been noted. Later, techniques involving measurement of the number and duration of fixations during reading allowed for quantitative comparisons. Poblano et al., investigated text reading time, and number of saccadic and regressive movements by means of EOG, to test if learning disabled children show altered strategies on text reading. Nineteen learning-disabled and thirteen control subjects were included in the study. Learning disabled children showed longer text reading time, and greater number of saccadic and regressive eye movements suggesting alteration in language system decoding used in eye movements for reading [27].

Hatzidaki et al., examined the impact of the effects of dyslexia on various processing and cognitive components (e.g., reading speed and accuracy) in a language with high phonological and orthographic consistency. Greek children with Dyslexia were compared with a chronological age-matched group on tasks that tested participants' phonological and orthographic awareness during reading and spelling, as well as their efficiency to detect a specific target-letter during a sequential visual search task. Children with dyslexia showed impaired reading and spelling that was reflected in slow reading speed and error-prone performance, especially for non-words. Eye movement measures of text reading also provided supporting evidence for a reading deficit, with dyslexic participants producing more fixations and longer fixation duration as opposed to non-dyslexic participants. The results of the visual search task showed similar performance between the two groups, but when they were compared with the results of text reading, dyslexic participants were found to be able to process fewer stimuli (i.e., letters) at each fixation than non-dyslexics. Their findings suggest that, although Greek dyslexics have the advantage of a consistent orthographic system which facilitates acquisition of reading and phonological awareness, they demonstrate more impaired access to orthographic forms than dyslexics of other transparent orthographies [28].

Overall, several studies carried-out by techniques provide support to our hypothesis, that Dyslexia is related to an alteration of the Central auditory processing, their results are in agreement with data from our observation.

CONCLUSION

Advances in developmental Dyslexia scientific research, had been multidimensional. Phonological and genetic basis of the alteration had generated several models that are in study. These models, and the high complexity of the work of the cortical areas engaged with normal reading, and in Dyslexia, highlights the co-morbidity relationships with language pathology in a first plane, but also, with other alterations in neurodevelopment of children. Central auditory processes and neural networks that support the activity, need consolidate evidence of the sensitivity and specificity of their tools, for a more useful practical research, and discover different sub-groups of Dyslexia.

REFERENCES

[1] Bishop D. The interface between genetics and psychology: lessons from developmental dyslexia. *Proc. R. Soc.* 2015; 282: 20143139.

[2] Norton SE, Beach DS, Gabrieli DEJ. Neurobiology of dyslexia. *Curr. Opin. Neurobiol.* 2015; 30: 73-78.

[3] American Psychiatric Association. Diagnostic and Statistical Manual of Mental Disorders, 4th edition (DSM-IV). Washington, American Psychiatric Association. 1994.

[4] American Psychiatric Association. Diagnostic and Statistical Manual of Mental Disorders, 5th edition (DSM-5). Washington, American Psychiatric Association. 2016.

[5] Lyon GR. The definition of dyslexia. *Ann. Dyslexia* 1995; 45: 1-27.

[6] Snowling M, Hulme C. The nature and classification of reading disorders-a commentary on proposals for DSM-5. J. Chil. Psychol. Psychiatry 2012; 53: 593-207.

[7] Peterson R, Pennington B. Developmental dyslexia. *Lancet* 2012; 379: 1997-2007.

[8] Fletcher MJ, Morris DR. Reading, laterality, and the brain: early contributions on reading disabilities by Sara S. Sparrow. *J. Autism Dev. Disord.* 2014; 44: 250–255.

[9] Boets B. Dyslexia: reconciling controversies within an integrative developmental perspective. *Trend Cogn. Sci.* 2014; 18: 501-503.

[10] Goswami U. Neuroscience and education: Can we go from basic research to translation? A possible framework from dyslexia research. *Psicol. Educ.* 2015; 21; 97-105.

[11] Boets B, Op de Beeck H, Vandermosten M, Scott S, Gillebert RC, Mantini D, Bulthé J, Sunaert S, Wouters J, Ghesquiere P. Intact but less accessible phonetic representations in adults with dyslexia. *Science*. 2013; 342:1251-1254.

[12] Finn SE, Shen X, Holahan MJ, Scheinost D, Lacadie C, Papademetris X, Shaywitz ES, Shaywitz AB, Todd-Constable R. Disruption of functional networks in dyslexia: A whole-brain, data-driven analysis of connectivity. *Biol. Psychiatry* 2014; 76: 397-404.

[13] Ramus F, Marshall C, Rosen S, van der Lely H. Phonological deficits in specific language impairment and developmental dyslexia: towards a multidimensional model. *Brain* 2013; 136: 630-645.

[14] Bishop D. Ten questions about terminology for children with unexplained language Problems. *Int. J. Lang Commun. Disord.* 2014; 49: 381–415.

[15] Siegel L. An evaluation of the discrepancy definition of dyslexia. *J. Lear Disab.* 1992; 25: 618-629.

[16] Taylor K, Regard M. Language in the right cerebral hemisphere: Contributions from reading studies. *News Physiol. Sci.* 2003; 18: 257-261.

[17] Jamison H, Watkins K, Bishop D, Matthews P. Hemispheric specialization for processing auditory nonspeech stimuli. *Cerebral Cortex* 2006; 16: 1266-1275.

[18] Tompkins CA. Right hemisphere communication disorders: theory and management. San Diego: *Singular Publishing Group* 1995.

[19] Murphy-Ruiz PC, Peñaloza-López YR, García-Pedroza F, Poblano A. Right hemisphere and central auditory processing in children with developmental dyslexia. *Arq. Neuropsiquiatr.* 2013; 71: 883-889.

[20] Shaywitz S, Shaywitz B. Dyslexia (specific reading disability). *Biol. Psychiatry* 2005; 57: 1301–1309.

[21] Olivares-García MR, Peñaloza-López YR, García-Pedroza F, Jesús-Pérez S, Uribe-Escamilla R. Identificación de la lateralidad auditiva mediante una prueba dicótica nueva con dígitos en español y de la lateralidad corporal y orientación espacial en niños con dislexia y en controles [in Spanish]. *Rev. Neurol.* 2005; 41:198-205.

[22] Noordenbos MW, Segers E, Wagensveld B, Verhoeven L. Aberrant N400 responses to phonological overlap during rhyme judgements in children at risk for dyslexia. *Brain Res.* 2013; 1537: 233-243.

[23] Maciejewska B, Wiskirska-Wosniaka B, Swidzinski P, Michalak M. Assessing auditory processing disorders in children with developmental dyslexia using auditory cognitive event related potentials. *Folia Phoniatr. Logop.* 2013; 65: 129-135.

[24] Salmelin R, Helenius P, Service E. Neurophysiology of fluent and impaired reading: a magnetoencephalographic approach. *J. Clin. Neurophysiol.* 2000; 17: 163-174.

[25] Wehner DT, Ahlfors ST, Mody M. Effects of phonological contrast on auditory word discrimination in children with and without reading disability: a magnetoencephalographic (MEG) study. *Neuropsychologia* 2007; 45: 3251-362.

[26] Paul I, Bott C, Heim S, Eulitz C, Elbert T. Reduced hemispheric asymmetry of the auditory N260m in dyslexia. *Neuropsychologia* 2006; 44:785-94.

[27] Poblano A, Cordova de Caballero B, Castillo I, Cortés V. Electro-oculographic recordings reveal reading deficiencies in learning disabled children. *Arch. Med. Res.* 1996; 27: 509-512.

[28] Hatzidaki A, Gianneli M, Petrakis E, Makaronas N, Aslanides AM. Reading and visual processing in Greek dyslexic children: an eye-movement study. *Dyslexia* 2011; 17: 85-104.

In: Dyslexia: Perspectives, Challenges and Treatment Options ISBN: 978-1-63485-328-6
Editor: Marilyn Frazier

Chapter 2

SOCIAL ASPECTS OF DYSLEXIA: A CASE OF TRANSPARENT ORTHOGRAPHY

Jiri Jost[1,*], Helena Havlisova[1], Iva Mrkvickova[2], Zuzana Bilkova[3] and Tomas Mrkvicka[4]

[1]University of South Bohemia, Faculty of Education, Department of Psychology, Ceske Budejovice, Czech Republic
[2]University of South Bohemia, Faculty of Education, Department of Czech Language and Literature, Ceske Budejovice, Czech Republic
[3]University of South Bohemia, Faculty of Education, Department of Psychology, Ceske Budejovice, Czech Republic
[4]University of South Bohemia, Faculty of Economics, Department of Statistics and Applied Mathematics, Ceske Budejovice, Czech Republic

ABSTRACT

Aim. To examine how dyslexia affects perception of academic performance in elementary school pupils and how it affects their sociometric position in the classroom.

Method. Participants consisted of more than 200 pupils from Grade 3 to 7 from five elementary schools in the Czech Republic (of whom 89 pupils had been diagnosed with dyslexia). Variables: reading test, IQ (Raven), phonological awareness test, morphological awareness test, SPAS (Student's Perception of Ability Scale measuring general abilities, mathematics, reading, spelling, graphomotor skills, and self-confidence), L-J sociometric test (Long-Jones), Locus of Control Test.

Results. The total score in self-esteem (SPAS) in dyslexics was lower than in controls. Dyslexics with higher intellectual performance achieved higher scores in self-esteem. Differences between dyslexics and controls were insignificant in the areas of mathematics and self-confidence.

Morphological awareness had a greater impact on academic self-concept in dyslexics than phonological awareness. This finding may be specific to the Czech language

* Corresponding author: Jiri Jost, Faculty of Education, Dukelska 9, 37001 Ceske Budejovice, Czech Republic, E-mail: jost@pf.jcu.cz, phone: +420 387 773 218, fax: +420 387 773 192.

environment as an environment which places moderate phonological but significantly higher morphological demands on the reader. Thus, reading level and spelling tend to be determined by morphological awareness.

Like tended to increase with reading performance across the entire sample of participants. Pupils who were liked and received recognition and awards were those who were all-round versatile performers. This is in line with Euro-American cultural values mediated via education and upbringing. However, reduced reading performance did not necessarily lead to reduced self-esteem or reduced like. Dislike correlated negatively with like. This finding was favourable since it reduced the likelihood of fragmented pupils, i.e., those who were assessed as being both liked and disliked. This ambivalence can be a sign of personality disorder or other disorders, the presence of which we considered unlikely in our dyslexic group.

In the Locus of Control Test, we found an insignificant difference in index internality between the dyslexics and controls. The result showed that dyslexics were developing in a desired direction towards self-regulation and did not perceive themselves as victims of fate.

Conclusion. Dyslexia affects self-concept, especially its academic component, and the sociometric status of students with the disorder at Czech elementary schools. Care for dyslexics must therefore be geared towards their own disorder and socialisation. Dyslexia does not probably constitute a serious risk to socialisation. Dyslexia becomes a risk if combined with other less favourable circumstances, e.g., inappropriate attitudes of teachers, classmates, or family dysfunction.

Keywords: dyslexia, self-concept, self-esteem, popularity, locus of control, transparent orthography

INTRODUCTION

Dyslexia research is focused primarily on identifying and treating root causes. Several theories about dyslexia were suggested over the years, such as cognitively oriented theories (phonological theory, double deficit theory) and neurobiologically oriented theories (magnocellular theory, cerebellar theory). Relatively less attention was paid to social aspects of dyslexia, i.e., how dyslexia affects social development in children, the social status of dyslexics among peers and schoolmates, how dyslexia affects parent-child or teacher-student relationships, the long-term satisfaction and quality of life in dyslexics from childhood to maturity, how dyslexics adapt to work and career, how they relate to work colleagues, dyslexic attitudes to marriage, and dyslexic self-concept, etc. Since social aspects of dyslexia are just as important as identifying and treating root causes of dyslexia, the present study attempts to address some of the previously mentioned issues. This study was conducted in the contemporary Czech environment which is unique for two reasons: 1. Totalitarian ideology is being replaced by democracy. However, this will be a long process since transformation will involve the education of new generations to respect their country, freedom and justice, to be willing to make sacrifices for these values, and to value themselves and their fellow citizens. It is no coincidence that John Dewey named his major literary work *Democracy and Education*. Schools have been allocated the important task of facilitating this transformation. The status of students with specific learning disabilities is changing, as are attitudes to such students. 2. Czech language is known to be phonologically "friendly" and easy to adopt.

Thus, the majority of 1st graders have no problems with sound-letter correspondence and initial reading. The unique characteristics of the Czech language affect the academic life of Czech dyslexics.

What Is Self-Concept?

Self-concept is the complex image an individual holds of themselves which fulfils a number of important functions:

- it allows the individuals to interpret and find meaning in life experiences, and to maintain a coherent image of themselves in relation to the external world;
- it helps to regulate social behaviour and contributes to self-regulation;
- it energises the individuals, allowing them to keep track of their targets and implement their plans;
- it allows the individual to identify with ideals and pursue self.

According to Harter (1999), a leading figure in Self Psychology, terminology related to self-concept can be divided into two groups: 1. self-descriptions (or self-perceptions), and 2. self-evaluations. Self-descriptions or descriptive terms are related to *who I am*. Self-evaluations are related to *what I am like*. Self-evaluations can be expanded to include, e.g., *Am I competent enough at school in general, or in which subjects or groups?* (when self-evaluating competencies in language and mathematics); *Am I popular in class?* (social self-evaluation); *Am I truthful and honest?* (moral self-evaluation); *Am I emotionally warm or cold?* (emotional self-evaluation); *Am I visually attractive and appealing?* (self-evaluation of physical appearance).

Self-Concept Models

In agreement with Harter (1999), there are two kinds of models: (1) one-dimensional, and (2) multi-dimensional. One-dimensional models were introduced in order to understand self-concept. These models operated with only one variable or factor, i.e., general self-concept or global self-esteem. Factor analysis gave rise to multi-dimensional models. In these, self-concept was seen as a multi-dimensional construct because it could be divided into various domains. Self-evaluations tend to be hierarchically organised and individual levels are autonomous. The highest position is occupied by the general self-concept, which behaves independently of lower domains of evaluation. At the lower level of generalisation are the properties of the self which are referred to as academic self-concept and non-academic self-concept. Academic self-concept affects various domains of school life, e.g., self-evaluation of success in mathematics, native language studies and natural sciences. Academic self-concept includes verbal and non-verbal academic self-concept. Non-academic self-concept is derived from the social, emotional and physical domain. Harter studied multi-dimensional self-concept from a developmental perspective, pointing out that high school students were able to distinguish between global self-evaluation and self-evaluation in the sub-domains of school performance. This finding was significant for the study of self-concept in children with learning disabilities because it allowed for a better understanding of their development in terms of socialisation. Multi-dimensional modelling of self-concept revealed a relatively low level of academic self-concept in dyslexics (see meta-analytical study by Zeleke, 2004). In contrast, the general self-concept in dyslexics was shown to be comparable with the control group. Less consistent were findings related to social self-concept, which is related to social status and shows how dyslexic individuals interpret their position among peers and classmates. It also shows how dyslexics feel about teachers and parents, whether dyslexics are made to feel like "outsiders" and whether they are ostracised, ridiculed, and so on. Some studies showed a negative self-concept in dyslexics (20% of studies; Zeleke, 2004), but most studies (70%; Zeleke, 2004) state significant difference between dyslexic and control groups.

Harter (1999) found that in 13 studies examining the relationship in adolescents between global self-esteem and sub-domains, an average correlation of physical self-esteem and global self-esteem (.65) was followed closely by academic performance (.48). Academic performance played a significant role in global self-esteem, and this finding was significant for people with dyslexia, making dyslexia a potential risk factor to self-concept and global self-esteem.

The additive model of self-esteem. Self-esteem has two major sources (Harter, 1999): (1) skills and abilities in a particular area which the individual interprets as important; (2) social recognition received from others viewed as important (e.g., parents, teachers, classmates, peers). Both sources have an accumulative effect on self-esteem (hence this is called the additive model). Harter (1999) found the lowest self-esteem in individuals with significantly reduced competence in a particular field and the absence of the support of others. The highest self-esteem was found in individuals who had a high level of competence in a particular field and also had a high level of support from social circles. Using the additive model, Harter suggested a typology for individuals building their self-esteem: (1) individuals who build their self-esteem using competencies as well as support from social circles; (2) individuals who build their self-esteem using competencies only, ignoring support from social circles; and (3) individuals who build their self-esteem using social circles, ignoring competencies.

The additive model can be successfully applied to self-esteem in dyslexics. Dyslexics are likely to fail in language competencies and orthography, and therefore seek to find self-worth in the support of others. According to the additive model, dyslexics experience difficulties achieving high levels of self-esteem in comparison to their typically developing peers. If social support is lacking, dyslexics will fall to lower levels of self-esteem more easily than the control group, with negative consequences on self-regulation. Dyslexics are more likely to develop learned helplessness and depression. Harter (1999) found high correlation (from .72 to .80) between self-esteem and depression in older children and adolescents in nonclinical samples. Low self-esteem was associated with overt manifestations of depression, while high self-esteem was associated with positive moods and joy. Reduced competencies together with poor social support increased the likelihood an individual would have low self-esteem which would result in depressive moods.

The looking-glass-self-model depicting the individual's opinions and evaluations of themselves and of people in their environment, has several domains: opinions and evaluations from (1) parents, (2) teachers, (3) classmates, and (4) friends. Not all of these sources of evaluation affect the formation of self-concept in the same way. According to Harter (1999), in younger children, the opinions and evaluations of their parents carry the most weight. In female and male adolescents, the opinions and evaluations of classmates and peers carry the greatest weight.

Locus of Control

The locus of control is related to the perceived source of control over one's own behaviour. The term was first used by Julian Rotter who distinguished dual source control: internal and external (Rotter, 1966). People with an internal source of control are strongly convinced their actions will lead to a set goal. The achievement of a goal is attributed to one's own behaviour and the amount of effort taken. People with an external locus of control, however, are convinced that effect is a result of chance, luck or the interference of others. Self-evaluation in people with an external locus of control is usually lower (Anderson et al., 2005; Ashby et al., 2002). These people believe they do not have control over their environment, so they become passive and wait, and they do not believe in themselves or others. They feel incompetent, skeptical, and have high levels of anxiety and depression. In contrast, people with an internal locus of control perceive themselves as responsible for their actions. Academically, they are more successful, more competitive and much more socially active. They also have a more positive feeling of self-perception, they feel healthier and have higher internal motivation. In terms of interpersonal relationships, people with an external locus of control are characterised as less competent and dexterous (Martin et al., 2005). When problems arise, people with an internal locus of control are more active, suggest possible solutions and create new relationships in order to solve their problems. People with an external locus of control, however, seek to escape problematic situations or wait, passively, without searching for solutions, until the situation resolves itself.

Many studies have shown how perception of self-control affects self-respect, motivation and academic results (Frederickson and Jacobs, 2001; Neff and Vonk, 2009). Students with a high internal locus of control achieve, on average, higher grades and have higher self-evaluation associated with feelings of happiness and optimism, than students with a high external locus of control.

Locus of control and self-handicapping. Some people are afraid of failure so they unconsciously protect their self-esteem by arranging things in ways so as to be able to attribute failure to a higher force. Their locus of control is external. This is the same as learned helplessness, i.e., perceived absence of control over the outcome of a situation. Dyslexia may cause dyslexic individuals to have an external locus of control. Continuous and long-term stress or disability in the form of a learning disability provokes an unconscious response in the dyslexic individuals during which their failures are attributed to a higher force, i.e., dyslexia. In this way the dyslexic individuals are freed from responsibility, from the obligations and expectations of important others (parents, teachers, classmates). They are also freed from their own aspirations (to succeed in competitions with others, to meet their own requirements and resolutions) and thus escape problematic life situations in which they find themselves through no fault of their own. They rid themselves of unpleasant tensions and do not feel threatened that their self-esteem will drop and that they will feel inferior in the eyes of others. Orientation towards the external locus of control has, in this sense, a positive effect on mental health: it protects the individual against chronically negative emotions that could jeopardise the integrity of his/her self-concept.

Social Aspects of Dyslexia from a Lifelong Perspective

Longitudinal studies focused on the longevity of dyslexics are few. They include a study by California's Frostig Centre (Raskind et al., 1998). Authors of this study observed the development of dyslexics in order to understand how dyslexia affects their personal lives and social status. The 20-year observational study began with a total of 206 children and ended with only 41 young adults of which 14 were women and 27 men. The average age of the examined persons at the end of the 20 year study was 32 years (age range 28-35 years). Development was evaluated using the score of psychosocial adaptation which contains the following aspects: 1. Work and education, 2. Family, 3. Health, and 4. A pro-social way of life (independent of social institutions, good behaviour, no addition to alcohol, drugs, gambling, etc., absence of criminality, prostitution and promiscuity). The authors divided the entire sample (N = 41) into two groups: successful (n = 21) and unsuccessful (n = 20). Members of the successful group outscored the other group in psychosocial adaptation. They had higher education, more qualified employment and felt happier; and were less frequently registered as unemployed. Existentially (finance, housing conditions), they were independent and tended to have their own families. In terms of health, both physical and psychological, both groups were comparable. Similarly, occurrences of substance addiction, including alcohol and criminal behaviour, were equal in both groups and occurred rarely. In terms of personality traits, the successful group was characterised by higher self-esteem, greater activity, perseverance, emotional stability, ability to plan and higher motivation to succeed. In contrast, the characteristics of the unsuccessful group were at the opposite end of the scale. The authors collectively dubbed the aforementioned characteristics as attributes of success. Their influence on psychosocial adaptation score was great - it was estimated they influenced variance to 75%.

Social and emotional problems in dyslexics are usually examined via cross-sectional studies, involving data collected from a population at one specific point in time. Unlike longitudinal studies, data in cross-sectional studies are not collected over a long period of time. The researchers do not need to wait until their subjects pass through a developmental stage during which an expected problem crystallises.

Scot et al. (1992) studied successful adult dyslexics and found the following to be crucial for successful adaptation: (a) early diagnosis and treatment, which encompasses reading, writing, spelling as well as social intervention, examining relationships with peers and parents; (b) identifying and developing abilities in which the child can excel and thus compensate for defective performance in reading and language, as well as education towards general confidence and self-esteem.

Hellendoom and Ruijssenaars (2000) interviewed 27 Dutch dyslexic adults aged 20 to 39 years. More than half reported feelings of strangeness and ostracism from school age until obtaining employment. They felt misunderstood by others who were non-empathetic to their problems. They were intensely self-conscious about their own social awkwardness.

McNulty (2003) conducted a 20-year study of socio-emotional development in 12 American adult dyslexics aged 25 to 45 years. All completed secondary education. Eight of them completed tertiary education. Despite their diagnosis of dyslexia, in some cases combined with ADHD, their academic history was good. And this was McNulty's intention - to examine the socio-emotional aspects of dyslexia in individuals who had more or less normal development. McNulty chose the difficult method of narrative analysis, combining narratives into a single, generalised narrative containing both positively and negatively perceived events. The structure of the narrative was similar to the structure of a theatrical work: exposition, collision, crisis, peripetia and epilogue. It was found that dyslexics began experiencing problems in relation to self-esteem much earlier than school age. The first awareness of feelings such as "there is something wrong with me" were formed alongside speech, impaired attention and impaired sensory-motor coordination during toddler and preschool age. At school age, participants had already experienced trauma associated with repeated failure in public (e.g., reading in front of the class), and all participants shared a feeling of inferiority and bitterness ("I'm stupid" or "I'm lazy"). Their social environment was experienced as either supportive and helpful (Pygmalion Effect) or as negative (ridicule from classmates and/or misunderstanding from teachers and parents, resulting in thoughts about transferring to a special needs school environment). Each participant tried to cope with the emotional experiences related to specific learning disabilities, sought compensation and adapted to school and extracurricular life. Despite the fact that all participants succeeded in their professional lives, they still carried persistant feelings of uncertainty and reduced self-confidence.

Significant contributions to research on the social aspects of dyslexia have been made by meta-analytic studies (Burden, 2008; Zeleke, 2004). Zeleke (2004) gathered together 28 analytical studies on self-concept in dyslexics and typically developing students. The studies pointed out the difference between general self-concept and academic self-concept. Academic self-concept represents a specific area of self-concept which is not necessarily generalised and included in the overall assessment of oneself. Zeleke compared academic self-concept in dyslexics and a control group and found significantly reduced values of academic self-concept in dyslexics in 80% of the comparative studies. In contrast, general self-concept in dyslexics was comparable to the control group in 70% of the studies compared. Similarly, Burden (2008) observed that academic self-concept was a function of educational strategies and significantly improved or worsened depending on the level of support the dyslexic individual received. Thus, academic self-concept can be expected to rise in children with learning disabilities if they learn coping strategies and receive sufficient socio-emotional support from teachers, parents and classmates. The growth of academic self-concept in turn enhances proficiency and performance.

Burden (2008) was concerned with surveying research on the relationship between dyslexia and self-concept in the last 20 years. His work shows that dyslexics have a higher number of emotional and behavioural problems than typically developing children. These problems include emotional withdrawal, anxiety, depression, anger, ostracism, ridicule to which they are exposed, aggressive reactions, and an impaired social position in peer groups. The relationship between dyslexia and emotional and behavioural problems, however, is not straightforward. Not all dyslexics experience the same problems to the same degree. Some dyslexics are in terms of psychosocial adjustment successful. Thus, understanding the relationship is imperative for effective prevention, intervention and proper treatment of dyslexic children.

Study by Matejcek and Vagnerova. The most comprehensive study addressing the social aspects of dyslexia is the work of the now deceased Z. Matejcek and his student M. Vagnerova (Matejcek and Vagnerova, 2006). Matejcek was the Vice President of the

International Academy for Research in Learning Disabilities, and the founder of care for dyslexics in the Czech Republic. Matejcek and Vagnerova divided problems into four areas: 1) subjective problems affecting dyslexic self-concept, 2) parental attitudes to dyslexic children, 3) attitudes of teachers to dyslexic students, and 4) attitudes of classmates to dyslexic students. PAQ (Rohner's Parental Acceptance Questionnaire) was used to measure the welfare of dyslexic children. It was found that there was a decrease in welfare in dyslexic children in comparison to the general population. Dyslexic children felt more hostile, pessimistic, inferior and emotionally liable. These findings were independent of the age and gender of the dyslexic child. In comparison with younger children, older children felt more pessimistic and more emotionally liable. However, they were less dependent on the support of others and assessed their own abilities in a less negative way. In girls and female adolescents with dyslexia, compared with boys and male adolescents with dyslexia, a greater tendency of negative self-esteem, emotional instability and pessimism was found. Using SPAS (Student's Perception of Ability Scale by F. J. Boersma and J. W. Chapman), age related differences were found. Younger individuals with dyslexia (2nd to 4th graders) perceived their academic success more positively than older individuals with dyslexia (6th to 8th graders). This finding was attributed to older individuals with dyslexia having been exposed to a greater number of negative experiences, and the presence of stronger self-criticism in older individuals. In both dyslexic groups, young and old, a characteristic dyslexic profile was observed: low self-evaluation of reading tasks compared to significantly better self-evaluation of mathematical ability. It was noted that male dyslexics overscored female dyslexics in global self-esteem. This finding was attributed to a more realistic concept of self-esteem in girls and female adolescents. It was shown that self-esteem in dyslexics expressed using SPAS was closely related to family upbringing. If dyslexic children perceived their parents' upbringing as emotionally warm and socially integrative, the children tended to exhibit higher self-esteem. In terms of the relationship of teacher-dyslexic student, it was found that senior teachers had less empathy and compassion towards dyslexic children, judging them rigidly as less adaptable. It was observed there were differences between upper and lower school teachers in their perception of students with dyslexia. Lower school teachers (1st to 5th grades) did not assess dyslexic students so strictly and their assessment was broader: in addition to qualities students needed for good academic results, they also appreciated qualities necessary for team work. It was found that Czech students, especially those who were younger, perceived classmates with dyslexia as lazy and stupid or morally impaired, and could not understand why such individuals should be provided extra assistance or "benefits." Upper school students, especially those who had completed elementary school (9th graders) already knew that dyslexia was a specific learning disability localised in linguistic performance, and that dyslexics can thrive in non-linguistic subjects, e.g., mathematics. On the basis of their study, Matejcek and Vagnerova argued strongly against the strategy of taboo, i.e., not talking about dyslexia, not disclosing the names of those with the diagnosis so as to protect dyslexic children, who are immature and unable to effectively deal with adverse environmental reactions, from trauma. They came to the same conclusion as other researchers that students with dyslexia are not necessarily immediately rejected by classmates and that their social status depends on how they behave rather than their Czech language ability.

Coping Strategy

Dyslexic students need to cope with repeated academic failure which can seriously compromise their academic self-concept. Coping strategies have a protective function in relation to self-concept. Some dyslexic students create their own beliefs about their own qualities and performance; while others simply demobilise.

According to Harter (1999), self-esteem forms in two ways. One of them is related to activities that are considered important. One such activity is education of which an important and key aspect is reading ability. The main objective of dyslexics in this respect is to bridge the gap between the desired level and reading, and the reading level actually reached. There are two basic strategies for coping with this conflict: (1) increase skill level to meet the required standards; (2) reduce performance standards to the level of current skills, e.g., downplay reading requirements and the importance of reading and education, or enrol at a special needs school. Both strategies are difficult for dyslexics. First of all, their efforts collide with a persistant long-term specific learning disability which is incurable. Secondly, dyslexics live in a culture represented by their parents, teachers and classmates in which reading and education are valued highly.

Self-esteem is also formed using the looking-glass-self-model, where self-evaluation is impacted significantly by the judgements of other people, in particular those on which the individual with dyslexia depends (classmates, friends, teachers and parents). In terms of this perspective, there are two possible coping strategies: (1) concealment of poor performance and failures, thereby preventing and avoiding the negative evaluation of others; (2) seek alternative activities in which they can succeed and achieve positive assessment from others.

Both strategies are in fact complementary. According to Singer (2008), children from approximately age 7 begin differentiating between self-esteem in specific school activities and self-esteem in general (global self-esteem). This is important for coping strategy: search for and develop skills and capabilities in alternative domains and thus achieve positive worth from others. Parental support is also important, as parents help dyslexic children differentiate between general human qualities and those which are more specific, e.g., being reliable and responsible vs. being not able to read properly. From the age of approximately 8, children begin comparing themselves to peers as a means to self-worth. Teachers use this ability to improve academic performance and to encourage competition. However, such an environment is less favourable for dyslexics. Singer (2008) found that for many dyslexics, the defence of self-concept was more important than academic performance. She found less desirable reactions, such as evasive behaviour and attempts to escape comparison with others, in more than half of the monitored dyslexics aged 9-12 years. This behaviour was motivated by the fear of reduced worth in the eyes of others as well as the fear of ostracism and feelings of inferiority. It was found that in more than 80% of monitored dyslexics, there was an enormous effort to stabilise self-esteem and maintain dignity, which as a value was preferred over and above achieving comparable academic level.

The Aim of the Study

The present study attempts to answer the following questions: What is the self-concept of contemporary Czech dyslexics? What is their sociometric status and locus of control in comparison to typically developing individuals? Additionally, whether self-concept in Czech dyslexics is affected by the particularities of the Czech language. In accordance with well-established prevailing findings outlined in the introduction, a working hypothesis was formulated. According to this hypothesis, generally speaking, the psychosocial adaptation of dyslexics will be lower in comparison with the control group, specifically: a) self-esteem of dyslexics will be lower in comparison with the control group, b) sociometric position of dyslexics will be worse in comparison with the control group, and c) the locus of control in dyslexics will be more external in comparison to the control group.

METHOD

Participants

The participants were more than 200 students from 3rd to 7th grade from five elementary schools in the Czech Republic, of whom 89 children were dyslexic. Diagnosis of dyslexia was made using DSM-5 (American Psychiatric Association, 2013). Intelligence was measured by means of the Raven Matrices Test. Reading scores on standardised tests were at least 1,5 standard deviation below the population mean for age. According to DSM-5, "reading problems had persisted for at least 6 months, despite the provision of interventions that target those difficulties. Learning difficulties had not been better accounted for by intellectual disabilities, uncorrected visual or auditory acuity, other mental or neurological disorders, psychosocial adversity, lack of proficiency in the language of academic instruction, or inadequate educational instruction" (American Psychiatric Association, 2013, pp. 66-67). Each dyslexic was assigned at least one classmate; dyslexics and control groups therefore shared a common school environment, i.e., shared curriculum, classmates and teachers.

The families of all children, dyslexics and controls, were functional, cooperating with the school, child counselling centre, paediatrician and/or other institutions dealing with children. None of the families was suffering from poverty or was under social workers' supervision, or involved in any judicial action. The mother tongue of all children and their parents were Czech. Bilingual families were excluded from the sample. Language particulars (bilingualism, naturalisation, or culturally different background) may cause reading or academic performance problems. All children were paediatrically evaluated as healthy; except for common children's diseases, they had no severe diseases. All children were enrolled in regular elementary school programs. All children participated voluntarily and parents gave their informed consent.

The whole sample of participants was divided into five groups according to reading ability. Reading was measured using a standardised test (Matejcek, Sturma, Vagnerova, and Zlab, 1992) and defined as a reading quotient (RQ). RQ is a standard score that is comparable to the IQ score and is based on the number of correctly read words per time unit. The speed and accuracy of reading in the Czech language environment (i.e., a phonetically highly consistent orthographic system) largely correlated to comprehension (Matejcek, 1998a, 1998b). For this reason, the comprehension test was not standardised in the Czech environment. Absence of the comprehension test was therefore not a substantial drawback, even though its application would have been enriching.

Group 1: working name “severe dyslexia”. This group included students whose reading ability expressed using standard score RQ ranged up to sten 3, i.e., RQ < 85; IQ – RQ ≥ 1.5 SD, which translates to a standard score of 23 or more.

Group 2: working name “mild dyslexia“. This group included students whose reading ability expressed using standard score RQ ranged up to sten 3, i.e., RQ < 85; IQ – RQ < 1.5 SD, which translates to a standard score less than 23.

Group 3: working name “below average reading”. This group included students whose reading ability expressed using standard score RQ ranged within sten 4, i.e., 85 ≤ RQ ≤ 92.

Group 4: working name “average reading”. This group included students whose reading ability expressed using standard score RQ ranged within stens 5 and 6, i.e., 93 ≤ RQ ≤ 107.

Group 5: working name “above average reading”. This group included students whose reading ability ranged in and above sten 7, i.e., RQ ≥ 108.

In comparison with group 2, group 1 is marked by IQ-reading discrepancy. Group 1 thus meets the requirements for a traditional, dyslexia discrepancy marker as per DSM-IV-TR (American Psychiatric Association, 2000); see also Keogh, Major, Omori, and Reid (1982). The discrepancy approach in diagnosing dyslexia became a subject of controversy and skepticism (e.g., Linan-Thompson, 2010). For this reason, we earmarked group 2 which was also characterised by below average reading ability, regardless of IQ-reading discrepancy.

The basic characteristics of the groups according to IQ (Raven), reading (RQ) and IQ-reading discrepancy are shown in table numbers 1, 2 and 3.

Table 1. IQ (Raven) in Groups

group	*n*	*M*	*SD*
1 severe dyslexia	48	111	9.2
2 mild dyslexia	21	94	6.8
3 below average reading	31	102	14.1
4 average reading	53	112	11.7
5 above average reading	35	114	13.1

Note. ANOVA: F = 15.16, Df = 187, p = 0.000.

Significant differences between means: group 1 vs. 2, 3; group 2 vs. 3, 4, 5; group 3 vs. 4, 5.

Table 2. Reading in Groups

group	*n*	*M*	*SD*
1 severe dyslexia	64	71	7.5
2 mild dyslexia	25	78	4.7
3 below average reading	35	89	1.9
4 average reading	77	97	4.1
5 above average reading	35	114	7.3

Note. M and SD express reading quotient. Average = 100±15.

ANOVA: F = 371.87, Df = 187, p = 0.000.

Significant differences between means: group 1 vs. 2, 3, 4, 5; group 2 vs. 3, 4, 5; group 3 vs. 4, 5.

Table 3. IQ-Reading Discrepancy in Groups

group	*n*	*M*	*SD*
1 severe dyslexia	48	38.1	10.9
2 mild dyslexia	21	16.3	5.9
3 below average reading	31	12.5	13.8
4 average reading	53	13.6	11.8
5 above average reading	35	0.3	15.0

Note. Reading is expressed by reading quotient. IQ – reading discrepancy ≥ 1.5 SD, which translates to a standard score of 23 or more (1.5 SD = 22.5 of standard score).

ANOVA: F = 53.74, Df = 187, p = 0.000.

Significant differences between means: group 1 vs. 2, 3, 4, 5; group 2 vs. 5; group 3 vs.5; group 4 vs. 5.

Group 1 had working name “severe dyslexia". Their average reading score measured by standardised testing was 1.93 below the population mean for age (i.e., 100 – 71 = 29 → z = 1.93). If IQ score is considered a measure of expected literacy level, then the average IQ-reading discrepancy was 38.1, i.e., $z = 2.54$.

Group 2 had working name “mild dyslexia”. Their average reading score was 1.46 below the population mean for their age (i.e., 100 – 78 = 22 → $z = 1.46$). Their average IQ-reading discrepancy was 16.3, i.e., $z = 1.1$).

Groups 3, 4 and 5 were controls.

Measurements

Intelligence. This was measured using Raven’s IQ test. It was administered individually with no time limit. The result was expressed as an IQ score.

Reading. This was measured using a standardised test and defined as a reading quotient (RQ), see above.

Morphological awareness. A test was constructed for this study and has not been standardised in the Czech Republic. In terms of content validity, we used Czech morphology from the standard elementary school curriculum. The test was administered individually with no time limit. Beside each question which tested one morphological phenomenon, there was a sample answer followed by the actual exam. The subject could obtain a maximum of 65 points where 1 point was equal to 1 correct answer. Split-half reliability: $r = .847$ ($N = 120$, $p = .000$).

Word analysis and synthesis test. This test was administered according to Matejcek (1993). In the analytical part, the researcher gave the child a real word and asked the child to divide the word into letters and maintain their correct order, e.g., pes (= *dog*) → p – e – s. In the synthetic part, the researcher divided a word into letters while maintaining their correct order, and the child was asked to say the word. In both parts, there was a total of 10 words, both monosyllabic and multisyllabic. Performance was evaluated in the following way: if the child reacted correctly during the first attempt (i.e., the child divided the word or re-combined the word without making any mistakes), it received 2 points. If the child failed during the first attempt, the researcher repeated the word. If the child divided or re-combined the word during the second attempt, it received 1 point. If the child failed during the second attempt, it received 0 points and the researcher moved on to the next word. The child could achieve a maximum of 20 points in the analytical part and 20 points in the synthetic part.

Phoneme deletion. This test consisted of two sets of one syllable pseudo words (Caravolas and Volin, 2005). Each set contained 10 pseudo words. In the first set, all the pseudo words had the structure CCVC, while in the second set CVCC. All pseudo words followed Czech phonetic rules and were easy to pronounce. The test was administered as follows: the child heard a pseudo word and was asked to repeat it. One letter was omitted and the child was to pronounce the new pseudo word. In the first set, the child had to omit the second letter (e.g., flin → fin), while in the second set it was the second last letter (e.g., rulp → rup). The maximum possible score was 20.

Spoonerism. This test was administered according to Caravolas and Volin (2005). In the test there were 10 pairs of one syllable pseudo words. The first two pairs of words had the structure CV, while the remaining eight pairs had the structure CVC. Pseudo words - similar to Phoneme Deletion - followed Czech phonotactic rules. The test was administered as follows: the child heard a pair of pseudo words and was to repeat them. The child was then required to transpose the first letters and pronounce the new words (e.g., nor - sep → sor – nep). The maximum possible score was 20.

SPAS (Student´s Perception of Ability Scale by F. J. Boersma and J. W. Chapman) restandardised by Matejcek and Vagnerova (1992).

Sociometric test by N. Long and E. Jones (Popeil, Hollinger, Loschi, and Crawford, 1983).

Locus control test (by S. Nowicki and B. R. Strickland) which was modified for use in the Czech environment by Kotaskova, Ekstromova, and Vajda (1981).

Results

Self-Perception of Scholastic Competence

The total SPAS score for each group is shown in Table 4.

Table 4. Total SPAS Score for Each Group

group	*n*	*M*	*SD*
1 severe dyslexia	64	4.4	2.12
2 mild dyslexia	25	4.2	2.22
3 below average reading	33	5.5	3.69
4 average reading	74	5.9	5.35
5 above average reading	35	7.0	2.29

Note. M a SD express sten scores.

ANOVA: F = 15.54, Df = 230, p = 0.000.

Significant differences between means: group 1 vs. 3, 4, 5; group 2 vs. 3, 4, 5; group 3 vs. 5; group 4 vs. 5.

Both groups of poor readers had lower total SPAS score than the controls. The control group was surpassed by the above average readers whose total SPAS score was significantly higher than others. Table 4 shows an association between reading performance and self-esteem of scholastic competence.

Comparison of the individual SPAS subtests between groups is shown in tables 5 to 10.

Table 5. Subtest General Abilities in SPAS for Each Group

group	*n*	*M*	*SD*
1 severe dyslexia	64	4.1	1.63
2 mild dyslexia	25	3.7	1.94
3 below average reading	33	5.1	2.34
4 average reading	75	5.5	2.29
5 above average reading	35	6.5	2.43

Note. M a SD express sten scores.
ANOVA: F = 10.32, Df = 231, p = 0.000.
Significant differences between means: group 1 vs. 3. 4, 5; group 2 vs. 3, 4, 5; group 3 vs. 5.

The finding in Table 5 is similar to the finding in Table 4. Both groups of poor readers had lower self-evaluation of general abilities in comparison with the controls. The control group was once again surpassed by the above average readers whose total self-evaluation was significantly higher than other groups.

Table 6. Subtest Mathematics in SPAS for Each Group

group	*n*	*M*	*SD*
1 severe dyslexia	64	5.9	2.41
2 mild dyslexia	25	5.1	2.70
3 below average reading	33	6.7	2.43
4 average reading	75	6.3	2.34
5 above average reading	35	6.9	2.13

Note. M a SD express sten scores.
ANOVA: F = 2.83, Df = 231, p = 0.025.
Significant differences between means: group 2 vs. 3, 4, 5.

Self-evaluation of mathematical performance in individuals with severe dyslexia was comparable to the control group. The whole sample of respondents was surpassed by the group with mild dyslexia whose self-evaluation of mathematics was considerably weaker.

Table 7. Subtest Reading in SPAS for Each Group

group	*n*	*M*	*SD*
1 severe dyslexia	64	3.3	1.59
2 mild dyslexia	25	3.6	1.71
3 below average reading	33	4.8	2.01
4 average reading	75	5.2	2.19
5 above average reading	35	7.2	1.37

Note. M a SD express sten scores.
ANOVA: F = 29.4, Df = 231, p = 0.000.

Significant differences between means: group 1 vs. 3, 4, 5; group 2 vs. 3, 4, 5; group 3 vs. 5; group 4 vs. 5.

Table 8. Subtest Orthography in SPAS for Each Group

group	*n*	*M*	*SD*
1 severe dyslexia	64	4.6	1.92
2 mild dyslexia	25	4.5	1.79
3 below average reading	33	5.6	1.81
4 average reading	75	6.1	2.10
5 above average reading	35	6.9	1.78

Note. M a SD express sten scores.
ANOVA: F = 10.69, Df = 231, p = 0.000.
Significant differences between means: group 1 vs. 3, 4, 5; group 2 vs. 3, 4, 5; group 3 vs. 5

The findings in Tables 7 and 8 are similar to those in Table 4. Both groups of poor readers had significantly lower self-evaluation of reading and orthographic performance in comparison with controls. The control group was surpassed by the above average readers whose self-evaluation was higher than all other groups.

Table 9. Subtest Writing in SPAS for Each Group

group	*n*	*M*	*SD*
1 severe dyslexia	64	5.8	1.89
2 mild dyslexia	25	5.3	1.98
3 below average reading	33	6.0	2.09
4 average reading	75	6.4	2.23
5 above average reading	35	6.4	1.59

Note. M a SD express sten scores.
ANOVA: F = 2.02, Df = 231, p = 0.092.
Significant differences between means: group 2 vs. 4, 5.

The group with severe dyslexia had similar results in self-evaluation of writing in comparison to the control group. The group with mild dyslexia did not differ significantly from the group with severe dyslexia, or from the group with below average readers; but lagged markedly behind the groups of average and above average readers.

Table 10. Subtest Self-Confidence in SPAS for Each Group

group	*n*	*M*	*SD*
1 severe dyslexia	64	5.0	1.89
2 mild dyslexia	25	4.6	1.59
3 below average reading	33	5.5	1.85
4 average reading	75	5.7	2.07
5 above average reading	35	5.9	1.83

Note. M a SD express sten scores.
ANOVA: F = 3.92, Df = 231, p = 0.004.
Significant differences between means: group 1 vs. 4, 5; group 2 vs. 3, 4, 5

The group with severe dyslexia had comparable self-evaluation of self-confidence to the group of below average readers, and lagged behind the average and above average readers. In contrast, the group with mild dyslexia lagged significantly behind all the controls.

Factor Analysis of SPAS

The SPAS questionnaire was analysed using factor analysis conducted separately for controls and dyslexics. The results are shown in Tables 11 and 12.

Table 11. Factor Loadings in Exploratory Factor Analysis with Varimax Rotation of Student´s Perception of Ability Scale in the Control Group

subtest	F1	F2
General abilities	**.799**	.352
Mathematics	**.831**	.017
Reading	.308	**.583**
Orthography	.159	**.819**
Writing	.111	**.774**
Self-confidence	**.817**	.355

Note. Factor loadings > .400 are in bold. Two factors were extracted which explain 67% of the total variance. Number of complete cases: 143.

Table 12. Factor Loadings in Exploratory Factor Analysis with Varimax Rotation of Student´s Perception of Ability Scale in the Dyslexic Group

subtest	F1	F2
General abilities	**.728**	.151
Mathematics	**.746**	-.190
Reading	.167	**.729**
Orthography	.023	**.746**
Writing	**.497**	.246
Self-confidence	**.735**	.185

Note. Factor loadings >.400 are in bold. Two factors were extracted which explain 53% of the total variance. Number of complete cases: 89.

Two factors were extracted from the controls and dyslexics. The characteristics of each factor varied in each group, probably due to the presence or absence of a learning disability. In both groups, Factor F1 was saturated with general skills, mathematics and self-confidence; and was given the working name of *general self-esteem factor*. Similarly, in both groups, Factor F2 was saturated with reading and orthography; and was given the working name of *specific verbal self-esteem factor*. In the control group, F2 also included writing, which in dyslexics was located in the more general factor F1. For more details, see Discussion.

Sociometric Position (Like vs. Dislike)

Both dyslexic groups displayed decreased popularity, especially in comparison with average and above average readers. The difference between dyslexics and below average readers was not statistically significant, see Table 13.

Table 13. Popularity Measured Using Test L-J for Each Group

group	*n*	*M*	*SD*
1 severe dyslexia	37	4.4	4.09
2 mild dyslexia	16	3.9	4.11
3 below average reading	21	5.7	3.82
4 average reading	45	6.3	4.16
5 above average reading	25	6.8	3.95

Note. M and SD mark the L-J weighted scores (0 indicates a markedly below average score, 1-5 indicates a slightly below average score, 6 indicates an average score, 7-12 indicates a slightly above average score, 13+ indicates a markedly above average score). The higher the score, the greater the popularity.

ANOVA: $F = 2.44$, $Df = 143$, $p = 0.049$.

Significant differences between means: group 1 vs. 4, 5; group 2 vs. 4, 5.

Table 14. Unpopularity Measured Using Test L-J

group	*n*	*M*	*SD*
1 severe dyslexia	37	9.4	12.19
2 mild dyslexia	16	9.4	9.54
3 below average reading	21	5.0	6.84
4 average reading	46	4.3	6.36
5 above average reading	25	3.2	3.84

Note. M and SD mark the L-J weighted scores (0 indicates a marked below average, 1-5 indicates a slight below average, 6 indicates average, 7-12 indicates a slight above average, 13+ indicates a marked above average). The higher the score, the greater the unpopularity.

ANOVA: $F = 3.35$, $Df = 143$, $p = 0.012$.

Significant differences between means: group 1 vs. 4, 5; group 2 vs. 4, 5.

The finding was similar to Table 13. Both dyslexic groups displayed increased unpopularity, especially in comparison with average and above average readers. The difference between dyslexics and below average readers was not statistically significant.

Locus of Control

Those with severe dyslexia had a comparable internality score with the control group. A lower internality score was found in the group with mild dyslexia, especially when compared with the groups of average and above average readers.

The impact of dyslexic age on internality. The entire sample of dyslexics was divided into two groups: younger (3rd and 4th graders, $n = 37$) and older (5th to 7th graders, $n = 20$). The difference was insignificant ($M_{younger} = 12.7 \pm 3.17$; $M_{older} = 13.6 \pm 2.64$; $t = -1.104$; $p = 0.274$). *M* and *SD* values represent raw scores.

Table 15. Locus of Control: Score of Internality

group	*n*	*M*	*SD*
1 severe dyslexia	41	13.3	2.93
2 mild dyslexia	16	12.4	3.18
3 below average reading	26	14.1	4.16
4 average reading	49	14.6	2.71
5 above average reading	31	14.3	2.54

Note. M and SD values represent raw scores. The higher the score, the higher the internality. ANOVA: F = 2.10, Df = 162, p = 0.083.

Significant differences between means: group 2 vs. 4, 5.

Table 16. Lie-Score in the Locus of Control Test

group	*n*	*M*	*SD*
1 severe dyslexia	41	3.8	1.58
2 mild dyslexia	16	3.1	1.62
3 below average reading	26	3.4	2.45
4 average reading	49	3.3	2.24
5 above average reading	31	2.7	1.98

Note. M and SD values represent raw scores. The higher the Lie-score, the higher the social desirability.

ANOVA: F = 1.41, Df = 162, p = 0.234.

Significant differences between means: group 1 vs. 5.

The highest Lie-score (and tendency towards social desirability) was found in those with severe dyslexia. In contrast, the lowest Lie-score was found in above average readers. The difference between these two groups was significant. The difference between the groups with severe dyslexia and mild dyslexia was insignificant, as was the difference between the group with mild dyslexia and the controls.

The Relationship between Self-Perception of Scholastic Competence (SPAS) and IQ, Reading, Phonological Awareness, Morphological Awareness, Sociometric Position, Internality, Age and Gender

In order to assess the impact of different variables on self-perception, linear stepwise regression was used. The dependent variable was the total SPAS score. The independent variables were IQ, reading quotient, gender, age, sociometric position (indexed using factor extracted via factor analysis of the sociometric test), Locus of control test result including internality score and Lie-score (indexed using factor extracted via factor analysis), morphological awareness and phonological awareness (indexed using factor extracted via factor analysis of already used phonological tests). Regression was conducted separately for groups with dyslexia (Table 17) and the control groups (Table 18) in order to be able to compare final models (see Discussion).

Table 17. Predictors of Dyslexic Self-Perception Measured by SPAS in the Final Linear Stepwise Regression Model

variable	*F*	*p*
IQ	4.79	0.035
Reading (RQ)	5.34	0.026
Gender	8.84	0.005
Like/dislike	3.58	0.066
Morphological awareness	2.82	0.102

Note. RQ = reading quotient.

The reduced phonological variable phono factor (55% of total variance), the like/dislike factor (74% of total variance) and the locus factor (56% of total variance) together with morphological awareness, IQ, reading quotient (RQ), grade, and gender were used in a linear stepwise regression to identify the model with the lowest Akaike Information Criterion (AIC) to examine the best predictive model for the total SPAS score. The final phase of the model included 3 highly significant variables and 2 slightly significant variables. The variable of morphological awareness played an important role in the model since it supported other variables in their significance – without this variable, the other variables were not as significant. Residual standard error: 1,460 on 38 degrees of freedom.

Table 18. Predictors of Control Self-Perception Measured by SPAS in the Final Linear Stepwise Regression Model

variable	*F*	*p*
Grade	47.66	0.000
Morphological awareness	21.52	0.000

Note. The reduced phonological variable phono factor (55% of total variance), the like/dislike factor (74% of total variance) and the locus factor (56% of total variance) together with morphological awareness, IQ, reading quotient (RQ), grade, and gender were used in a linear stepwise regression to identify the model with the lowest Akaike Information Criterion (AIC) to examine the best predictive model for the total SPAS score. Residual standard error: 2,513 on 75 degrees of freedom.

The impact of age on total SPAS score in dyslexic group was insignificant. The groups with severe and mild dyslexia were divided according to age: younger (3rd and 4th graders) and older (5th to 7th graders). In the group with severe dyslexia, the following total SPAS score was found (sten values): $M_{younger} = 4.7 \pm 1.4$ ($n = 33$); $M_{older} = 4.1 \pm 1.8$ ($n = 11$). In the group with mild dyslexia, the following total SPAS score was found (sten values): $M_{younger} = 4.1 \pm 1.5$ ($n = 31$); $M_{older} = 4.2 \pm 1.3$ ($n = 14$). ANOVA: $F = 1.29$; $Df = 88$; $p = 0.281$; No differences between means were significant.

The finding in Table 17 is that morphological awareness played an unusual role in self-evaluation in dyslexic individuals. An attempt to explain this role was conducted by constructing a matrix of different variables which were analysed using factor analysis (Table 19). See Discussion.

Table 19. Factor Loadings in Exploratory Factor Analysis with Varimax Rotation of Self-Perception Measured by SPAS, Sociometric Position, Internality, IQ, Reading, and Phonological and Morphological Awareness in the Dyslexic Group

variable	F1	F2	F3	F4
SPAS	-.109	.087	-.017	**.769**
IQ	**.427**	-.129	.054	**.727**
Reading (RQ)	.312	-**.562**	.297	-**.479**
Like	.160	.163	**.695**	.160
Dislike	-.344	-.291	-**.556**	.027
Lie-score	.152	.050	-**.716**	.379
Internality	-.056	-.170	**.564**	**.552**
Word analysis	.284	**.852**	.085	.045
Word synthesis	.182	**.843**	.251	-.145
Phoneme deletion	**.855**	.045	-.012	-.012
Spoonerism	**.807**	.302	.130	-.027
Morphological awareness	**.552**	.198	**.467**	.222

Note. RQ = reading quotient. Factor loadings > .400 are in bold. Four factors were extracted which explain 68% of the total variance. Number of complete cases: 44.

Self-Perception of Scholastic Competence and Gender

Table 20 shows the general difference between genders: females had lower self-evaluation than males, in both dyslexic and control groups. The presence of dyslexia exacerbated this difference. Female dyslexics had the overall lowest self-evaluation in the entire sample, and lower self-evaluation than the female controls. Male dyslexics had significantly lower self-evaluation than the male controls who had the overall highest self-evaluation in the entire sample. Male dyslexics had significantly lower self-evaluation than the female controls.

Table 20. Total SPAS Score According to Gender

group	*n*	*M*	*SD*
1 Males in dyslexic group	63	4.7	1.24
2 Females in dyslexic group	26	3.5	1.65
3 Males in control group	78	6.6	1.91
4 Females in control group	62	5.5	2.22

Note. M a SD express sten scores.

ANOVA: F = 23.81, Df = 228, p = 0.000.

Significant differences between means: group 1 vs. 2, 3, 4; group 2 vs. 3, 4; group 3 vs. 4.

Discussion

Self-Perception of Scholastic Competence

The self-perception of dyslexics, represented by groups 1 (severe dyslexia) and 2 (mild dyslexia), turned out to be markedly lower than in the controls, represented by groups 3-5 (see Table 4). Self-perception tended to increase with increasing reading ability. Of all groups, those with mild dyslexia (Group 2) scored the lowest in terms of self-perception. However, the difference between groups 1 and 2 was not statistically significant. The results of Group 2 may have been influenced by intelligence, which was lowest in this group, see Table 1. In addition to reading performance, intellectual performance also impacted significantly on academic performance as reflected in SPAS. In those with severe dyslexia (Group 1), it was relatively high intelligence, comparable with the above average readers, which probably contributed to compensating for lowered reading ability.

Similar distribution of total SPAS score, i.e., an increasing trend, from the dyslexic groups to Group 5, was also found in individual subtests (see Tables 5 to 10). Dyslexics had significantly lower self-perception of general abilities, reading and spelling. Dyslexics also had lower self-confidence. The smallest differences between dyslexics and the controls were found in self-perception of writing. Graphic layout in workbooks and written exercises are generally viewed in contemporary Czech schools as “irrelevant” and this is reflected in teacher evaluation. In contrast, reading and spelling are viewed as highly demanding and are therefore closely monitored. A positive finding was in the self-perception of mathematics, where the differences between dyslexics and controls were reduced. Mathematics is a school subject in which dyslexics can succeed and thus compensate their otherwise reduced self-perception of reading and spelling. In the SPAS test battery, differences were observed between the two groups with dyslexia identified as “severe” and “mild”. The group with severe dyslexia had self-perception of mathematics on a par with the control group. In contrast, the group with mild dyslexia had lower self-perception of mathematics than the control group. A probably cause of this was IQ (see Table 1). The IQ of the group with severe dyslexia was comparable to the control group, while the IQ of the group with mild dyslexia was the lowest of all other groups. The group with severe dyslexia was characterised by greater self-confidence, partially comparable with the controls. In terms of self-perception of writing, differences between the group with severe dyslexia and the controls disappeared, i.e., did not reach significance level.

In the factor analysis of SPAS (see Table 11) administered to the control group, two factors were extracted: F1 as a general factor related to assessment of general abilities, mathematics and confidence, and F2 as a specific factor related to the assessment of reading, spelling and grapho-motor performance. Factor analysis of SPAS administered to the dyslexic groups yielded similar results (see Table 12). However, there were some differences. In dyslexics, perception of general abilities was sharply separated from specific linguistic performance; the saturation of factor F2 in dyslexics was 0.151, and 0.352 in the controls. Similar results were obtained for confidence. In dyslexics, F2 was less saturated at 0.185 compared to 0.355 in the controls which indicates the different impacts reading, spelling and writing performance have on the perception of confidence in both dyslexics and controls. The control group perceived reading as part of specific academic performance as well as part of general ability. Dyslexics perceived reading as specific academic performance only, quite distinct from general abilities. This finding was most likely due to a defence mechanism which allows dyslexics to better adapt to school life - they limit their problems to certain school subjects and performances which allows them to live a normal life and be competitive outside the school environment. Writing was perceived by the controls as specific academic performance, quite distinct from general skills. In dyslexics, however, writing shifted from factor F2 to factor F1, thus acquiring the status of general ability, perhaps as compensation for impaired reading abilities. Mathematics was perceived as being part of general abilities in both dyslexics and controls.

Sociometric Position

The trend in popularity score (see Table 13) was dependent on reading performance: a rise in reading performance saw a corresponding rise in general group popularity. The lowest popularity was observed in Group 2 (mild dyslexia). This was probably due to lower IQ. The apparent weakening of reading performance along with lower intellectual performance caused a decline in popularity at primary school. Recognition, appraisal and popularity were reserved for students who were versatile performers, and this is the general value orientation propagated in the Western world. At high school and university, the relationship between popularity and performance is generally not as strong; peers or classmates are judged according to popularity as well as personality traits (e.g., affability, kindness, friendliness, sincerity and willingness to help) and performance characteristics are separate and distinct to personality traits.

A similar trend was observed in dislike (see Table 14). Dyslexics were differentiated from most of the controls, and their average score in dislike was significantly higher. It is an important finding because dislike score includes actively expressed antipathy. It would have been more favourable if dyslexics had obtained a lower like score and a dislike score on a par with the controls. It is not clear to what extent sociometric findings in Tables 13 and 14 were influenced by situational factors (i.e., students with impaired reading performance and/or impaired IQ were disliked) or whether the findings were influenced by deeper, personality characteristics. The question still remains as to whether dyslexia has a formative effect on character traits for which a child is assessed as less popular, and whether this formative effect occurs after the child begins school, or whether dyslexia as a neurobiological unit contains within itself changes to personality. Another matter for discussion is whether dyslexia is separate and distinct to the personality of a person who is already, e.g., unpopular. This would indicate comorbidity of dyslexia and unpopularity. Our findings revealed a markedly close relationship between dyslexia and unpopularity in which coincidence played no role. Dyslexics in our sample came from different schools and different locations in the Czech Republic. Therefore, local relationship problems between dyslexics and their teachers or classmates were less likely. It is unlikely that only individuals with a certain sociometric position, e.g., those who were unpopular, would be predisposed to dyslexia. The most likely explanation is that within a performance-oriented culture, dyslexia induces unpopularity, which could be ontogenetically transitory, or that dyslexia facilitates personality traits due to which the individual becomes less popular. Large variance in our sociometric findings can be explained by the high heterogeneity of dyslexia and its varied typology; Professor Matejcek at the annual seminar of the Czech Dyslexia Association was cited as saying: "There are as many types of dyslexia as there are dyslexics." Unfortunately, our findings did not yield reliable enough results to resolve the question concerning the relationship between dyslexia and sociometric position (like/dislike). This would require longitudinal study of individuals in our sample and may be a subject for further research.

Locus of Control

Table 15 shows reduced internality in Group 2 (mild dyslexia). The trend towards externality in this group could be explained by the combination of impaired reading performance with reduced intellectual performance. The impact of intelligence on internality is probably stronger in dyslexics than the impact of reading ability. Dyslexics characterised by significantly higher IQ and markedly lower reading ability (Group 1) had the same level of internality as the controls. This finding shows that at least a portion of dyslexics were comparable to the controls in terms of auto regulation and that it is possible for dyslexic individuals to develop without developmental delay. The group with mild dyslexia was characterised by significantly lower average IQ (see Table 1). Those with mild dyslexia displayed a higher reading level than those with severe dyslexia (see Table 2). And yet their level of internality was the lowest and significantly differentiated from most of the controls. The impact of age on internality in dyslexics was not significant. The tendency towards internality in young dyslexics (3rd and 4th graders) was comparable to the group of older dyslexics (5th to 7th graders).

In terms of Lie-score (Table 16), there was an increase in value among a portion of dyslexics characterised throughout the sample as having relatively high IQ, the lowest reading ability and highest IQ-reading discrepancy (Group 1). This Lie-score value suggested increased social desirability which probably helped dyslexics in this group to compensate for their disability. The source of increased social desirability within this group of dyslexics could have been induced by the tension between the ideal self and the real self. Dyslexics in this group, characterised by higher IQ, may have been more vulnerable to comparisons with classmates as they were keenly aware of their own disability. The lowest Lie-score was found in the group of above average readers whose intellectual performance was also well above average. Lie-score values in this group could be considered a sign of high developmental maturity reflected in a realistic outlook on oneself, and their self-concept could be defined as being an educational aim for dyslexics.

The Relationship between Self-Perception of Scholastic Competence (SPAS) and IQ, Reading, Sociometric Position, Internality, Gender, Age, and Phonological and Morphological Awareness

Regression analysis, where the dependent variable was the total dyslexic SPAS score (Table 17) identified three strong predictors (IQ, reading and gender) and two weaker, but not weak, predictors (gender and morphological awareness). The same analysis in the controls (Table 18) identified two strong predictors (age and morphological awareness). In the dyslexics, however, age played an insignificant role in their self-concept. Younger dyslexics

(3rd and 4th graders) had comparable total SPAS scores with older dyslexics (5th to 7th graders). However, Matejcek and Vagnerova (2006) found a significant difference when younger dyslexics, comparable in age with the groups in the present study, obtained higher scores than the older dyslexics, also comparable in age with the groups in the present study. This statistical disagreement between our results and those of Matejcek and Vagnerova could have been coincidental. However, Matejcek and Vagnerova conducted their study after the Velvet Revolution (1989) at the turn of the 21st century, while the present study was conducted more than 10 years later. Czech education changed significantly in the time between studies. Thanks to the research conducted by Matejcek and his successors, educators changed their approach to students with dyslexia. Those with dyslexia began to be treated with respect, and special attention was given to their educational needs. They were offered support in order to promote a positive mindset and integrate them into the school environment. Additionally, Professor Matejcek founded child counselling centres which were focused on early diagnosis of dyslexia and its long-term treatment. Part of his work was also to provide support to schools and parents of dyslexic children. It is highly likely that this transformation in pedagogy had a positive impact on the development of self-concept in Czech dyslexics. As a result, older dyslexics were no longer exposed to negative school experiences so their self-concept was comparable to younger dyslexics.

The relationships between self-perception of scholastic competence (SPAS), IQ and reading were characterised in Tables 4 to 10. Of particular interest was the role morphological awareness played in self-perception in Czech students (with and without dyslexia) which is why it will be discussed in greater detail.

The Role of Morphological Awareness in Self-Perception of Scholastic Competence in Czech Dyslexics

Phonological skills in Czech readers are quite different to those in English readers. In the Czech environment, the predictive value of phonological skills in relation to reading was examined by Matejcek and his colleagues (Matejcek and Halamova, 1988). Matejcek and Halamova (1988) replicated a study by Bradley and Bryant (1985) examining the abilities of alliteration and rhyme in preschool children (N = 80, 40 boys and 40 girls). The test was administered twice, with a year between testing. It was found that the order of children in both examinations remained almost unchanged - this result correlated with the findings of Bradley and Bryant (1985), pointing to the high stability of phonological skills over time. The phonological skills test result was then compared with literary performance during school age. The relationship was much weaker than in the Bradley and Bryant study.

An as yet unpublished cross-sectional study by Jost, Mrkvickova, Havlisova, and Mrkvicka investigated the relationship of morphological and phonological skills to reading in Czech students. The sample consisted of typically achieving primary school students in their 3rd and 8th grades. In the study, the students were tested on their phonological awareness, morphological awareness, IQ, and reading ability. The results were processed using hierarchical regression. It was found that morphological awareness had a comparable if not higher impact on reading ability than phonological awareness, and this impact increased with age.

The reason for the different impact of phonological skills on reading ability in Czech students in comparison with English students could be explained by the distinct characteristics of each language (see Matejcek, 1998a, 1998b). Czech is a transparent language in which the spoken and written forms of the language are very similar. Phonological skills required for reading are acquired by most Czech children at preschool age or during 1st grade primary school. As a result, most Czech children in 2nd semester of 1st grade are able to fluently read text appropriate to their mental age. Despite being phonologically easy, the Czech language is morphologically challenging. For this reason, morphological awareness has a comparable if not greater impact on reading ability than phonological awareness.

In the controls (Table 18), it was evident that morphological awareness contributed significantly to self-perception of scholastic competence or academic self-concept. In dyslexics, the finding was "hidden" and morphological awareness contributed to self-perception of scholastic competence implicitly. Phonological awareness in dyslexics receded into the background in terms of its impact on self-perception of scholastic competence or academic self-concept. The most likely explanation is the aforementioned characteristic of the Czech language.

In order to understand the unusual impact of morphological awareness on self-perception in dyslexics, it was necessary to produce a matrix of different variables and analyse it using factor analysis (Table 19). Morphological awareness often behaved as a linguistic characteristic. Additionally, morphological awareness together with phonological tests (Phoneme Deletion and Spoonerism) saturated factor F1. However, at the same time, morphological awareness separated itself from phonological tests and, together with sociometric characteristics and the Locus of control test, saturated factor F3. This analysis allowed the role of morphological awareness in self-perception of scholastic competence or academic self-concept to be explained in two ways:

1) Morphological awareness contributed to reading performance in certain language environments, and this reading ability impacted on the social status of the students in question. Thus, morphological awareness strengthened self-perception of scholastic competence (total SPAS score). In this way, morphological awareness was similar in importance to phonological awareness, however morphological awareness was more important due to the specific characteristics of the Czech language environment which is highly morphologically challenging.
2) Morphological awareness may have its own special function related to personality traits, upon which *like/dislike* is based in the school environment or those which impact on internality/externality. Hypothetically, morphological awareness could contribute to the ability in social interaction to "read" verbal and non-verbal language, allowing the individuals to orientate themselves better in social relationships as well as within themselves, and to better adapt to themselves and social circles, thereby strengthening popularity within their social group and the tendency towards auto regulation (growth of intentionality). All this was reflected according to the hypothesis in self-perception of scholastic competence or academic self-concept of dyslexics in the sample. The link between morphological awareness and sociometric variables (like/dislike), internality/externality and social desirability (expressed using factor F3) allowed dyslexics to build a positive self-esteem which

was relatively independent from reading; factor F4 - self-perception of scholastic competence (SPAS), IQ and internality correlated negatively with reading.

The Role of Sociometric Characteristics (Like/Dislike) and Internality/Externality in Self-Perception of Scholastic Competence

Four factors were extracted using factor analysis (Table 19). Two of these (F3 and F4) could be seen as personality traits. Factor F3 was oriented towards like and internality. A rise in F3 corresponded with a rise in like and a fall in dislike, a stronger tendency towards internality, and a fall in Lie-score, i.e., there was a trend towards a realistic evaluation of oneself. Liked were also those who relied on themselves, were goal-oriented and believed they were in control of their own fate. In contrast, those who perceived themselves as pawns of fate, and waited with patience without attempting to take control, were not liked - just as those who were pretentious, pretending to be better than they truly were, were also not liked. A high Lie-score in dyslexics was probably seen by other classmates as an expression of arrogance and egoism, and provoked within classmates feelings of dislike and antipathy. A high Lie-score in dyslexics was interpreted as compensatory to help dyslexics adapt psychosocially.

F3 correlated positively with like and negatively with dislike; an increase in like corresponded with a decreased likelihood of an increase in dislike. This finding was positive because it reduced the likelihood of the occurrence of a significantly fragmented student, who would be assessed by others as liked and disliked at the same time. This ambivalence is often a sign of personality disorders, the presence of which was unlikely in the present sample of dyslexic children.

Factor F4 was oriented towards self-perception of scholastic competence or academic self-concept. A rise in F4 corresponded with a rise in self-esteem expressed by total SPAS score. F4, like F3, was also saturated with internality/externality. The personality regulator which directed the performance capabilities of the student was the internal locus of control, i.e., the belief in one's own abilities, that one is in control of one's own fate, and that efforts will positively impact on future success. Students who were able to perform successfully strengthened their self-esteem and gained like more easily from other classmates than pupils who were not as strong. These relationships are found within a particular sociocultural environment which values goal-orientation, perseverance and success. This framework for relationships may, however, present some risk for dyslexics who are unable to compete in reading and may therefore fall into the trap of reduced self-esteem, a decline in like, and an undesirable orientation towards an external locus of control. Positive correlation of internality with factor F4 shows that dyslexics in the present sample were led to this positive belief in themselves and positive thinking in general. F4 was also the factor related to cognitive characteristics, intelligence and reading. F4 correlated negatively with reading which is seen as a positive finding: a decline in reading ability does not have to result in a decline in self-esteem or internality. Saturation of F4 with intelligence identified intelligence as significantly impacting self-perception. Individuals most at risk of forming a weak self-perception of scholastic competence or self-esteem were dyslexics whose intelligence was below average. In the factor matrix, like and self-perception of scholastic competence were relatively independent characteristics to reading ability, where reduced reading ability did not necessarily cause reduced self-esteem and/or reduced like. It was a positive finding for dyslexics and supports the Czech school environment.

Self-Perception of Scholastic Competence and Gender

Dyslexic boys had significantly higher self-esteem (total SPAS score) than dyslexic girls (Table 20). The same trend was found in the control group: boys had significantly higher scores than girls. This could suggest that there were differences between genders in the sample of 3rd to 7th graders in how they saw themselves as individuals. Girls tended to be more modest, less arrogant and more self-critical regardless of whether they were dyslexic or not. Boys, on the other hand, regardless of whether they were dyslexic or not, tended to exaggerate. Boys probably find it easier to resolve their problems using escapist strategies, escaping into fantasy, downplaying or rationalising ("a bad mark here, a bad mark there, it's not the end of the world"). Girls tended to experience a problem more deeply and felt more responsible, which resulted in increased depression, pessimism and negative self-evaluation. The same finding was observed by Matejcek and Vagnerova (2006). It can be assumed that these gender-related differences in self-perception have a deeper, neuropsychiatric source and are therefore stable and resistant to environmental influences than attitudes of the public and schools (teachers and classmates) to dyslexics.

CONCLUSION

Dyslexia affects self-concept, especially its academic component, as well as the sociometric position of a student among classmates in Czech elementary schools. Care for dyslexics should therefore be aimed both at the condition itself and socialisation. Dyslexia does not probably present a serious risk for socialisation. Dyslexia is a risk only when it is combined with other less favourable circumstances, e.g., inappropriate attitudes of teachers and/or classmates, or a dysfunctional family environment. The present study observed a turn for the better in the self-perception or self-esteem in Czech dyslexics. This change was attributed to new attitudes of teachers who began respecting the special educational needs of students with dyslexia. Self-perception of scholastic competence and popularity of students with dyslexia were associated in Euro-American culture with reading performance. In the Czech language environment, known to be phonologically simple but morphologically challenging, self-perception or self-esteem of reading performance was affected more by morphological rather than phonological skills.

REFERENCES

American Psychiatric Association (2000). *Diagnostic and Statistical Manual of Mental Disorders*, Fourth Edition, Text Revision. Washington, DC: Amerian Psychiatric Association.

American Psychiatric Association (2013). *Diagnostic and Statistical Manual of Mental Disorders*, Fifth Edition. Arlington, VA: Amerian Psychiatric Association.

Anderson, A. Hattie, J. and Hamilton, R. J. (2005). Locus of control, Self-efficacy, and Motivation in Different Schools. *Educational Psychology, 25*, 517-535.

Ashby, J. S., Kottman, T. and Draper, K. (2002). Social Interest and Locus of Control: Relationship and Implications. *Journal of Individual Psychology, 58*, 52-61.

Bradley, L. and Bryant, P. (1985). *Rhyme and Reason in Reading and Spelling*. Ann Arbor: The University of Michigan Press.

Burden, R. (2008). Is Dyslexia Necessarily Associated with Negative Feelings of Self-worth? A Review and Implications for Future Research. *Dyslexia, 14*, 188-196.

Caravolas, M. and Volin, J. (2005). Baterie diagnostickych testu gramotnostnich dovednosti [The Diagnostic Battery of Literacy Skills]. Praha: IPPP. [In Czech]

Frederickson, N. and Jacobs, S. (2001). Controllability attributions for academic perfomance and the perceived scholastic competence, global self-worth and achievement of children with dyslexia. *School Psychology International, 22*(4), 401-416.

Harter, S. (1999). *The Construction of the Self: A Developmental Perspective*. New York: The Guilford Press.

Hellendoorn, J. and Ruijssenaars, W. (2000). Personal experiences and adjustment of Dutch adults with dyslexia. *Remedial and Special Education, 21*, 227-239.

Keogh, B., Major, K., Omori, G. and Reid, H. (1982). *A System of Marker Variables for the Field of Learning disabilities*. New York: IARLD.

Kotaskova, J., Ekstromova, H. and Vajda, I. (1981). Lokalisace kontroly [Locus of Control]. *Psychologia a patopsychologia dietata, 16*, 483-499. [In Czech].

Linan-Thompson, S. (2010). Response to instruction, English language learners and disproportionate representation: the role of assessment. *Psicothema, 22*, 970-974.

Martin, R., Thomas, G. and Charles, K. (2005). The Role of Leadermember Exchanges in Mediating the Relationship between Locus of Control and Work Reactions. *Journal of Occupational and Organizational Psychology, 78*, 141-147.

Matejcek, Z. (1993). *Dyslexie*. Praha: H+H.

Matejcek, Z. (1998a). Reading in Czech. Part I: Test of Reading in a Phonetically Highly Consistent Spelling System. *Dyslexia, 4*, 145-154.

Matejcek, Z. (1998b). Reading in Czech. Part II: Reading in Czech Children with Dyslexia in a Phonetically Highly Consistent Spelling System. *Dyslexia, 4*, 155-168.

Matejcek, Z. and Halamova, A. (1988). Zkouska rymovani na pocatku skolni dochazky [Test of Rhyme in the Beginning of School Attendance]. *Psychologia a patopsychologia dietata, 23*, 541-548. [In Czech]

Matejcek, Z. and Vagnerova, M. (1992). *SPAS* [Student´s Perception of Ability Scale]. Brno: Psychodiagnostika [In Czech].

Matejcek, Z. and Vagnerova, M. (2006). *Socialni aspekty dyslexie* [Social aspects of dyslexia]. Praha: Karolinum [In Czech].

Matejcek, Z., Sturma, J., Vagnerova, M. and Zlab, Z. (1992). *Zkouska cteni* [Test of Reading]. Brno: Psychodiagnostika. [In Czech]

McNulty, M.A. (2003). Dyslexia and the Life Course. *Journal of Learning Disabilities, 36*, 363-381.

Neff, K. D. and Vonk, R. (2009). Self-Comparison versus Global Self-Esteem: Two Different Ways of Relating to Oneself. *Journal of Personality, 77*, 23-50.

Popeil, P.S., Hollinger, J.D., Loschi, G.A. and Crawford, D.R. (1983). A Sociometric Approach to Understanding Interpresonal Relationships In a Classroom For Emotionally Disturbed Pupils. *The Pointer, 27*, 5-12.

Raskind, M. H., Higgins, E.L., Goldberg, R.J. and Herman, K.L. (1998). Patterns of Change and Predictors of Success in Individuals with Learning Disabilities: Results from a Twenty-Year Longitudinal Study. *Thalamus, 16*, 40-64.

Rotter, J. B. (1966). General expectancies for internal versus external control of reinforcement. *Psychological Monographs, 80*, 1-28.

Scott, M. E., Scherman, A. and Phillips, H. (1992). Helping individual with dyslexia succeed in adulthood: Emerging keys for effective parenting, education, and development of positive self-image concept. *Journal of Instructional Psychology, 19*, 197-204.

Singer, E. (2008). Coping with Academic Failure: A Study of Dutch Children with Dyslexia. *Dyslexia, 14*, 314-333.

Zeleke, S. (2004). Self-concepts of students with learning disabilities and their normally achieving peers: A review. *European Journal of Special Needs Education, 19*, 145-170.

Reviewed by Jaroslav Sturma, Ph.D., the President of the Czech Psychological Society and Director of the Child Centre of Mental Health, Sestajovicka 19, 19800 Prague, Czech Republic, E-mail: jaroslav.sturma@gmail.com

Biographical Sketches

Jiri Jost, PhD

Jiri Jost, born on 1950, completed his PhD studies in educational psychology at Charles University, Prague, Czech Republic. Currently is a faculty at University of South Bohemia, Czech Republic. Professional appointments: head of special educational department at University of South Bohemia. A pupil of prof. Zdenek Matejcek (who is well-known as a founder of the care in individuals with dyslexia in Czech Republic and a former vicepresident of the International Academy for Research in Learning Disabilities, IARLD). His major interests are in learning disabilities and their early diagnosis including eye/gaze tracking methods. He cooperates with Czech Technical University, Prague in the field of development of advanced eyetrackers designed for application in the field of learning disabilities and other neurodevelopmental diagnostical categories. He conducted longitudinal studies concerning predictors of reading development and its deviations. He is a member of the Czech Dyslexia Association, a branch of the International Dyslexia Association. Professional correspondence and personal contacts with foreign experts in the field of learning disabilities, e.g., prof. William Cruickshank, a founder of the IARLD; prof. Dirk Bakker, a head of neuropsychological research in learning disabilities in the Netherlands; prof. George Th. Pavlidis, a former head of Dyslexia and Eye Movement Project at University of Medicine and Dentistry-Rutgers Medical School, New Jersey, USA; prof. Magda Bogdanowicz, University of Gdansk, Poland, a founder of the care in dyslexics in Poland. He worked as a school psychologist for twenty years. Since 2001 he has taught at University of South Bohemia, Czech Republic.

Publications last three years:

Jost, J. (2014). Could pre-school eye movements contribute to diagnostics of reading and/or dyslexia? A longitudinal case study. *Asia Pacific Journal of Developmental Differences* (Chiefeditor: prof. Angela Fawcett), *1*, 224-236.

Brabcova, D., Krsek, P., Kohout, J., Jost, J. and Zarubova, J. (2015). Academic self-concept in children with epilepsy and its relation to their quality of life. *Neurological Research, 37*, 288-294.

Brabcova, D., Zarubova, J., Kohout, J., Jost, J. and Krsek, P. (2015). Effect of learning disabilities on academic self-concept in children with epilepsy and on their quality of life. *Research in Developmental Disabilities, 45-46*, 120-128.

J. Jost, A. Nohavova, and H. Havlisova (Eds.) (2015). *Pedagogicko psychologicka diagnostika* (In Czech) [Diagnostics in Educational Psychology]. Prague: Eduko.

Jost, J., Havlisova, H. and Bilkova, Z. (2015). Ocni pohyby predskolnich deti a diagnostika cteni/dyslexie (In Czech) [Pre-school Eye Movements and Reading/Dyslexia: A Six-year Longitudinal Study]. In J. Jost, A. Nohavova, and H. Havlisova (Eds.), *Pedagogicko psychologicka diagnostika* (In Czech) [Diagnostics in Educational Psychology] (pp. 66-80). Prague: Eduko.

Jost, J., Thein, R., Havlisova, H., Brabcova, D. and Petraskova, V. (2015). Subdeprivace a její obraz ve školním vývoji dítěte (In Czech) [Social-emotional Neglect and Its Image in School Development of the Child]. In J. Jost, A. Nohavova, and H. Havlisova (Eds.), *Pedagogicko psychologicka diagnostika* (In Czech) [Diagnostics in Educational Psychology] (pp. 21-37). Prague: Eduko.

Correspondence address: jost@pf.jcu.cz
Pedagogicka fakulta, Dukelska 9, Ceske Budejovice, Postal code: 37001, Czech Republic

Helena Havlisova, PhD

Helena Havlisova born on 1958, completed her PhD studies in special education at Charles University, Prague, Czech Republic. Currently is a faculty at University of South Bohemia, Czech Republic. Her major interests are in reading development and learning disabilities and their early diagnosis and remedy. She conducted longitudinal studies concerning precursors of reading development and its deviations. Professional Appointment: executive secretary of special educational department at University of South Bohemia.

Publications last three years:

J. Jost, A. Nohavova, and H. Havlisova (Eds.) (2015). *Pedagogicko psychologicka diagnostika* (In Czech) [Diagnostics in Educational Psychology]. Prague: Eduko.

Jost, J., Havlisova, H. and Bilkova, Z. (2015). Ocni pohyby predskolnich deti a diagnostika cteni/dyslexie (In Czech) [Pre-school Eye Movements and Reading/Dyslexia: A Six-year

Longitudinal Study]. In J. Jost, A. Nohavova, and H. Havlisova (Eds.), *Pedagogicko psychologicka diagnostika* (In Czech) [Diagnostics in Educational Psychology] (pp. 66-80). Prague: Eduko.

Jost, J., Thein, R., Havlisova, H., Brabcova, D. and Petraskova, V. (2015). Subdeprivace a její obraz ve školním vývoji dítěte (In Czech) [Social-emotional Neglect and Its Image in School Development of the Child]. In J. Jost, A. Nohavova, and H. Havlisova (Eds.), *Pedagogicko psychologicka diagnostika* (In Czech) [Diagnostics in Educational Psychology] (pp. 21-37). Prague: Eduko.

Correspondence Address: havlis@pf.jcu.cz
Pedagogicka fakulta, Dukelska 9, Ceske Budejovice, Postal code: 37001, Czech Republic

Zuzana Bilkova, PhD

Zuzana Bilkova, born on 1980, completed her PhD studies in psychology of education at Charles University, Prague, Czech Republic. Currently works at Faculty of Education of University of South Bohemia, Czech Republic. Her major interest is in psychology and education of children with ADHD.

Publications last three years:

Jost, J., Havlisova, H. and Bilkova, Z. (2015). Ocni pohyby predskolnich deti a diagnostika cteni/dyslexie (In Czech) [Pre-school Eye Movements and Reading/Dyslexia: A Six-year Longitudinal Study]. In J. Jost, A. Nohavova, and H. Havlisova (Eds.), *Pedagogicko psychologicka diagnostika* (In Czech) [Diagnostics in Educational Psychology] (pp. 66-80). Prague: Eduko.

Correspondence address: bilkova@pf.jcu.cz
Pedagogicka fakulta Jihoceske univerzity, Dukelska 9, Ceske Budejovice, Postal code: 37001, Czech Republic

Tomas Mrkvicka, PhD

Tomas Mrkvicka, born on 1975, completed his PhD studies in probability and statistics at Charles University, Prague. His major interest is in spatial statistics and application of statistics for all kinds of sciences. He organized an invited session from the topic of "Testing in spatial statistics" on the Spatial statistics conference in Avignon, 2015. Currently he works on Faculty of Economics at University of South Bohemia, Ceske Budejovice, Czech Republic.

Publications last three years:

Myllymäki, M., Mrkvicka, T., Seijo, H., Grabarnik, P. and Hahn, U. (2016). Global envelope Tests for spatial processes. *JRSSB* (In print).

Mrkvicka T. (2014). Distinguishing different types of inhomogeneity in Neyman-Scott point Processes. *Methodology and Computing in Applied Probability, 16*(2), 385-395.

Mrkvicka T., Muska M., Kubecka J. (2014). Two step estimation for Neyman-Scott point process with inhomogeneous cluster centers. *Statistics and Computing 24*(1), 91-100.

Correspondence address: mrkvicka.toma@gmail.com

Ekonomicka fakulta, Studentska 13, Ceske Budejovice, Postal code: 37001 Czech Republic.

Iva Mrkvickova, PhD

Iva Mrkvickova, born on 1977, completed her PhD studies in bohemistics at Charles University, Prague. Her major interest is in didactics of Czech language. She also worked as a teacher of Czech language for the Deaf. Since 2009 she has taught at University of South Bohemia, Ceske Budejovice, Czech Republic. She participates in organization of regular sessions of university didactics of Czech language. Her publications treat of teaching Czech language and literature.

Correspondence address: iva.mrkvickova@post.cz

Pedagogicka fakulta, Dukelska 9, Ceske Budejovice Postal Code: 370 01, Czech Republic

In: Dyslexia: Perspectives, Challenges and Treatment Options ISBN: 978-1-63485-328-6
Editor: Marilyn Frazier

Chapter 3

UNDERSTANDING DYSLEXIA FROM AN EDUCOLOGICAL PERSPECTIVE

Arnold Chee Keong Chua
SPD Early Intervention Programme for Infants and Children, Singapore

ABSTRACT

Dyslexia is a reading disability in which speed and accuracy in word decoding is impaired. It is usually accompanied by spelling and/or arithmetic difficulties. Many researchers have postulated their own terms and findings on dyslexia. Right until now, there is still no agreed-upon operating definition of dyslexia as it varies from country to country. In this chapter, the author has proposed using an educological framework to define dyslexia and establish appropriate intervention. The term "educological" is derived from the word "educology" which means "the fund of knowledge about the educational process." Educology comprises of warranted assertions, valid explanatory theories and sound justificatory arguments about the educational process. The educological framework consists of five different perspectives: (1) historical, (2) praxiological, (3) scientific, (4) philosophical, and (5) jurisprudential respectively. Each of the five educological perepectives is further elaborated by its respective models.

Keywords: definition, dyslexia, educology, intervention, theories

INTRODUCTION

The mastery of any language is not easy as it involves four different languaging sub-processes: oracy sub-process: listening and speaking; and literacy sub-process: reading and writing (Thomas, Lawrence, Robert, Glenn, and James, 1974). In almost every country, there is a significant number of children struggling to master the skill of reading, failing which it would result in difficulties in word recognition. Such difficulties, without appropriate intervention given, usually persist into adulthood (Buttner and Hasselhorn, 2011). The term frequently used to describe this phenomenon is usually referred to as developmental reading disability. In the field of learning disabilities, reading disability is the most common condition (Buttner and Hasselhorn, 2011). According to Fletcher et al. (2007), about 80-90% of children have reading difficulties in the special education programmes. This could be attributed to the high demand in reading skills in modern societies (Buttner and Hasselhorn, 2011).

In Singapore, one of the pressing concerns is the growing number of children diagnosed with dyslexia. This rapid increase can be attributed to better awareness among parents and educators and better screening procedures. A big part can also be attributed to the mass media such as television and newspaper reports to raise the awareness of dyslexia. According to the Dyslexia Association of Singapore (DAS, 2009), there is an average of one to two students who could have dyslexia in a class of 40 students with a 10-15% increment in the number of enrolment of individuals with dyslexia. It has been estimated there are about 23000 students with dyslexia, though not all have been diagnosed with this reading disability.

Reading and writing skills are essential in Singapore mainstream education as the examination components include reading comprehension and composition writing. The Singapore Ministry of Education introduced the Learning Support Programme (LSP) since 1992 to Primary One and Primary Two pupils with language learning difficulties so that they do not lag behind their peers. In 2016, all will benefit from School-based Dyslexia Remediation Programme (SDR). SDR was first piloted in 2012 as a two-year intervention programme for Primary 3 and 4 students with weak language and literacy skills at Primary 1 through LSP. For those whose literacy difficulties persist, they would be referred for further assessment and diagnosis by the end of Primary 2. Students who are diagnosed with dyslexia would receive SDR programme when they reach Primary 3 and 4.

Over the decades, there has been a multitude of definitions of dyslexia. Researchers in this field are facing the issue as every country has its own definition. There is still no agreed-upon definition of this reading disability. Perhaps, one of the main difficulties to come to a consensus on the anomaly concerning the definition of dyslexia is the question of inclusivity (Elliott and Grigorenko, 2014). General definitions often invite criticism, which seems to be too inclusive by some while it is considered as too exclusive by others. Since there is no agreed-upon operating definition of dyslexia, this author proposes using an educological framework to define dyslexia and establish appropriate intervention.

The term *educological* is used to refer to a *fund of knowledge about the educational process* and this fund of knowledge is rich in meaning about dyslexia and the intervention strategies (see Harding, 1956, for more details). From the perspective of educology, studying is the set of activities one undertakes to learn something (Fisher, 1996). In other words, educology is not used to study education because educology is not an activity. To study educology, one needs to undertake activities in order to acquire knowledge about education (Christensen, 1981). Educology means "the fund of knowledge about the educational process and it consists of warranted assertions, valid explanatory theories and sound justificatory arguments about the educational process" (see Harding 1951, 1956, 1964, 1965, for detail).

The educological perspective includes five different perspectives: (1) historical (what has been done about dyslexia currently?), (2) praxiological (how effective is the current intervention for dyslexia?), (3) scientific (what evidence to show the existence of dyslexia?), (4) philosophical (what is good, desirable, ethical and sound about the different intervention on dyslexia?), and (5) jurisprudential (what is legally permitted, prohibited and/or required for the different interventions for dyslexia?). The next section of this chapter provides a brief account of these five different educological perspectives on dyslexia.

DEFINING DYSLEXIA FROM THE EDUCOLOGICAL PERSPECTIVE

From the educological perspective, the process of education is a process of teaching and studying some contents within some particular setting with the objective that something valuable will be learned. The author of this chapter would like to adopt the educological perspective as a framework to define dyslexia and establish appropriate intervention as it provides a more holistic and deeper understanding of dyslexia. Figure 1 below shows the five different perspectives based on the framework of educology on dyslexia.

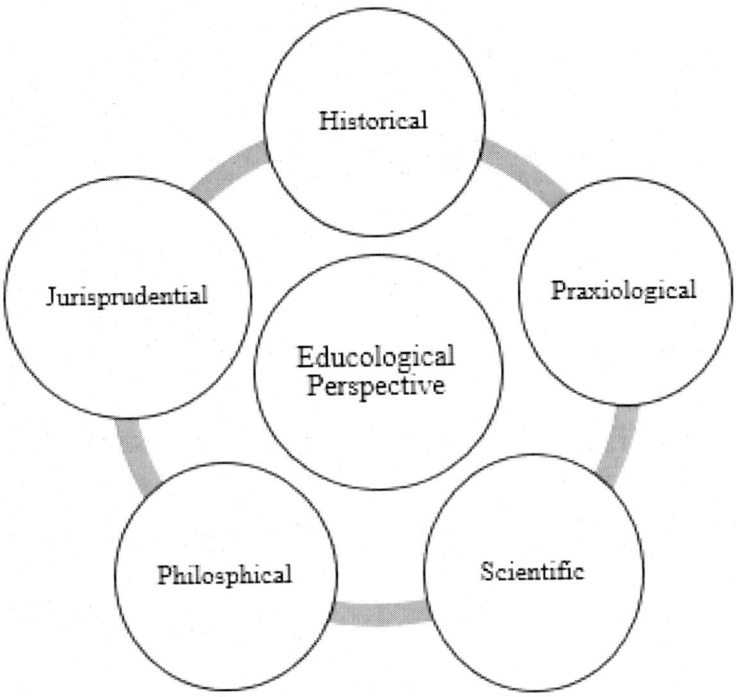

Figure 1. The Five Perspectives of Educological Framework.

Historical Educological Perspective

The historical educological perspective asks what research has been done so far on dyslexia. To understand this better, there are three different perspectives to be considered (see Figure 2):

(1) Medico-historical
(2) Neuropsycho-educational-historical
(3) Sociocultural-historical

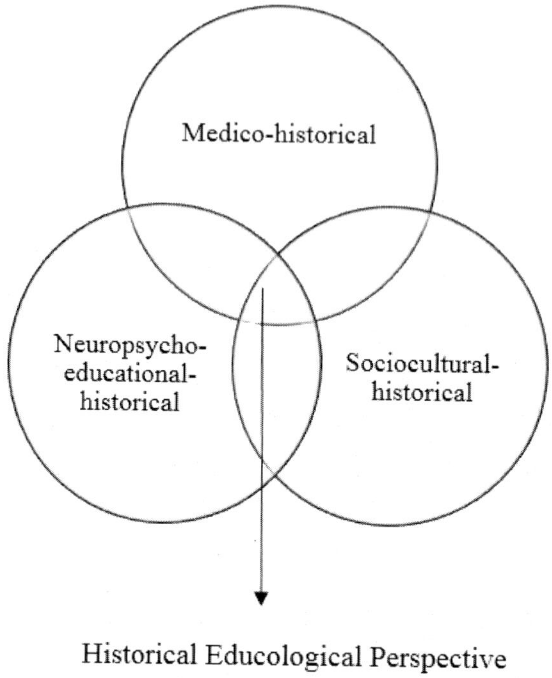

Figure 2. Model of Historical Educological Perspective.

Medico-Historical

The concept of dyslexia was first studied by ophthalmologists and neurologists who described the case of an adult with acquired dyslexia (i.e., loss of reading ability due to a brain lesion). Shortly, another German neurologist, Kussmaul (1877), suggested the term "word blindness" to describe an adult patient with aphasia who had lost his ability to read. Similarly, the term “alexia” was coined by Charcot in 1887 to denote a total loss of reading ability while Bateman (1890) defined alexia as a form of verbal amnesia whereby patients have lost the memory of the conventional meaning of graphic symbols (Soler, Fletcher-Campbell, and Reid, 2009).

The medical perspective of reading challenges continued into 1900. Morgan (1896) wrote a paper on “congenital word-blindness” that described a fourteen years old child who failed to learn to read despite good vision and normal intelligence. Though the boy was good in arithmetic, he was very poor in writing (made mistakes in his own name without noticing until his attention was called for more than once) and spelling and even had poor visual memory (Morgan, 1896). In his paper, Morgan wrote: “The schoolmaster who has taught him for some years says that he would be the smartest lad in the school life if the instruction were entirely oral” (Morgan, 1896, p.1378). Another six cases with two generations of one family were also described by Morgan with strikingly similar symptoms of poor reading and spelling and defective visual memory of letters and words.

Morgan’s work acts as a platform for Dr. James Hinshelwood (b.1859-d.1919), an ophthalmologist and eye surgeon, where Hinshelwood reported two cases of word-blindness in 1902. He described a ten-year old boy with normal vision who could not read words by sight but able to spell words letter by letter. He attributed his reading difficulty to defective visual memory of letters and words (Hinshelwood, 1902). An autopsy on a patient whom he observed for several years, Hinshelwood found that the cause of reading disability was located in the angular gyrus of the brain and he suggested that the core deficit of the disability was visual memory for letters and words. He then advocated that intervention should be focussed to increase visual memory (Hinshelwood, 1902). Both Morgan and Hinshelwood further their research on acquired word-blindness in adults to congenital word-blindness in children.

Neuropsycho-Educational-Historical

An American neurologist, Dr. Samuel Orton, (b.1879-d.1948) was probably the first to recognize that children with reading difficulties often reversed letters and he coined it as *strephosymbolia* (twisted symbols). In addition, he also introduced the term *developmental alexia* to describe these children with reading difficulties (Orton, 1925). A multisensory-type of reading intervention was designed by Samuel Orton and Anna Gillingham in the 1930s known as the Orton-Gillingham (OG) based instruction. This form of intervention was believed that individuals with specific reading difficulties would reap benefits from a more structured teaching using components of sensorial modalities that include visual, auditory and tactile-kinaesthetic elements. Hypothesized by Orton (1937), the OG-based multisensory intervention was believed to circumvent and compensate for "optical reversibility" (seeing letters backwards) and other types of visual perceptual deficits. He theorized that reading difficulties was caused by developmental delay in hemispheric dominance. When evidence started to suggest that most reading difficulties are likely caused by language-based deficits (e.g., weak phonological processing) instead of visual perceptual deficits, the OG-based multisensory interventions requires overcoming for language-based deficits and other visual perceptual deficits.

There has been a substantial advancement in neuroscience and genetics of reading disabilities over the past decade and work in this field offers great assistance in the resolution of the dyslexia debate. An article by Galaburda (1993) reviewed that the neuroanatomic and neuropathologic bases of developmental dyslexia are present in individuals with the reading difficulties. This is evident from the observations of the autopsy brains and experimental animal models that showed problems with cerebral asymmetry, focal developmental disorder that affected the cerebral cortex, and abnormalities in the magnocellular pathway of the visual system (Galaburda, 1993).

Sociocultural-Historical

Many professionals disagree to use dyslexia as a neurological reading disorder as they believed that the label on children might do more harm to them. One of them is Dr. Thomas Armstrong who does not believe in learning disabilities, instead he emphasized on learning differences in which adults should not blame the children for their learning failure due to their neurological impairments. Hence, he used the term "*dysteachia*" to attribute the cause of reading difficulties to poor teaching of educators who tend to focus on the deficits of the children (where they should be looking at their strengths) and adults' stubbornness to adapt their teaching practices to suit the needs of the children (Armstrong, 1987). Children learn best when they do not feel anxious or stressful. If they are being labelled and blamed for their inability to read, write, and spell, then emotional conflicts or fears set in.

However, poor teaching does not necessary cause dyslexia. This author would like to use the term "psychologically induced dyslexia" or "pseudo dyslexia" based on the sociocultural perspective. These terms can be better understood from Manzo's (1987) seminal work on "Conversion Reaction Syndrome (CRS)" which refers to a subconscious process by which deep emotional conflicts or fears which otherwise would give rise to considerable anxiety are put aside by converting them into an external expression of some type" (Manzo and Manzo, 1993, p. 409). CRS originates from a type of somatic disorder known as the conversion reaction. The authors classified conversion into two forms: somatic and physiologic. Somatic conversions generally result in loss of control due to involuntary muscles (Laughlin, 1967). For example, a child with dyslexia will ask to be excused for having stomachache, headache and various complaints from class whenever instructed by his English teacher to read aloud in front of his peers or taking an oral English test with the examiner. Physiologic conversions lead to involuntary muscles control and bodily functions. Children who struggle to read may shows symptoms of poor learning or academic achievements in school which will lead teachers suspecting them of having developmental disabilities. Manzo and Manzo (1993) concurred that "the student, in his preteen whose life is largely influenced by parental rather than peer pressures, wins considerable attention from his parents while reducing his preoccupation with his true emotional conflict and this is achieved at a relatively small cost: namely, not being able to read" (p. 410). In Singapore, societal stress and high expectations placed children to perform well academically from parents and peers could also result in such a pseudo-form of dyslexia. According to Chia (2009), he used the term "*compound term dyslexia-of-idiopathic-origin*" to describe this condition caused by socio-emotional stress.

Praxiological Educological Perspective

It is crucial to assess children at the earliest possible age for any reading and writing disabilities in order to discover dyslexia. Possible and suspected symptoms of dyslexia could be rectified with the provision of early intervention from professionals. Over the years, there are many different intervention approaches in dyslexia such as phonics instructional approach, whole language approach, Fernald approach, Singerland approach, Orton-Gillingham (OG) approach, Response-to-Intervention (RtI), and others.

The praxiological educological perspective focuses on the current intervention strategies and their respective efficacies of dyslexia. Over the years, there has been a wide range of intervention strategies for dyslexia including, but not limited to, Lindamood-Bell Program, Response-to-Intervention (RtI), Alphabetic Phonics, the Orton-Gillingham approach and Project Read, and many others. Among these approaches, the phonics approach which includes the OG-based instruction is the commonly used intervention for dyslexia.

Designed to strengthen both word reading skill and spelling accuracy, the phonics approach is used to help individuals with dyslexia. There has been conclusive evidence to support that phonologically based interventions can help to improve the accuracy of word decoding of individuals with poor word reading (Snowling and Hulme, 2011). The type of instruction differs for both young and old readers with reading difficulties as it depends on the age and current level of reading skills. According to Mather and Wendling (2012), there are five different instructional approaches to teach phonics and they are:

1) Analogy – use of word families to teach unfamiliar words containing rimes (e.g., using *–at* to teach *cat*),
2) Analytic – uses a whole-to-part approach where a known word is used to analyze letter-sound relations and applies to an unknown word (e.g., Using *ou* letter-sound relations from the word "house," unfamiliar words like mouse, cloud, loud, proud is being taught),
3) Embedded - an implicit and unstructured approach within text reading,
4) Phonics through spelling - teach word segmentation into phonemes and select letters that represent each phoneme to spell the word phonetically and write it down
5) Synthetic - uses an explicit part-to-whole approach to teach association between sounds and letters by pronouncing a word by blending sounds together

One example of analytic phonics approach is the Orton-Gillingham program developed by Dr Samuel Orton, Anne Gillingham and Bessie Stillman in the 1930s. The philosophy of the OG-based instruction believes that learners with specific reading difficulties would benefit from a more systematic, multisensory learning using visual, auditory and tactile-kinaesthetic elements and the bottom-up approach in learning to read (Rose and Zirkel, 2007). Foorman and Torgensen (2001) also accentuated the importance of providing an explicit reading instruction with repetitive reading of words with accuracy and fluency for learners at-risk of reading difficulties (Foorman and Torgensen, 2001). These elements are important principles of the OG-based reading methodology and it is believed that learners with reading difficulties can achieve success in learning how to read if they are taught the appropriate reading strategies (Torgensen, 2006).

To date, there has been limited validation of its effectiveness in the evidence-based research studies on the OG-based instruction. Twelve quasi-experimental and experimental studies of OG-based reading instruction yielded positive results in word identification and reading as compared to the control groups of other approaches used (e.g., Wilson Reading System, Project Read, Dyslexia Training Program, Alphabetic Phonics) (Chia and Houghton, 2011; Henry, 1998; Ritchey and Goeke, 2006; Rose and Zirkel, 2007).

Regardless of which phonics instructional approach being used, the instruction given has to be intensive and structured for effective intervention. According to Uhry and Clark (2005), the instructions follow three core principles:

(1) Explicit teaching of letter-sound associations,
(2) Use of preplanned procedures of letter-sound associations, and
(3) Practice letter-sound associations in text and in isolation.

Based on the above three principles, this author has proposed a framework for the praxiological educological perspective on dyslexia (see Figure 3).

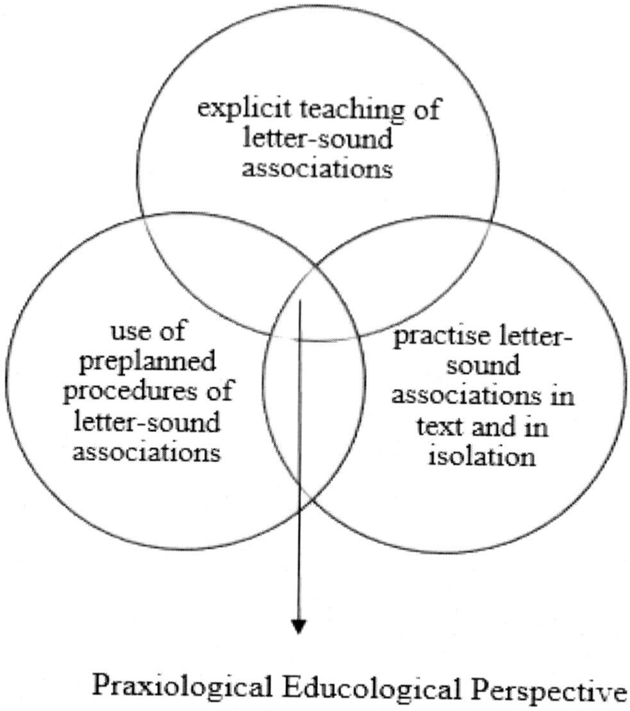

Adapted from Uhry and Clark, 2005

Figure 3. Model of Praxiological Educological Perspective

Scientific Educological Perspective

The scientific lens of the educological perspective seeks to establish the basis of empirical evidence of dyslexia. Over the years, there is a huge body in the establishment of empirical research evidence of dyslexia based on the various theories proposed by different researchers. However, operationally defining dyslexia is essential and crucial as it guides assessment and appropriate intervention for practitioners (Pennington, 2009). In other words, having known the operating definition of any disorder can lead to more targeted intervention. The scientific educological perspective looks into three different areas (see Figure 4):

(1) Symptomatological
(2) Nosological
(3) Etiological

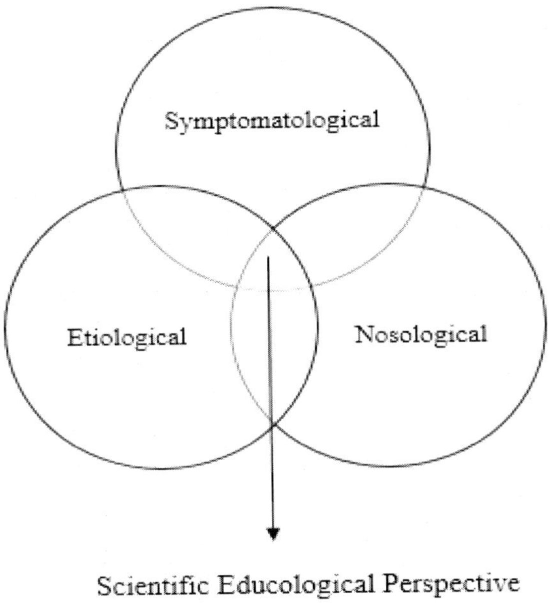

Figure 4. Model of Scientific Educological Perspective.

Symptomatological

The primary difficulty in dyslexia is in written language, not spoken language (Pennington, Peterson, and McGrath, 2009). Individuals with dyslexia generally encounter problems in auditory processing, visual processing, poor organizational skills, attention deficits and written output difficulties (Chia, 2009). The list below shows some of the diagnostic symptoms of dyslexia (IDA, 2008; Hallahan and Kauffman, 2006; Lerner, 2005):

- trouble learning the letter names of the Alphabet and rhyming words
- may not understand what is being read
- difficulties in spelling
- may have difficulties following instructions
- may confuse math symbols and misread numbers
- poor organizational skills

Though dyslexia varies from person to person, the core deficits are weaknesses in the manipulation of sounds in words (phonological processing), spelling and rapid response in visual-verbal modality (National Institute of Neurological Disorders and Stroke, 2005). Though the underlying problem of dyslexia is weakness in phonological processing, there are also consequential (secondary) symptoms resulted from the core symptoms. In the case of dyslexia, the consequential symptoms include problems in reading comprehension and reduced reading experience of individuals with dyslexia (IDA, 2008). Dyslexia can co-exist with other types of learning disorders. Prior studies (e.g., Bental and Tirosh, 2007; Willcutt and Pennington, 2000) have found that dyslexia can co-exist with attention deficit/hyperactivity disorder and developmental coordination disorder (Rochelle and Talcott,

2006), dyspraxia (Dewey, 1995), language disorders such as specific language disorder and speech sound disorder (Catts and Kamhi, 1999, 2005; Kamhi and Catts, 1986).

It is hard to establish a collective operating definition for learning disabilities, and the same goes to defining dyslexia (Siegel and Lipka, 2008). Terms such as specific reading retardation, reading difficulties, specific reading difficulties, learning disability, reading disability, reading disorder, specific learning difficulties, and unexpected reading difficulty have been used interchangeably by researchers during studies. Hence, this give rise to the enigmatic nature of Learning Disabilities (LD) in the field of special education. According to Hammill (1990), there are 11 different definitions of LD from various researchers all over the world. These discrepancies in definitions have given rise to various operationalization procedures when specifying diagnostic criteria, thereby affecting planning and designing appropriate intervention for individuals with dyslexia (Proctor and Prevatt, 2003).

Operationalization simply means a process of defining a phenomenon that is not directly measurable though its existence is indicated by other observable distinctive features. In summary, operationalization refers to a process of specifying the extension of a concept by describing what is and what is not part of that concept. According to Chia (2015), there are three basic components of an operating definition: (1) to identify a phenomenon through establishing a theoretical concept, (2) validate with appropriate tests to determine its existence, duration and quantity, and (3) procedure should be replicable by others. Among all the components, the two important factors under the scientific educological perspective is the validation and verification of the condition of dyslexia (Chia, 2015).

Validation simply refers to accuracy of a construct or phenomenon being measured with appropriate tests so as to determine its existence, duration and quantity (Chia, 2015). In other words, validation concerns the concept of dyslexia, which means the symptoms must be valid to indicate that the exhibited symptoms are the triad of impairments in dyslexia (i.e., the core symptoms are (1) difficulties in accurate word recognition, (2) poor decoding ability, and (3) poor spelling ability). According to Chia (2015), there are four different categories of symptoms in any learning disorders and they are (1) core (primary) symptoms and they are the definite non-variant traits present and are usually observable, (2) causal (correlated) symptoms and these are the underlying neurological/genetic traits, (3) consequential (secondary) symptoms and these are the traits that result from the core and/or causal traits, and (4) co-existing (co-morbid) symptoms where there are other traits found to be occurring with the existing core and/or causal traits of the disorder (see Table 1 below for a classification of symptoms in dyslexia based on the IDA definition).

Table 1. Classification of Symptoms in Dyslexia using the IDA definition (Chia, 2015)

Core (Primary)	**Causal (Correlated)**	**Consequential (Secondary)**	**Co-existing (Comorbid)**
difficulties with accurate and/or fluent word recognition poor spelling ability poor decoding ability	deficit in the phonological component of language	problems in reading comprehension reduced reading experience	impeded growth of vocabulary impeded growth of background knowledge

Another factor under the scientific educological perspective is verification. Verification requires quantitative evidence-based findings to support the definition and the existence of dyslexia through demonstrated symptoms of the reading disorder. The existence of dyslexia was researched more than three centuries ago with the first case of loss of reading ability reported in 1676 by John Schmidt. However, many of the published work appeared later in the nineteenth century where the inability to read became a concern in the medical field (Campbell, 2011). In 1887, dyslexia was first used by a German ophthalmologist, Rudolf Berlin, to describe a form of word blindness in adults caused by brain lesions. He used the term alexia to describe a total loss of reading ability due to severe brain damage whereas dyslexia refers to difficulty in decoding written symbols caused by partial brain damage (Berlin, 1887). The existence of dyslexia is substantiated by many conceptual frameworks and theories such as magnocellular theory, phonological deficit hypothesis, vision deficit theory, and others. Each of these phenomena has the backing of evidence-based research studies. One of the theories that gain prominence is the phonological deficit hypothesis. Studies with preschool children to determine the best predictors of pre-reading skills found that phonological awareness – the ability to detect and manipulate the sounds of spoken English, is one of the important factors for future reading and writing ability (Bishop and Snowling, 2004; Bradely and Bryant, 1983; Ecalle, et al., 2009; Olson, 1985; Scarborough, 1998; Rack, Snowling, and Olson, 1992; Vellutino et al, 2004). While the phonological deficit hypothesis is popular, emphasis has also been placed on the magnocellular theory. This theory postulates that reading is primarily a visual process and it requires visual attention and eye control during reading that is controlled by the magnocellular system (Stein, 2008). Studies have found that both the visual and auditory magnocellular systems are impaired in individuals with dyslexia (Stein and Talcott, 1999; Stein and Walsh, 1997). Other studies (e.g., Lovegrove et al, 1986; Livingstone et al. 1991; Galaburda and Livingstone, 1993) found that difficulty in reading is caused by a slow or irregular functioning of the magnocellular pathway of the visual system. Findings of the magnocellular hypothesis remain highly controversial as there is insufficient empirical evidence to support this theory (Stein, 2012).

Nosological

Dyslexia is learning disability that does not exist on a single symptom, rather a syndrome with multiple manifestations (Orton, 1925). Just like other types of learning disabilities, there are different subtypes of dyslexia. According to Chia (2000, p.11), dyslexia is a multi-faceted spectrum syndrome which comprises of signs and symptoms that characterize a form of psychological or abnormal condition. Chia (2000) grouped dyslexia syndrome into four main types: (1) developmental dyslexia (inherited), (2) acquired dyslexia (due to external insults to the brain), (3) induced dyslexia (also known as pseudo-dyslexia or conversion reaction syndrome), and (4) and idiopathic dyslexia (of unknown origin or causation). Developmental dyslexia can be further divided into three primary subtypes:

1) *Dyseidesia* (also known as visual-spatial dyslexia) – where individuals with this subtype of dyslexia have poor sight-word recognition and rely heavily on using word attack skills (e.g., phonics) to decode words (Boder, 1971)
2) *Dysphonesia* (also known as auditory-linguistic dyslexia) – where individuals have problems in phonetic skills when decoding unfamiliar words (Boder, 1971), and

3) *Dysnemkinesia* – very high frequency of letter reversals (e.g., misread *dog* as *bog* (i.e., changes in rotation in letters), *war* as *raw* (kinetic reversals), misread or misspell words (e.g., *tragedy* as *tradegy*) or commit mirror-image reversals involving both letters rotation and direction in the words during writing or spelling (e.g., *bump* as *qmud*).

In addition, there are other secondary subtypes of dyslexia resulting from the combination of the above three primary subtypes and they are: dysphoneidesia, dysnemkineidesia, dysnemkinophonesia, and dysnemkinphoneidesia (see Table 2).

Table 2. Subtypes of Dyslexia (adapted from Chia, 2000)

Types of Dyslexia	Primary Subtypes	Secondary Subtypes
Developmental Dyslexia	Dyseidesia	Dysphoneidesia and dysnemkineidesia
	Dysphonesia	Dysphoneidesia and dysnemkinophonesia
	Dysnemkinesia	Dysnemkineidesia and dysnemkinphoneidesia

Etiological

Due to the advancement in both behavioural and molecular genetics of reading and reading disability, the understanding of the etiology of dyslexia has gain prominence in the last two decades. The etiologies of dyslexia include, but not limited to, genetics, brain mechanisms, phonological deficits, rapid naming and the double deficit, visual processing difficulties, auditory processing difficulties, and others. It is not the purpose of this chapter to discuss all the etiologies of dyslexia. As such, the author only selects four (genetics, brain mechanisms, phonological deficits, and visual processing difficulties) for a brief discussion.

Genetics

Genes play a crucial role in any individual's development of both reading and spelling skills and the aim of studying genetic influences on dyslexia is to tease apart the effects of nature (role of genes) and the environment (nurture) (Hulme and Snowling, 2009). There is sufficient evidence that dyslexia runs in families (Bishop and Snowling, 2004; Grigorenko, 2004; Hallgren, 1950; Muter and Snowling, 2009; Pennington and Olson, 2007). Supporting the evidence of familial transmission of dyslexia is also evident from studies and case reports (e.g., Bakwin, 1973; DeFries, Singer, Foch, and Lewitter, 1978; Hallgren, 1950). Family history is one way to predict potential risk for dyslexia so that early assessment and intervention can be prescribed. Studies have shown that between 30-50% of children will develop reading disorder if their parents also have dyslexia (Pennington and Lefly, 2001; van Bergen et al., 2011). Children are also predisposed to having reading difficulties if their close relative also has dyslexia (Muter and Snowling, 2009).

Although genetic studies are unable to provide a definite answer to the actual cause of dyslexia, it is hoped that greater understanding of the genetic bases of the reading disability can ultimately help educators to predict risk of reading failure more accurately and provide specific and structured intervention early.

Brain Mechanisms

The reading systems of children and adults with dyslexia have been studied using functional brain imaging. There is converging evidence that shows inefficient functioning of left posterior brain systems during reading (Richlan, Kronbichler, and Wimmer, 2009; B. Shaywitz, et al., 2002; S. Shaywitz and B. Shaywitz, 2005). Studies using functional neuroimaging of reading and language tasks found reduced activation of left occipitotemporal (Badian, 1997; Brunswick, McCrory, Price, Frith, 1999; Paulesu et al., 2001; Shaywitz, et al., 2003). Other researchers (e.g., Dehaene, Cohen, Sigman, and Vinckier, 2005; McCandliss, Cohen, and Dehaene, 2003; Vinckier et al., 2007) argued that the left occipitotemporal region is a "visual word form area" responsible for orthographic processing of words during reading. Inefficient functioning in this area has important practical implication pertaining to the provision of accommodations for individuals with dyslexia (i.e., extra time provided during assessment and school test).

Brain imaging studies provide evidence in neurobiology that help to clarify the current understanding of the nature of dyslexia. Comparison of brain functions and differences have been studied between typical readers and readers with dyslexia with converging evidence to suggest that dyslexia is real with the existence of brain differences.

Phonological Deficits

The phonological deficit hypothesis has been the dominant cognitive explanation of dyslexia (Goswami, 2000; Miles and Miles, 1999; Ramus, 2003; Stanovich, 1988; Stanovich and Siegel, 1994; Vellutino et al., 2004). This theory is a universal neurological explanation for the cause of reading difficulties and dyslexia. It suggests that individuals with dyslexia are weak in constructing, maintaining, and retrieving of phonological information.

There is converging evidence (Brady and Shankweiler, 1991; Rack et al., 1992) to suggest that dyslexia can be characterized by one of several phenotypic manifestations of a phonological deficit (e.g., phonological awareness, phonological short-term memory, and rapid automatized naming). Research indicated that individuals with dyslexia were impaired on a variety of phonological awareness skills (Bruck and Treiman, 1990; Joanisse et al., 2000; Swan and Goswami, 1997). A study to examine phonological awareness and spelling skills among controls and dyslexics by Bruck and Treiman (1990) found that children with dyslexia performed worse on tasks of phonological awareness and spelling than the controls.

Visual Processing Difficulties

The visual dysfunction occurs on the division of the visual system into two distinct pathways that have different roles and properties: the magnocellular and parvocellular pathways. The visual processing theory postulates that the magnocellular pathway is selectively disrupted in individuals with dyslexia, leading to deficiencies in visual processing (Hari et al., 2001) During reading, the visual magnocellular system is responsible for timing visual events and the magnocellular pathway helps control eye movement. This system is also sensitive to visual motion, and direction of movement and gaze. Researchers (e.g., Lovegrove et al., 1986; Livingstone et al., 1991) suggested that the development of the visual magnocellular system is impaired in individuals with dyslexia with abnormal magnocellular layers of the lateral geniculate nucleus in individuals with dyslexia. This finding is further supported by Galaburda and Livingstone (1993) where a postmortem study of five brains with dyslexia found that the magnocells were disordered and more than 20% of the cells were smaller as compared to normal brains.

Philosophical Educological Perspective

This perspective asks about what is desirable, ethical and sound about the different interventions on dyslexia. To understand this, there are three different viewpoints to be considered (see Figure 5):

(1) Epistemological perspective
(2) Analytical perspective
(3) Contemporary perspective

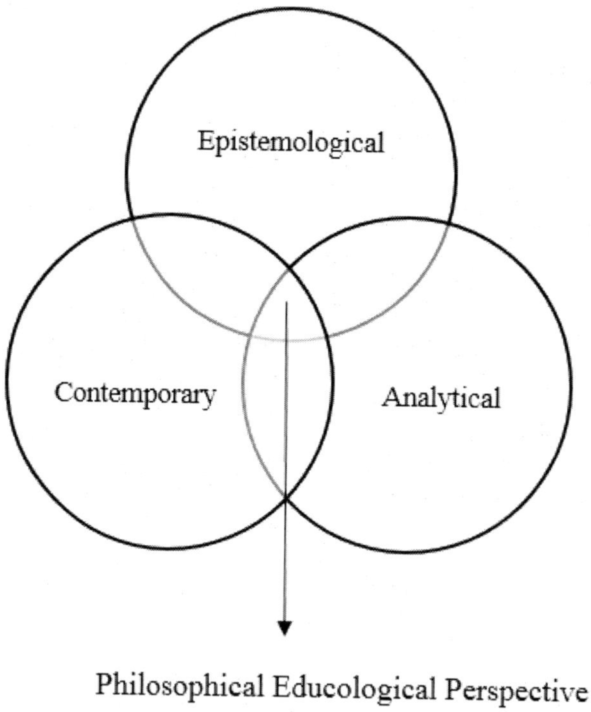

Figure 5. Model of Philosophical Educological Perspective.

Epistemological

Like attention-deficit hyperactivity disorder (ADHD), dyslexia has also been questioned on its existence. Questions such as "Does dyslexia really exist? Is dyslexia a man-made disorder?" are still a debatable controversy. With more than fifty years of academic and clinical experience in the practice of behavioral neurology and development, Saul (2014) argued that ADHD does not exist and reiterated that the definition of ADHD is wrong and that the disorder stems from a cluster of symptoms that include more than twenty other conditions such as vision problems, hearing problems, sleep disorders, sensory processing disorders, seizure disorders, Asperger Syndrome, and many others (Saul, 2014). He went on to stress that the DSM is flawed and that it has overlooked many other conditions that may better explained ADHD (Saul, 2014, p.15).

Levinson (1994) in his book on "Scientific Watergate Dyslexia: How and why countless millions are deprived of breakthrough medical treatment?" stirred a major controversy about dyslexia. With his more than 25 years of research and experience with dyslexia, he showed convincing evidence of a new theory of dyslexia which he hypothesized and presented empirical evidence that dyslexia was caused by a cerebellar-vestibular dysfunction resulting in dysmetric dyslexia and dyspraxia (Frank and Levinson, 1973). In his book, Levinson backed up his theory of inner-ear dysfunction in people with dyslexia by providing their names, pictures, and writing portfolios of his patients he has treated for dyslexia. After evaluation, he employed medical treatment and has used "inner-ear enhancing drugs," such as antihistamines, stimulants, antidepressants, and anti-motion sickness medications. Levinson's studies on his research found that 80% of his patients experience some improvement through one or more medications that he personally recommends. Even his own son, Justin (who has dyslexia), showed a dramatic improvement when resorted to medical treatment within 48 hours after Levinson's recommendation (Levinson, 1994).

After studying thousands of students with reading disabilities, Levinson was surprised to find that none had any neurological evidence of linguistic impairment (which was mistakenly assumed to be present by most experts) and that over 95% had evident balance and/or coordination difficulties, a clearly inner-ear/cerebellar dysfunction. With these empirical data, he refuted the traditionally held brain damage and language disordered theories of dyslexia, postulating his own theory of the inner-ear dysfunction that triggers dyslexia.To explain his theory, Levinson (1994) hypothesized that the inner-ear serves as a cortical 'fine-tuner' in a similar way like sensory signals like the controls of a TV set. When there is a fine-tuning dysfunction in any specific channel, sensory signals will become mixed up. And thus the quality and intensity of all the dyslexia-related symptoms as well as depends on three major factors: (1) the unique pattern of inner-ear circuits, (2) the degree of signal mix up, and (3) the capability of the normal thinking process and therapies used to intervene these mixed up signals.

For almost a century, the underlying cause of dyslexia is still an ongoing debate. A British television programme known as "*Dispatches Programme*" on *The Dyslexia Myth*" gained prominence when an ongoing debate on dyslexia went widespread. The programme asserts that there are many myths on the nature of dyslexia and its interventions. Elliott (2005) saw no difference between a child with dyslexia and a child labelled as "poor reader," i.e., there is far too many children with dyslexia so much so that there is no actual basis to the label at all. He believes that the term *dyslexia* is not helpful at all as the reading difficulties are so wide-ranging (Elliott, 2005). He also believed that it is too expensive and a waste of time spending too many resources as more can be done to help all children with reading difficulties. Instead, Elliott (2005) proposed to conduct early intervention for children at-risk of reading problems early instead of focusing on expensive assessments, and also questioned on the rigor, utility and added value of a clinical diagnosis of dyslexia without a uniform test used by all psychologists. For example, some may look at memory, some at sounds and words, while others look at visual processing in making a diagnosis. As a result, researchers are unable to arrive at a mutual agreement on what the underlying problems constitute dyslexia are. Finally, there is a big misconception that dyslexia is associated with IQ. He stated that reading does not require a high level of intelligence as there are children who struggle to read possess different IQ profiles from low, middle, and high levels of intellectual capacity (Elliott, 2005).

However, the debate of the mythology of dyslexia continues with Rod Nicolson, a psychologist in UK, commented that dyslexia is not a myth. In his paper, he quoted: "The fact that 50 per cent of the variance in dyslexia is genetic means that dyslexia does have a clear and distinct basis and hence cannot be a 'myth' (Nicolson, 2005, p. 658). On the issue of definition, he mentioned that Elliott (2005) has chosen to focus more on exclusionary diagnosis of dyslexia while he viewed secondary symptoms to be informative in addition to the primary symptoms (i.e., difficulties with accurate and/or fluent word recognition, poor spelling ability, and poor decoding ability). These secondary symptoms such as attention deficit/hyperactivity disorder and developmental coordination disorder (Rochelle and Talcott, 2006), motor coordination, dyspraxia (Dewey, 1995), specific language disorder and speech sound disorder (Catts and Kamhi, 1999; Catts, Adlof, Hogan, and Weismer, 2005; Kamhi and Catts, 1986) can co-exist with dyslexia. When the co-existing symptoms are taken into account, it will lead to a different classification system of dyslexia.

Analytical

The analytical perspective is defined as the characterization of the meaning of dyslexia. In other words, it asks what actually dyslexia is. Based on a pathogenic perspective, dyslexia may be viewed as a disease that is caused by a neurological disorder. However, dyslexia is not a disease but it can be inherited or acquired (due to external insults to the brain). Just like autism spectrum disorder, the severity of dyslexia can range from mild to severe on a spectrum. Individuals can be either neuroatypical (i.e., dyslexic) or neurotypical (i.e., adyslexic) on a continuum (see Figure 6 below).

Neuroatypical (Dyslexic) ⟷ Continuum ⟷ Neurotypical (*a*dyslexic)

Figure 6. A continuum of neuroatypical to neurotypical.

The above analogy can be further explained by pathogenesis (the development of a disease) which is one end of the continuum to salutogensis (the origin and the maintenance of health, stress, and coping) on the other. In other words, pathogenesis focuses on *dis-ease* while salutogenesis on *ease* (see Figure 7).

Pathogenesis (*Dis*-ease) ⟷ Continuum ⟷ Salutogenesis (Ease)

Figure 7. A continuum of pathogenesis to salutogenesis.

Hence, the focus of providing interventions on dyslexia should focus on the strengths and needs of every individual based on the human genome, and not on the pathogenic perspective.

Contemporary

Most of the terms used to describe dyslexia are deficit-based such as specific reading *retardation*, specific reading *difficulties*, reading *disability*, unexpected reading *difficulty*, and specific learning *difficulties*. Just like autism spectrum disorder, some individuals possessed splinter skills and talents related to working with systems (e.g., mathematical systems, machine manuals, computer languages, database management, etc.), a term known as *systemizing* coined by Baron-Cohen (2006). Systemizing is the power to analyze or construct systems with organized rules to govern the entire system so as to forecast how the system works (Baron-Cohen, 2006). Individuals with dyslexia do also possess special talents and giftedness such as Alexander Graham Bell (inventor and scientist), Orlando Bloom (actor), Richard Branson (entrepreneur), Tom Cruise (actor), Steve Jobs (co-founder of Apple), Lee Kuan Yew (first Prime Minister of Singapore), and many more.

If dyslexia is being viewed as a disability, then only the deficits (e.g., poor word decoding, difficulty in spelling and writing) will gradually take over the strengths of the individuals diagnosed with dyslexia. Hence, it is important for educators to identify abilities, strengths, and intelligences rather than focused on the weaknesses of the reading disability. In other words, rather than looking at the deficits of the individuals, viewing dyslexia as learning differences rather than learning disabilities through their strengths will eventually change the attitudes of people towards the field of special education. According to a survey of U.S. business people by Warren (2008), results found that one-third of entrepreneurs were reported to have dyslexia, compared with only one percent of middle managers in large organizations.

In order to develop respect for each individual with learning differences, this author would like to introduce *neurodiversity*, a term first used in the autistic community by Judy Singer, an Australian disability activist, in the late 1990's. According to Armstrong (2011), all human brains are wired differently and we have different learning styles. His concept of neurodiversity looks at *learning differences* instead of learning disabilities, where every individual has their unique learning styles. Educators embracing a neurodiversity perspective can show respect for individuals' differences and find ways to provide interventions based on strengths rather than their weaknesses of the individuals.

Jurisprudential Educological Perspective

This perspective looks from a viewpoint pertaining to the characterization of what is legally allowed, prohibited and required within that jurisdiction. Many developed countries (e.g., US and UK) have mandatory laws to protect the interests and rights of persons with disabilities. This author considers the jurisprudential educological perspective from three viewpoints (see Figure 8):

(1) Jurisdiction
(2) Prudence
(3) Therapy

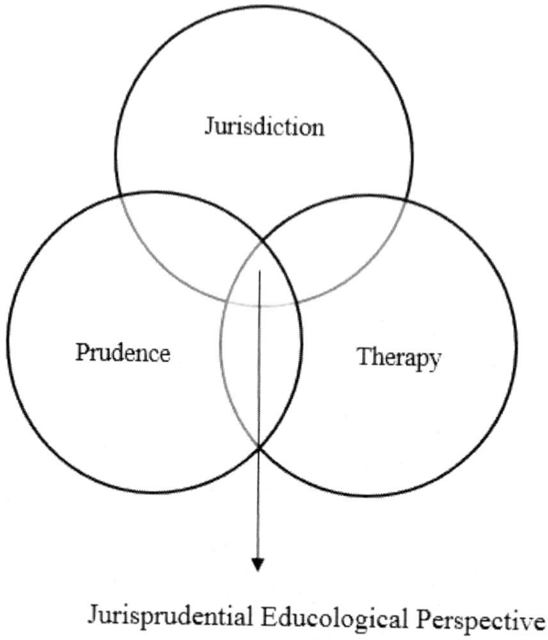

Figure 8. Model on Jurisprudential Educological Perspective.

Jurisdiction

The special education programme in the US were made compulsory in 1975 when the Congress passed the Education for All Handicapped Children Act (EAHCA). In order to protect students with disabilities, EAHCA was later revised to Individuals with Disabilities Education Act in 2004 (IDEA, 2004) which requires all states to provide special education and related services to all individuals with disabilities to receive federal funding. Under the IDEA, Section 504 of the Rehabilitation Act 1973, every student is entitles to a Free and Appropriate Public Education (FAPE). FAPE protects the rights of individuals with where there will be a regular provision of regular or special education and relevant aids and services designed to meet the educational needs of every individual. All school-age children with disabilities as defined by Section 504 and IDEA are entitled to FAPE. States like Texas, California, Colorado, New Jersey, Hawaii, and Washington have statewide dyslexia laws that require public schools to conduct screening for children with dyslexia during the first or second grade in kindergarten.

Currently, there is no compulsory special education programme stipulated by law in Singapore. According to the Compulsory Education Act in 2003, all school-age children must attend at least six years of primary education in mainstream schools. However, there are three groups of children who are exempted if they are: (1) attending Muslim religious schools, (2) receiving home-schooling, and (3) diagnosed with learning disabilities. Children with mild learning disabilities and are able to cope with mainstream curriculum will also continue to attend these schools. As for those diagnosed with moderate to profound learning disabilities, they are required to attend special education schools to learn basic self-help skills and vocational skills so as to secure jobs in open employment.

Singapore joined 132 other countries in 2012 and ratified the UN Convention on the Rights of Persons with Disabilities to ensure persons with disabilities are treated equally with dignity and respect and their rights are protected. The Singapore Government also introduced several Acts to support and protect persons with disabilities such as:

1) Mental Capacity Act enacted in 2010 to safeguard the interest of those who lose their mental capacity, including persons with intellectual disabilities.
2) Central Provident Fund (CPF) Act amended in 2011 to provide Special Needs Savings CPF monies.
3) A data protection law, the Personal Data Protection Act (PDPA) 2012, consists various rules that governs the collection, use, disclosure and care of personal data. PDPA protects both the rights of individuals on their personal data (includes rights of access and correction, and the needs of organizations to collect, use or disclose personal data for legitimate and reasonable purposes).
4) The Building Construction Authority's Code on Accessibility 2013 to mandate buildings to incorporate building designs (e.g., ramps, wheelchair stair lifts, handrails, grab bars, etc.).
5) Appropriate Adult (AA) Scheme provides assistance to people with intellectual or mental disabilities (PWIDs) who are required to give a statement to the Police during investigation. Currently, the AA Scheme is not covered under any act in the Singapore law.

Peer group influences can easily cause children and teenagers to commit crime. Individuals with neurodevelopmental impairments are prone to be victims to fall into committing crime. According to Conti-Ramsden and Botting (2004), children with speech and language impairment are three times higher to be 'regular targets for victimization.' This finding suggests that young people with neurodevelopmental impairments may be readily targeted and manipulated by peers, instigating them to commit crimes. The prevalence rate among young people with dyslexia has been reported by Siegel (2007) to range from 5-10% while the rate was 43-57% who was in custody (Snowling, Adams, Bowyer-Crane, and Tobin 2000).

Prudence

This perspective looks into exercising good judgment with care and caution by professionals to individuals with dyslexia. Diagnostic assessment is a crucial phase before any appropriate intervention can be designed. However, it must be noted that there is no one-size-fits-all approach when it comes to assessing individuals suspected with dyslexia. Professionals need to be aware that no two individuals with dyslexia are alike as the reading disability exists on a continuum. Hence, this author would like to use the term *profiling* (an educational term), rather than *diagnosis* (medical term) as diagnosis involves some kind of IQ test.

Specific interventions are crucial as there are different subtypes mentioned in the nosology of dyslexia under the scientific educological perspective. The same approach should not be used for all individuals with dyslexia. Hence, a more descriptive identification of individuals with dyslexia is needed. In order to accomplish this, the Educator's Diagnostic Manual of Disabilities and Disorders (EDM) (Pierangelo and Giuliani, 2007) can be used to ensure a detailed description of any disability. The EDM provides a five-level diagnostic coding system and they are:

1) Level 1: IDEA 2004 disability classification where codes of disability are categorized (e.g., LD for specific learning disability)
2) Level 2: Specific disorders based on Level 1 (e.g., dyslexia is coded as LD 4.00)
3) Level 3: Specific types of disorders (e.g., dysphonetic dyslexia is coded as LD 4.07)
4) Level 4: Specific subtypes of disorders (e.g., as there is no Level 4 code for dysphonetic dyslexia, this level can be classified as Not Applicable)
5) Level 5: Degree which the disability adversely affects the child's educational performance (members in the Individualized Educational Plan (IEP) decides if child needs: (1) modifications, (2) classroom accommodations, (3) assistive technology, (4) related services, and (5) external agencies (e.g., special education school, residential classroom, etc.)

Table 3 below shows an example of the multilevel coding system of EDM of a student classified with a specific learning disability having difficulties that are associated with reading (i.e., dyslexia).

There is no gold standard and agreed-upon diagnostic tool that professionals can use when determining whether a child meets the criteria for a specific disability. The importance of the EDM is a quick and useful reference book as it provides information, guidelines, and examples created specifically for professionals in the field of special education. Definitions, symptoms, characteristics, types, and subtypes for disabilities as specified by IDEA 2004 can also found in the manual.

Table 3. EDM Multilevel Coding System of Dyslexia (Pierangelo and Giuliani, 2007)

Level	Description	Code Number
1	Specific Learning Disabilities	LD
2	Dyslexia	LD 4.00
3	Dysphonetic Dyslexia	*LD 4.07
4	No specific subtypes of disorders	Not applicable
5	Degree which the disability adversely affects child's educational performance	**Moderate

*usually diagnosed through a multidisciplinary assessment by professionals
**decided by IEP team members

Therapy

Before any therapy is provided, a thorough diagnostic assessment is crucial to determine the underlying cause of dyslexia and other co-existing disabilities. As dyslexia constitutes a wide spectrum, there are possibilities of comorbidity and the inclusion of subtypes in relation to the primary disability. Professionals need to exercise caution not to depend on a single diagnostic assessment tool or procedure to arrive at a definitive diagnosis. Hence, a differential diagnosis is strongly recommended to assess possibilities of comorbidities with dyslexia or constitution of possible subtypes. Dyslexia should be assessed using a differential diagnosis through comprehensive assessments by professionals as this can provide targeted intervention strategy to meet the needs of that individual. For example, dysgraphia (difficulties in writing) should be considered when assessing individuals for dyslexia as they may have weak fine motor skills which make writing difficult. Thus, professionals conducting diagnostic assessments need to be aware that there is currently no one foolproof assessment tool or procedure. In addition, interventionists should also be aware that not all with dyslexia will benefit with the same intervention approach. For example, a cognitive approach using phonemic-morphemic method may benefit someone with mild dyslexia, but not for individuals with Conversion Reaction Syndrome as the priority is to address their socioemotional issues.

An intervention tool that has gained considerable support lately in the US is the Response to Intervention (RTI) model which typically consists of three or four tiers with increasing levels of intervention. According to Pennington (2009), children who are struggling with below-average progress will receive additional and supplemental instruction in small settings (Tier 2). If they still fail to respond to interventions, they will be evaluated individually and given one-to-one instruction (Tier 3). Mather and Wendling (2012) suggested that RTI models can help students overcome their academic problems by providing early intervention but do not explain the causes of students' failure as it does not provide diagnosis.

One often neglected aspect when discussing therapy perspective is the term *Therapeutic Jurisprudence (TJ)*. First coined by Professors David Wexler and Bruce Winick in 1987, TJ studies the extent in which substantive rules, legal procedures and the role of lawyers and judges produced therapeutic consequences for people involved in the legal process (Wexler and Winick, 1991). According to Wexler and Winick (1991), TJ tells us how impactful the justice system can have on people's psychological and physical well-being. In other words, the law itself can be observed to act as a therapist or therapeutic agent (Wexler and Winick, 1991).

The implementation of TJ requires an awareness of the intellectual and socio-emotional needs of young people within the youth justice system. Such awareness can be done through an improvement during the initial screening and diagnostic assessment process of dyslexia. Timely diagnostic assessment and therapy are essential to the successful identification and intervention of dyslexia and associated intellectual, socio-emotional and behavioral needs of all individuals.

CONCLUSION

In order to understand dyslexia holistically, it is essential to take a multiple dimensional approach involving both macro- and micro-educological perspectives. In summary, the educological framework in understanding dyslexia explores the following five macro perspectives and three micro perspectives (in brackets):

1) Historical (medico-historical, neuropsycho-educational-historical, sociocultural-historical);

2) Praxiological (explicit teaching of letter-sound associations, use of pre-planned procedures of letter-sound associations, and practise letter-sound associations in text and in isolation);
3) Scientific (symptomatological, nosological, etiological);
4) Philosophical (epistemological, analytical, contemporary);
5) Jurisprudential (jurisdiction, prudence, therapy).

REFERENCES

Armstrong, T. (1987). In Their Own Way: Discovering and Encouraging your Child's Personal Learning Style. CA: Los Angeles, J.P. Tarcher.

Armstrong, T. (2011). The power of neurodiversity: Unleashing the advantages of your differently wired brain. Cambridge, MA: DaCapo Lifelong/Perseus Books.

Badian, N. A. (1997). Dyslexia and the double deficit hypothesis. *Annals of Dyslexia,* 47, 69-87.

Bakwin, H. (1973). Reading disability in twins. Developmental Medicine and Child Neurology, 5, 184-187.

Baron-Cohen, S. (2006). The hyper-systemizing, assortative mating theory of autism. *Progress in Neuropsychopharmacology and Biological Psychiatry,* 30(5), 865–872.

Bateman, F. (1890). On aphasia, or a loss of speech, and the localization of the faculty of articulate language (2nd ed.). London: J. and A. Churchill.

Bental, B. and Tirosh, E. (2007). The relationship between attention, executive functions and reading domain abilities in attention deficit hyperactivity disorder and reading disorder: A comparative study. *Journal of Child Psychology and Psychiatry*, 48, 455-463.

Berlin, R. (1887). Eine besondre Art der Wortblindheit.

Bishop, D.V.M. and Snowling, M.J. (2004). Developmental dyslexia and specific language impairment: Same or different? *Psychological Bulletin,* 130, 858-888.

Boder, E. (1971). Developmental dyslexia: Prevailing diagnostic concepts and a new diagnostic approach. In H.R. Myklebust (Ed.), *Progress in learning disabilities,* 2 (pp. 293-321). New York, NY: Grune and Stratton.

Bradley, L. and Bryant, P.E. (1983). Categorizing sounds and learning to read-A causal connection. *Nature,* 301, 419-421.

Brady, S.A. and Shankweiler, D.P. (1991). Phonological processes in literacy: A tribute to Isabelle Y Libermann(1st ed.). Lawrence Erlbaum, ISBN: 080580501X, pp: 37-45.

Bruck, M. and Treiman, R. (1990). Phonological awareness and spelling in normal children and dyslexics: The case of initial consonant clusters. *Journal of Experimental Child Psychology,* 50, 156-178.

Brunswick, N., McCrory, E., Price, C.J., Frith, C.D. and Frith, U. (1999). Explicit and implicit processing of words and pseudowords by adult developmental dyslexics: A search for Wernicke's Wortschatz? *Brain,* 122, 1901-1917.

Buttner, G. and Hasselhorn, M. (2011). Debates on definitions, causes, subtypes, and responses. *International Journal of Disability, Development and Education,* 58(1), 75-87.

Campbell, T. (2011). From aphasia to dyslexia, a fragment of genealogy: An analysis of the formation of a "medical diagnosis." *Health Sociology Review*, 20, 450-461.

Catts, H.W. and Kamhi, A.G. (1999). Language and reading disabilities. MA: Allyn and Bacon, Needham Heights.

Catts, H.W., Adlof, S.M., Hogan, T.P. and Weismer, S.E. (2005). Are specific language impairment and dyslexia distinct disorders? Journal of Speech, Language, and *Hearing Research*, 48, 1378-1396.

Chia, N.K.H. (2000). Dyslexia the multi-faceted syndrome. *Health Digest,* 11(1), 10-22.

Chia, N.K.H. (2009). Dyslexia and reading-related anomalies. Series on special educational needs in mainstream schools paper no. 4. Prentice Hall: Pearson Education South Asia.

Chia, N. K. H. and Houghton, S. (2011). The effectiveness of Orton-Gillingham-based instruction with Singaporean children with specific reading disability (dyslexia). *British Journal of Special Education,* 38(3), 143-149.

Chia, N.K.H. (2015). Learning disabilities: From operating definition to operational application. Plenary paper presented at the UnITE SpLD Conference, Toa Payoh HDB Hub Auditorium, Singapore, 26 June.

Christensen, J.E. (1981). Educology and some related concepts. In Christensen, J.E. *Perspectives on Education as Educology*. Washington, DC: University Press of America (pp. 121–158).

Conti-Ramsden, G. and Botting, N. (2004). Social difficulties and victimization in children with SLI at 11years of age. *Journal of Speech, Language, and Hearing Research,* 47, 145– 161.

DeFries, J.C., Singer, S.M., Foch, T.T. and Lewitter, F.I. (1978). Familial nature of reading disability. *British Journal of Psychiatry*, 132, 361-367.

Dehaene, S., Cohen, L., Sigman, M. and Vinckier, F. (2005). The neural code for written words. A proposal. *Trends in Cognitive Sciences,* 9, 335-341.

Dewey D. (1995). What is developmental dyspraxia? [Review*]. Brain Cognition,* 29, 254–74.

Dyslexia Association of Singapore (2009). A practical approach to learning: An exclusive workshop series – 18 to 20 November. Retrieved from http://www.das.org.sg/dyslexia-myths.html.

Ecalle J., Magnan A., Bouchafa H. and Gombert, J.E. (2009). Computer-based training with ortho-phonological units in dyslexic children: new investigations. *Dyslexia: The Journal of the British Dyslexia Association 15*(3), 218-238.

Elliott, J.G. (2005). The dyslexia debate continues. *The Psychologist,* 18, 728-729.

Elliott, J.G. and Grigorenko, E.L. (2014). The dyslexia debate. NY: Cambridge University Press.

Fisher, J.E. (1996). The domain of educology. *International Journal of Educology,* 10(1), 66-43.

Fletcher, J.M., Lyon, G.R., Fuchs, L.S. and Barnes, M.A. (2007). Learning disabilities: From identification to intervention. New York, NY: Guilford Press.

Foorman, B. R. and Torgesen, J. (2001). Critical Elements of Classroom and Small-Group Instruction Promote Reading Success in All Children. *Learning Disabilities Research and Practice*, 16(4), 203-212.

Frank, J. and Levingson, H.N. (1973). Dysmetric dyslexia and dysgraphia: Hypothesis and study. *Journal of American Academy of Child Psychiatry*, 12, 690-701.

Galaburda, A.M. (1993). Neuroanatomic basis of developmental dyslexia. *Neurology Clinic,* 11, 161-173.

Galaburda, A. M. and Livingstone, M. (1993). Evidence for a magno-cellular defect in developmental dyslexia. Annals of the New York Academy of Sciences, 682, 70-82.

Goswami, U. (2000). Phonological representations, reading development and dyslexia: towards a cross-linguistic theoretical framework. *Dyslexia,* 6, 133-151.

Grigorenko, E.L. (2004). Genetic bases of developmental dyslexia: A capsule review of heritability estimates. *Enfance,* 3, 273-287.

Hallahan, D.P. and Kauffman, J.M. (2006). Exceptional learners: Introduction to special education (10th ed.). Needham Heights, MA: Allyn and Bacon.

Hallgren, B. (1950). Specific dyslexia (congenital word-blindness): A clinical andgenetic study. *Acta Psychiatrica et Neurologica Supplement*, 65, 1-287.

Hammill, D.D. (1990). On defining learning disabilities: an emerging consensus. *Journal of Learning Disabilities,* 23, 74-84.

Harding, L. W. (Ed.) (1951). Anthology in educocology. Dubuque, IO: Wm C. Brown.

Harding, LW. (1956). Essays in educology. Dubuque, IO: Wm C. Brown.

Harding, L. W. (Ed.) (1956). Essays in educology. Dubuque, IO: Wm C. Brown.

Harding, L. W. (1964). More essays in educology. Columbus, OH: Association for the Study of Educology.

Hardling, L. W. (1965). Educology: The fourth collection. Columbus, OH: Association for the Study of Educology.

Hari, R., Renvall, H. and Tanskanen, T. (2001). Left mini neglect in dyslexic adults. *Brain, 124,* 1373–80.

Henry, M. K. (1998). Structured, Sequential, Multisensory Teaching: The Orton Legacy. Annals of Dyslexia, 48, 3-26.

Hinshelwood, J. (1902). Congenital word-blindness, with reports of two cases. *Ophthalmology Review,* 21, 91-99.

Hulme, C. and Snowling, M.J. (2009). Developmental disorders of language learning and cognition. West Sussex, United Kingdom: Wiley-Blackwell.

Joanisse, M.F., Mania, F.R., Keating, P. and Seidenberg, M.S. (2000). Language deficits in dyslexic children: Speech perception, phonology and morphology. *Journal of Experimental Child Psychology*, 77, 30-60.

Kamhi, A.G. and Catts, H.W. (1986). Toward an understanding of developmental language and reading disorders. *Journal of Speech and Hearing Disorders,* 51, 337-347.

Kussmaul, A. (1877). Word deafness and word blindness. In H. von Ziemssen and J. A. T. McCreery (Eds.), Cyclopedia of the practice of medicine. (pp. 770–778). New York: William Wood.

Laughlin, H.P. (1967). The neuroses. Washington, DC: Butterworths Press.

Lerner, J.W. (2005). Learning disabilities: Theories, diagnosis, and teaching strategies (10th ed.). Boston: Houghton Mifflin.

Levinson, H.N. (1994). A solution to the riddle dyslexia. New York: *Springer-Verlag.*

Livingstone, M.S. et al. (1991). Physiological and anatomical evidence for a magnocellular defect in developmental dyslexia. *Proceedings of the National Academy of Sciences,* 88, 7943-7947.

Lovegrove, W. et al. (1986). A theoretical and experimental case of a visual deficit in specific reading disability. *Cognitive Neuropsychology,* 3, 225-267.

Manzo, A.V. (1987). Psychologically induced dyslexia and learning disabilities. *The Reading Teacher*, 40(4), 408-413.

Manzo, A.V. and Manzo, U.C. (1993). Literacy disorders: Holistic diagnosis and remediation (1st ed). Orlando: Florida. Wadsworth Publishing.
Mather, N. and Wendling, B.J. (2012). Essentials of dyslexia assessment and intervention. Hoboken, N.J: Wiley.
McCandliss, B.D., Cohen, L. and Dehaene, S. (2003). The visual word form area: Expertise for reading in the fusiform gyrus. *Trends in Cognitive Sciences,* 7(7), 293-299.
Miles, T.R. and Miles, E. (1999). Dyslexia a hundred years on (2nd ed.). Buckingham: Open University Press.
Morgan, W. P. (1896). "A case of congenital word-blindness." *British Medical Journal* 11, 378.
Muter, V. and Snowling, M.J. (2009). Children at familial risk of dyslexia: Practical implications from an at-risk study. *Child and Adolescent Mental Health*, 14, 37-41.
National Institute of Neurological Disorders and Stroke (2005). Dyslexia. Retrieved February 10, 2016, from http://www.ninds.nih.gov/disorders/ dyslexia/dyslexia.htm.
Nicolson, R. (2005). Dyslexia: Beyond the myth. *The Psychologist,* 18(11), 658-659.
Olson, R.K. (1985). Disabled reading processes and cognitive profiles. In D.B. Gray and J.F. Kavanagh (Eds.), Biobehavioral measures of dyslexia (pp. 197-216). New York: Psychology Press.
Orton, S.T. (1925). Word-blindness in school children. *Archives of Neurology and Psychiatry,* 14, 582-615.
Orton, S.T. (1937). Reading, writing, and speech problems in children. New York: Norton.
Paulesu, E., Demonet, J.F., Fazio, F., McCrory, E., Chanoine, V., Brunswick, N., et al. (2001). Dyslexia: Cultural diversity and biological unity. *Science,* 291, 2165-2167.
Pennington, B.F. and Lefly, D.I. (2001). Early reading development in children at family risk for dyslexia. *Child Development,* 72, 816-833.
Pennington, B.F. and Olson, R.K. (2007). Genetics of dyslexia. In M.J. Snowling and C. Hulme (Eds.), The science of reading. A handbook (pp. 453-472). New York, NY: Blackwell.
Pennington, B. F. (2009). Diagnosing learning disorders: A neuropsychological framework (2nd ed.). New York, NY: *Guilford Press.*
Pierangelo, R. and Giuliani, G. (2007). EDM: The educator's diagnostic manual of disabilities and disorders. San Francisco, CA: *John Wiley and Sons.*
Proctor, B. and Prevatt, F. (2003). Agreement among four models used for diagnosing learning disabilities. *Journal of Learning Disabilities*, 36, 459-467.
Rack, J.P., Snowling, M.J. and Olson, R.K. (1992). The nonword reading deficit in developmental dyslexia-a review. *Reading Research Quarterly,* 27, 28-53.
Ramus, F. (2003). Developmental dyslexia: Specific phonological deficits or general sensorimotor dysfunction? *Current Opinion in Neurology*, 13, 212-218.
Richlan, F., Kronbichler, M. and Wimmer, H. (2009). Functional abnormalities in the dyslexic brain: A quantitative meta-analysis of neuroimaging studies. *Human Brain Mapping*, 30, 3299-3308.
Ritchey, K.D. and Goeke, J.L. (2006). Orton-Gillingham and Orton-Gillingham: Based reading instruction. A Review of the Literature. *The Journal of Special Education,* 40(3), 171-183.

Rochelle, K.S.H., Talcott, J.B. (2006). Impaired balance in developmental dyslexia? A meta-analysis of the contending evidence. *Journal of Child Psychology and Psychiatry,* 47, 1159-1166.

Rose, T. E. and Zirkel, P. (2007). Orton-Gillingham methodology for students with reading disabilities: 30 years of case law. *The Journal of Special Education*, 41(3), 171-185.

Saul, R. (2014). ADHD does not exist (1st ed.). NY: *HarperCollins Publishers.*

Siegel, L.S. (2007). Perspectives on dyslexia. *Paediatrics and Child Health*, 11, 581–588.

Siegel, L.S. and Lipka, O. (2008). The definition of learning disabilities: Who is the individual with learning disabilities? In G. Reid, A. Fawcett, F. Manis and L. Siegel (Eds.), *The Sage handbook of dyslexia* (pp. 290-307). London: Sage.

Scarborough, H.S. (1998). Predicting the future achievement of second graders with reading disabilities: Contributions of phonemic awareness, verbal memory, rapid naming, and IQ. *Annals of Dyslexia,* 48, 115-136.

Shaywitz, B.A., Shaywitz, S.E., Pugh, K., et al. (2002). Disruption of exterior brain systems for reading in children with developmental dyslexia. *Biological Psychiatry*, 52(2), 101-110.

Shaywitz, S.E., Shaywitz, B.A., Fulbright, R., et al. (2003). Neural systems for compensation and persistence: Young adult outcome of childhood reading disability. *Biological Psychiatry,* 54(1), 25-33.

Shaywitz, S.E., Shaywitz, B.A. (2005). Dyslexia (specific reading disability). *Biological Psychiatry*, 57(11), 1301-1309.

Snowling, M. J., Adams, J. W., Bowyer-Crane, C. and Tobin, V. (2000). Levels of literacy among juvenile offenders: the incidence of specific reading difficulties. *Criminal Behaviour and Mental Health,* 10(4), 229-241.

Snowling, M. J. and Hulme, C. (2011). Evidence-based interventions for reading and language difficulties: Creating a virtuous circle. *British Journal of Educational Psychology,* 81, 1-23.

Soler, J., Fletcher-Campbell, F. and Reid, G. (2009). Understanding difficulties in literacy development: issues and concepts. Open University. *SAGE Publications.*

Stanovich, K.E. (1988). Explaining the differences between the dyslexic and the garden variety poor reader: the phonological-core variable-difference model. *Journal of Learning Disabilities*, 21, 590–612.

Stanovich, K.E. and Siegel, L.S., (1994). The phenotypic performance profile of reading-disabled children: a regression-based test of the phonological-core variable-difference model. *Journal of Educational Psychology*, 86, 1-30.

Stein, J. (2008). The neurobiological basis of dyslexia. In H. Reid, A. Fawcett, F. Manis, and L. Siegel (Eds), *The Sage handbook of dyslexia* (pp. 53-76). London: Sage.

Stein, J. (2012). The magnocellular theory of dyslexia. In A.A. Benasich and R.H. Fitch (Eds.), Developmental dyslexia: Early precursors, neurobehavioral markers, and biological substrates (pp. 32-45). Baltimore, MD: Paul H. Brookes Publishing.

Stein, J. and Talcott, J.B. (1999). Impaired neuronal timing in developmental dyslexia-The magnocellular hypothesis. *Dyslexia,* 5, 59-77.

Stein, J. and Walsh, V. (1997). To see but not to read: The magnocellular theory of dyslexia. *Trends in Neuroscience*, 4, 209-211.

Swan, D. and Goswami, U. (1997). Phonological awareness deficits in developmental dyslexia and the phonological representations hypothesis. *Journal of Experimental Child Psychology*, 66, 18-41.

Thomas, S.G., Lawrence, B.J., Robert, H.N., Glenn, K.M. and James, J.H. (1974). Auding and reading: A developmental model. Human Resources Research Organization. Alexandria: Virginia.

Torgesen, J. K. (2006). Recent discoveries from research on remedial interventions for children with dyslexia. In Snowling, M. and Hulme, C. (Eds.). The Science of Reading: A Handbook. Oxford: Blackwell Publishers.

Uhry, J.K., Clark, D.B. (2005). Dyslexia: Theory and Practice of instruction (3rd ed.). Austin, TX: PRO-ED.

van Bergen, E., de Jong, P.F., Regtvoort, A., Oort, F., van Otterloo, S. and van der Leij, A. (2011). Dutch children at family risk of dyslexia: Precursors, reading development, and parental effects. *Dyslexia*, 17, 2-18.

Vellutino, F.R., Fletcher, J.M., Snowling, M.J. and Scalon, D.M. (2004). Specific reading disability (dyslexia): what have we learned in the past four decades? *Journal of Child Psychology and Psychiatry*, 45(1), 2-40.

Vinckier, F., Dehaene, S., Jobert, A., Dubus, J. P., Sigman, M. and Cohen, L. (2007). Hierarchical coding of letter strings in the ventral stream: Dissecting the inner organization of the visual word-form system. *Neuron,* 55, 143-156.

Wexler, D.B. and Winick, B.J. (1991). Essays in therapeutic jurisprudence. Durham, NC. Carolina Academic Press.

Willcutt, E.G. and Pennington, B.F. (2000). Comorbidity of reading disability and attention deficit/hyperactivity disorder: Differences by gender and subtype. *Journal of Learning Disabilities,* 33. 179-191.

In: Dyslexia: Perspectives, Challenges and Treatment Options ISBN: 978-1-63485-328-6
Editor: Marilyn Frazier

Chapter 4

The Views of Parents of Pupils with Dyslexia on Their Collaboration with Teachers: Ethnographic Case Study

Maria Rontou [*]
University of Athens e-learning Programme, Greece

Abstract

This chapter investigates the views of parents of pupils with dyslexia concerning their collaboration with teachers. Data analysed in this chapter includes fieldnotes from observations and interviews with six parents and two EFL teachers from two state secondary schools conducted during a school year. Taking a Vygotskian approach to learning, activity theory (Engeström, 2001) is applied to analyse the contradictions that emerge around the issue of teachers' collaboration with parents. The analysis shows that contradictions are created when teachers and parents try to achieve their goal of collaboration by the lack of teachers' knowledge and training on dyslexia, the unclear Ministry's policy, the timetable and parents' work commitments. Suggestions are made regarding teachers' training, the arrangement for parents' meetings with teachers and information to parents.

Keywords: parents, dyslexia, collaboration, teachers, contradictions

Introduction

This chapter investigates parents' perspectives on dyslexia support. Parents of pupils with dyslexia who participated in this study expressed their concerns about teachers' knowledge on dyslexia and teachers' collaboration with parents. Activity theory and ethnographic methods

[*] EFL teacher in Korinthia; Associate at University of Athens e-learning Programme, Greece 149 Ivikou St; Loutraki 20300; Korinthia; Greece; Email: mariarontou720@hotmail.com.

are used to show the contradictions in dyslexia support and parents' collaboration with teachers.

Dyslexia is also referred to as 'specific learning difficulties.' 'The nature and relationship of both concepts and their relationship remains controversial.' What is referred to as dyslexia could be considered as a variety of 'dyslexias' which could be included under the term specific learning difficulties (Pumfrey and Reason 1991). The term 'dyslexia' is used in this chapter as it is 'embedded in popular language' (Reason 2002).

Pupils with dyslexia in Greece are assessed at Centres for Diagnosis, Assessment and Support of people with special needs in order to receive support at school. These centres are supposed to create adapted individualised programmes of support in collaboration with teachers and special educational staff (Ministry of National Education and Religion 2008). Pupils diagnosed with dyslexia are entitled to be examined orally during the school year, at final exams and at university entrance exams (MNER 2009; 2006). School advisers are also responsible for providing in-service training to teachers (Ifanti 1995).

Collaboration between Teachers and Parents

According to Mackay (2004), dyslexia-friendly schools enjoy the trust of parents. A key element that leads to parental trust is a quick response to issues raised and the dialogue maintained between the school and the parents. When parents raise the issue that their child might have dyslexia, teachers can agree to teach the child differently, offer advice to parents about how to help children at home, offer to seek further advice, set agreed improvement targets and ask for a teaching assistant to support the child. Parents can also be consulted about effective approaches and the effectiveness of approaches used with their children.

One of the SENCO's interviewed in Hunter-Carsch's (2001) study described the provision of an 'open day' in his school which involved study skills workshops for all students and interested parents. Parents' meetings in groups were also found to be helpful for explaining to parents ways of helping with students' work. Hunter-Carsch (2001) and Pollock and Waller (2003) suggest that parents are members of a local dyslexia support group and meet other parents of students with dyslexia at local meetings at which they can hear informed guest speakers and see new resources. Constantopoulou (2002) has found that in the Greek context such seminars or workshops for parents do not exist. She attributes this to the lack of support departments at schools. Kirby et al. (2008) examined the use of a message centre, a forum where parents of children with specific learning difficulties discussed their concerns with other parents and which provided support, information and advice.

Griffiths et al. (2004) conducted a two-year evaluation project with in-depth interviews of parents across five Local Education Authorities (LEAs) on the communication between parents and professionals on dyslexia provision for children in mainstream schools. The study showed that parents tried to talk to the school and teachers and if they found no support they by-passed schools and they asked for private assessments and had private tuition for their children. Griffiths et al. (2004) endorse a more inclusive 'extended professionalism' in which teachers are sensitive to parents' concerns, appreciate their knowledge and respond to their concerns with sensitivity and respect. In this study, interviews with parents are used to investigate parents' collaboration with teachers and the school, the strategies they adopt and whether the concept of 'extended professionalism' is evident in teachers-parents' collaboration.

THEORETICAL FRAMEWORK

A theoretical framework that studies human learning within organizational systems in a collective way was needed for this study. Activity theory and the work of Engeström (2001) provided one such framework. Socio-cultural activity theory was initiated by Vygotsky (1978; 1987). Vygotsky believed that human activity happens when the subjects, those whose actions are analysed, resolve a shared problem, an 'object' by using 'tools' to achieve a goal (Martin 2008).

Engeström (2001) describes how the current understanding of activity theory has evolved through three generations of research. The first generation contributed to activity theory the idea of 'mediation' which was represented in Vygotsky's (1987) triangular model (Figure 1) linking the subject and the object through mediating artefacts (Engeström 2001).

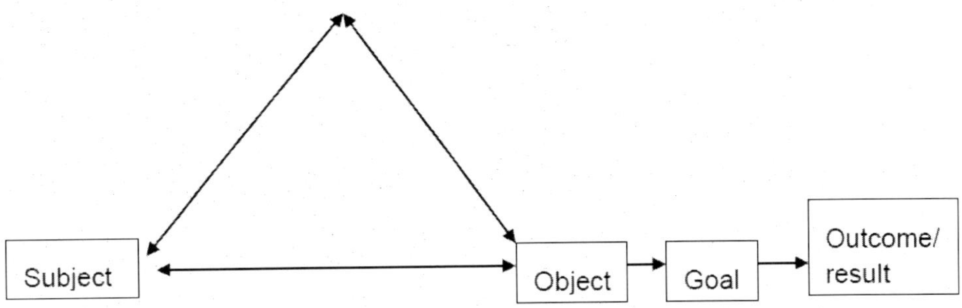

Figure 1. The principal relationship in an activity system.

In the second generation, which was developed from Leont'ev's writing, (Leont'ev 1978; 1981; Engeström 2001) Engeström expanded the triangular representation of an activity system to enable the examination of activity systems at an organizational level as opposed to a focus on the individual actors operating with tools (Daniels 2004). This expansion of the Vygotskian triangle represents the social or organizational elements in an activity system through the addition of the elements of community, rules and division of labour (see Figure 2).

Activity theory was chosen as a theoretical framework for the data collection and analysis of this study because it allowed the inclusion of different groups of participants: teachers, students and parents and the investigation of their relationship. It also afforded the investigation of the factors that influence their relationship: 1) the tools that participants can use to achieve their objects, that is, what they are working on, 2) the wider community, that is, the context and the wider socio-cultural influences and 3) rules, the principles regulating the actions of the participants that can be both written and unwritten (policy and common practices).

Engeström directs his analysis towards contradictions and tensions with emphasis on the object and the outcomes of the activity (Daniels 2004). Contradictions are tensions or dilemmas that arise from the processes within and between the elements of the activity system and become the object of collaborative learning (Martin 2008). Contradictions between elements of the activity system are indicated in the figures by lightning shaped arrows (Engeström et al. 1999).

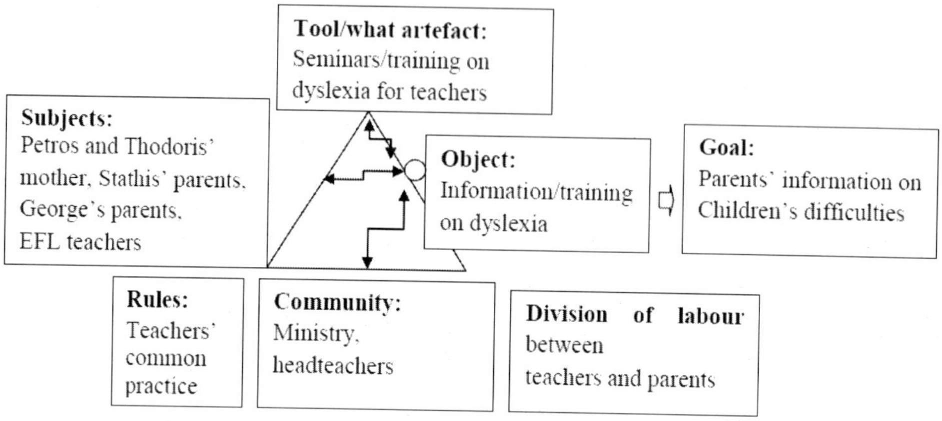

Figure 2. Second generation activity theory.

The subjects of learning of the activity system in school 1 and 2 are EFL teacher 1 and 2, George's parents (Mo1 and F1), Stathis' parents (Mo2, F2), Peter's mother (Mo3) and Thodoris' mother (Mo4) (see figure 2). A possible object of learning, that is, what the subjects are working on, is teachers' training on dyslexia (Daniels 2004). The goal in an activity system is the result of the 'creative effort' that can be achieved when the problems are resolved (Davydov 1999). A possible goal in this study is parents' information on dyslexia issues.

The subject-object interaction is mediated by tools (Bedny and Harris 2005). Cole (1996) and Engeström (1999a) suggest that tools are a subcategory of artefacts. Engeström (1999a) suggests four types of artefacts referring to different ways of using artefacts: what, how, why and where to artefacts. In this study, 'what' and 'how' artefacts were used. 'What' artefacts describe objects and 'how' artefacts refer to processes and procedures within or between objects. A 'what' artefact in this study is knowledge on dyslexia while the EFL teacher's collaboration with parents is a 'how' artefact.

The community includes the context of the activity, that is, the people who are concerned with the same object: the headteachers of the schools, the other pupils and teachers, the Local Education Authority and the Ministry of National Education, Lifelong learning and Religion (Leadbetter 2004; Daniels 2004). Therefore, the activity is a collective one and not an individual action of the teachers only (Engeström 2001).

The division of labour in this study refers to the division of tasks between the EFL teacher and teachers. The rules are the national policies on dyslexia and their interpretations by the headteacher of the school (Daniels 2004) as well as the routines and professional practices of the teachers.

Leadbetter (2004) has used activity theory to analyse different types of artefacts that can be useful in planning and structuring meetings between teachers and educational psychologists. She also explores the use of consultation within educational psychology practice associated with multi-agency working using 2nd generation activity theory (Leadbetter 2006).

METHODOLOGY

Context and Participants

The data for this study come from two state secondary schools in Athens. The study was first carried out at an upper secondary school in borough 1 (see figure 3). The second school was a lower secondary school in borough 2. Both schools belong to the same LEA, called Athens C.

The data used in this chapter from School 1 involved a student's with dyslexia (George) mother and father (Mo1, F1) and their son's EFL teacher, EFL teacher 1. EFL teacher 1 had 19 years of teaching experience, 6 out of which were at the state sector. The data used in this chapter from School 2 involved four parents of students with dyslexia, Stathis' mother and father, Peter's and Thodoris' mother and their children's EFL teacher, EFL teacher 2. EFL teacher 2 had 19 years of teaching experience, eight of which were at the state sector.

The wider study included a 17-year-old student with dyslexia in School 1, George, three 12-13 year-old students with dyslexia in School 2, Stathis, Peter and Thodoris and the headteachers of the schools. The diagnostic report was the same for all students in the study; they all had normal I.Q. and faced difficulties in spelling, handwriting and dyscalculia according to their diagnostic reports. Diagnoses that Greek state schools accept are produced in state diagnostic centres that give an I.Q. test to pupils and tests that assess pupils' reading, writing, spelling, reading comprehension, maths, phonological skills, speech etc.

The selection of schools was guided by convenience, that is, the accessibility from where the researcher lived and the availability of individuals in them due to professional contacts (Cohen et al. 2007; Fine and Shulman 2009). The headteachers had also given the researcher the information that there were students with dyslexia in the schools. The EFL teachers selected were the ones working in the schools selected who had students diagnosed with dyslexia in their classes and who agreed to participate in the study after being informed about its aims and procedure. The parents selected were the ones who gave their consent for their children's and their own participation in the study. In order not to identify the school and the participants, pseudonyms were used for the pupils and the teachers' names were replaced with codes like EFL teacher 1 and 2, mother 1 (Delamont 2002). The researcher was not a teacher at the schools in which the research was conducted but was a teacher permanently employed by the Greek Ministry of Education working in another LEA but had lived in the area where the research was carried out and had knowledge of the local services.

Since activity theory is deeply contextual and studies specific local practices it is often linked with the use of case study (e.g., Engeström 1999a; 1999b; 2001) that takes context and its details into account (Denscombe 2003). An appropriate design for this study using activity theory as a theoretical framework was a case study. A case study was suitable for this study as it aimed to go into sufficient detail and explore the complexities of dyslexia provision and multiple sources were necessary for the collection of data (Denscombe 2003).

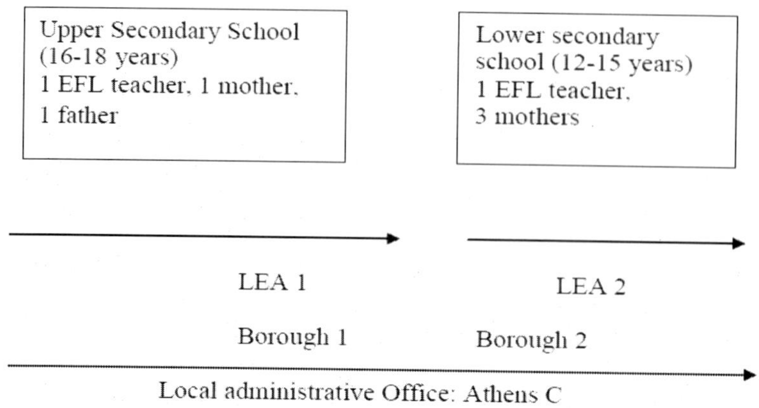

Figure 3. Research design.

Methods

Before starting the main study the methods were piloted in a secondary school in Greece for a period of two weeks. The main study included multiple methods for triangulation purposes which is a characteristic of case studies (Robson 2002): semi-structured and unstructured ethnographic interviews with two EFL teachers and six parents and field notes from lesson observations. The wider study included interviews with the four pupils with dyslexia mentioned above, the two headteachers of the schools, three more teachers and a collection of documents.

The interviews with participants were conducted in the Greek language and they were transcribed and translated into English. This process involved construction of meaning and interpretations by the transcriber and translator (Marshall and Rossman 2010).

The case studies in this chapter are ethnographic because this study had a longitudinal element as it involved contact with participants in a setting over a prolonged period of time (Brewer 2000). The researcher spent 13 weeks collecting data with School 1 participants and 16 weeks collecting data with School 2 participants.

The data were analysed using activity theory in order to investigate the following research questions:

1) What kind of provision do parents of pupils with dyslexia need and are offered by teachers and the school?

Subquestions:

a) Are the parents of the pupils with dyslexia in this study informed about the nature of dyslexia by the headteacher or the teachers?

b) Do teachers collaborate with parents?

c) Are parents satisfied with the provision offered to them?

2) What issues or factors cause systemic contradictions between the subjects, tools, rules, community and objects?

The data were analysed using activity theory in order to investigate the perspective of the different groups of participants and the relationship between them as well as the relationship between the participants and the tools, the rules, the community and the division of labour and how these influence the achievement of participants' goals. Patterns in teachers,' pupils' and parents' needs became the focus of the analysis as well as the contradictions in the achievement of the participants' goals. Therefore, the analysis aims at identifying the contradictions that arise when the teachers and parents try to work on their object of collaboration with each other as well as the factors that caused these contradictions.

DATA ANALYSIS

Collaboration between Teachers and Parents

The issues of information to parents and meetings between parents and teachers are dealt with in this section. These issues are discussed using evidence from interviews with all participating mothers, Stathis' father and EFL teacher 2 from School 2 and EFL teacher 1 and George's parents from School 1.

Information to Parents: School 2

Stathis' mother said that they take Stathis to a private centre where they pay for dyslexia support but only for emotional support:

M: Is there enough information on dyslexia, about what you should do, where you can take the child?
Mo2: Nothing, we go somewhere else separately and we pay.
Extract 1/Interview with Stathis' parents

They do this because at the primary school where Stathis went teachers were unaware of what dyslexia is. They never informed Stathis' parents about what Stathis did:

F2: ... in schools I'm telling you with certainty teachers are completely ignorant, especially in primary school
Mo2: In primary school nobody told us what Stathis was doing ...
F2: They rather did harm in primary school ...
Extract 2/Interview with Stathis' parents

For this reason, Stathis' father (F2) wanted teachers for his son who knew their students' difficulties and what to do about students with dyslexia:

F2: the most important thing is for the teacher to know what [difficulty] the student has.
M: Yes.
F2: to know and be conscious as an educator ...

Extract 3/Interview with Stathis' parents

Petros' mother (Mo3) also complained about the lack of information for teachers on dyslexia. She reports what a specialist from a state diagnostic centre told her (Extract 4, lines 374-6) and then she talks about the teachers in the local primary school and in School 2 (lines 379-380):

374 Mo3: ... 'teachers are not informed and they cannot be informed with just
375 one seminar or two,' she says. And neither do they learn it [about
376 special needs], they are not in the position to
377 M: Haven't these people done an MA or something like that? Do they
378 just attend a seminar?
379 Mo3: Yes all of them ... from the primary and the secondary school
380 teachers to EFL teacher 2 ..., have no special [training on Special Needs], all of them.

Extract 4/Interview with Mo3

Petros' mother like Stathis' mother also complained about the lack of information from the primary school to parents. The only information she obtained was from a leaflet by a private centre that she found in the schoolyard of the primary school which Petros attended:

M: Now, what about seminars?

Mo3: [There is] no seminar, there is no information at school at all. I told you about some leaflets only like those handed for pizza or those for the English language centres that exist. Some leaflets like that made from the private [educational] sector though.

Extract 5/Interview with Mo3

Thodoris' mother (Mo4) also complained about teachers' lack of knowledge and training on dyslexia. She said that secondary school teachers do not know the difficulties that students may face and for this reason they did not believe that her daughter had dyslexia (Extract 6, lines 90-3). Therefore, these teachers did not show 'extended professionalism,' that is, they did not respond to parents' concerns with sensitivity and respect (Griffiths et al. 2004). In primary school they did not even know what dyslexia is (lines 100-101):

90 Mo4: Many [teachers] don't know exactly the difficulty that the child may have.
91 For example, for my Evi they said 'ah her aunt did something and she
92 gave [Evi] the paper' [diagnosis] … they can't understand that the
93 child has received enough support, she has done well, she has a good
94 intelligence test…

96 M: They [teachers] don't know about it [dyslexia diagnosis],
97 unless the parent goes to tell them.
98 Mo4: Yes, and when you go and tell them
99 M: Again
100 Mo4: They are ignorant, they haven't studied. I don't know, in primary
101 school they don't know at all what it [dyslexia] means.

Extract 6/Interview with Mo4

Thodoris' mother believes nursery and primary school teachers should be informed about dyslexia in order to inform parents that their children need a diagnosis so that they can start a program early (extracts 7, 8). Otherwise, she believes it is too late if they get the diagnosis at secondary school because there would not be enough time to cover the program (extract 8). Thodoris' mother has this experience and knowledge on special needs issues because she works at a private centre for special needs.

Mo4: Even in nursery you can identify the children that face difficulty... Neither is [the nursery school teacher] informed to be able to understand. Because if they [nursery school teachers] knew, parents would be helped, they could find it [dyslexia] earlier.
Extract 7/Interview with Mo4

Mo4: In primary school where the children are younger they [teachers] should identify it [dyslexia], because, if teachers identified it at a very young age then the child would follow a good program starting in year 1 or 2. This child would have many chances to do very well afterwards ... they [children] come in the first year of secondary school, the second year of secondary school and they [parents] say 'dyslexia diagnosis' and parents take their children to start a program. How many school years can s/he make up for my girl?
Extract 8/Interview with Mo4

In Figure 4 the activity system of the primary school where Stathis, Petros and Thodoris went is presented. Stathis,' Petros' and Thodoris' mothers (community) would have liked their children to have trained teachers (object) so that they could have information on their children's difficulties and they would have liked to have this information from teachers early enough to take the children for assessment (goal). Mothers are not in the subject position as they do not collaborate with teachers on the issue of training. Their object and goal were not met by the primary school teachers who were not informed or trained on dyslexia.

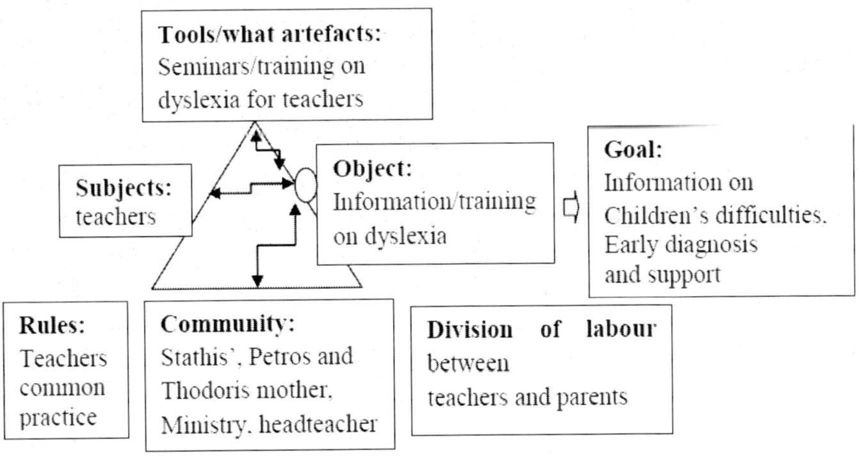

Figure 4. Primary school's activity system.

On the other hand, both Stathis' mother and father seemed to be pleased with the collaboration they had with EFL teacher 2 as she showed interest in informing them and showed them Stathis' work:

M: How do you collaborate with her ... has she informed you on his difficulties?
Mo2: She brings us his work ...
F2: She looks for exams he has written, generally we could say she was good, she talked, she showed interest when we went for the grades as well.
Extract 9/Interview with S2's parents

Stathis' mother and father also said they were happy with the other teachers in School 2 but they were not happy with the teachers in the primary school:

M: What about the provision that the school offers?
Mo2: Well, about school provision, we are now talking about the secondary school, right?
M: Yes yes.
Mo2: Because in primary school we were not happy.
F2: It is a good school...
Mo2: Ok he [Stathis] has just started, we don't have any problem, the teachers I have talked to are truly excellent.
Extract 10/Interview with Stathis' parents

However, Stathis' father got angry with a teacher who disagreed with Stathis' diagnosis and did not show 'extended professionalism,' that is sensitivity to parents' concerns (Griffiths et al. 2004). He thinks teachers should accept students' diagnoses because they come from specialists:

F2: Not every teacher should give his/her own opinion as if they have specialised in everything. 'I think' she says. What do you think? I would be abrupt if I talked to this teacher ... we took a paper [diagnosis] from the specialists and do you still have an opinion? She will accept it, she can't have such opinions, 'I think he [Stathis] has no such thing [as dyslexia],' I'm just giving an example.
Extract 11/Interview with Stathis' parents

Therefore, the object of Stathis' parents was to have teachers for their son who would inform them about his progress. This teacher was probably not informed about what dyslexia is and was probably not sensitive enough to Stathis' difficulties, which means that mother and father 2's object was not met by a teacher in the community of School 2.

The object of Petros' mother is also to have teachers who are more informed on dyslexia so that students with dyslexia are not seen as students of low intelligence: '*and more training, so that they are not seen as mentally retarded*' (Interview with Mo3).

Petros' mother said she is happy with EFL teacher 2 because she shows understanding which is something that she wants from teachers:

Mo3: Well, I have nothing to say about the specific teacher, up to now she has a lot of understanding. That is, [I want] this, each teacher to have understanding...
Extract 12/Interview with Mo3

Thodoris' mother is also happy with Thodoris' teachers because she talked to them about Thodoris' difficulty and they understood:

M: Are the teachers good then?
Mo4: Yes, I am pleased, that is, whenever I saw them and when I went and talked about Thodoris' difficulty they understood. Thodoris has never complained about anything, if he wants, he does well.
Extract 13/Interview with Mo4

Therefore, Thodoris' mother has gone to School 2 to give her son's diagnosis and to inform the teachers about his difficulties but she does not discuss dyslexia issues with teachers in the school (extract 14) as she believes they do not have the knowledge to answer her questions (extract 15). Instead she goes to the centre where she works to ask these questions (extract 15).

M: Have you been to the school, have you seen them?
Mo4: I have given them the paper [diagnosis], I have talked to them... If I have a question or if I should do something I won't refer to the school.
Extract 14/Interview with Mo4

Mo4: if I have some questions, I can find the answers myself at work… nobody can answer my questions at school ... they don't have the [required] knowledge...
Extract 15/Interview with Mo4

EFL teacher 2 said that she has answered parents' questions on students' difficulties when they have showed interest but she cannot tell them what they can do for their children as she does not know (extract 16), which is what Thodoris' mother said in extracts 14 and 15.

M: Have you informed them on what problems their children have?
T2: Yes, of course. What they have asked me yes of course, when they are interested.
M: About what they can do?
T2: I don't know what they can do.
Extract 16/Interview with T2

Therefore, the object of all mothers was to have teachers for their children who are informed or trained on dyslexia so that they are informed about their children's difficulties and progress (Stathis' mother and father), so that they understand the students' difficulties and are sensitive to them (all mothers) and they can inform them about dyslexia issues (all mothers, see figure 5). The object of having sensitive teachers who could understand the children's difficulties and inform parents about them was met by EFL teacher 2 (extracts 12 and 16) and some other teachers in School 2 but not by the teacher in extract 11. Therefore, some teachers in the community of the activity system of School 2 might have created a contradiction in the realization of this object. The object of receiving information and provision on dyslexia issues was probably not met by any of the teachers as all mothers have mentioned teachers' lack of knowledge and training.

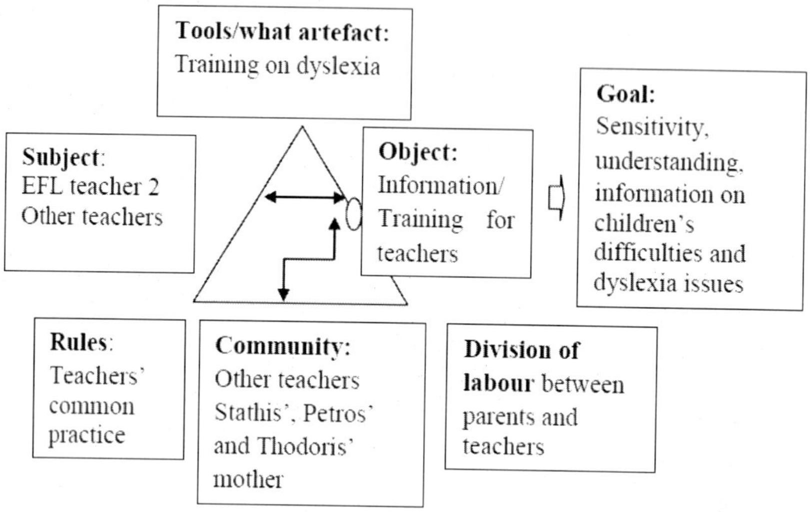

Figure 5. Training for teachers in School 2.

Information to Parents: School 1

During the interview with George's parents they said that they were never informed by his school of the examination process, that is, the fact that the students with dyslexia go to a different school from their own to take their entrance exams for university and that the examiners there have qualifications in special needs:

> M: And the treatment they receive is different, you go to a different examination centre with people who know more
> Mo1: Ah they don't take exams in the school; they take exams in another place.
> M: In another place yes.
> Mo1: We didn't know that. To tell you the truth we didn't know about this process at all.
> Extract 17: Interview with Petros' parents/19-01-07

This is evidence that the headteacher did not inform the parents about this issue. In fact, in a conversation with headteacher 1 the researcher understood that he did not intend to inform parents and students about the examination way of students with dyslexia:

I went to the headteacher's office again and I said I found a circular I wanted to give to George about these students' examination way from last year that other parents may want to see. He looked at it ... I asked if he wanted me to copy the circular and he said 'what do we have to do with it?' I said parents were stressed about these exams and the fact they had to go elsewhere. He said it would come to them. I think he didn't want to be involved in informing the parents about this.
Extract 18/Field notes

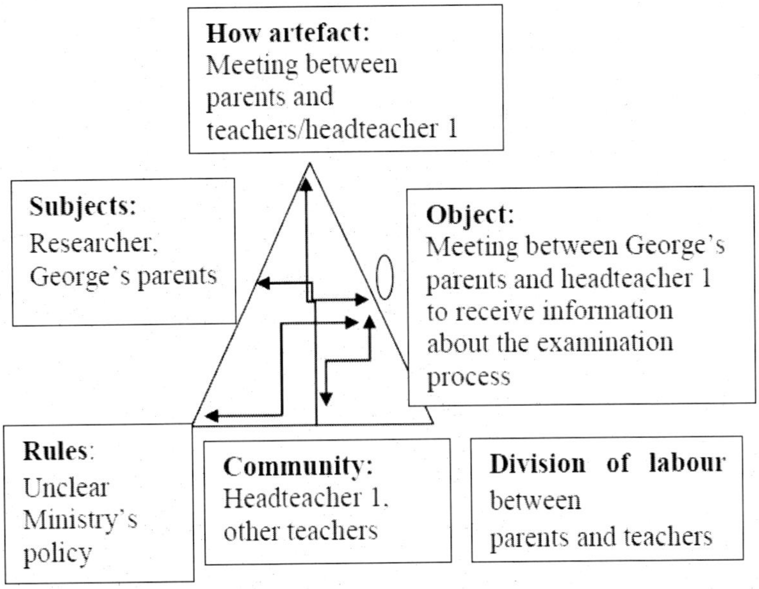

Figure 6. Meeting between parents and headteacher 1.

George's parents object of meeting with headteacher 1 to receive information about the examination process is presented in figure 6 below. It was not carried out during the study because the headteacher thought it was not part of his role to carry out such a meeting. The rules, that is, the Ministry's policy, were not clear about this issue, thus creating a contradiction. The researcher is in the subject position as she worked with parents on the issue.

Meeting between Parents and Teachers

Contradictions emerged around the meeting and collaboration of teachers and parents in both schools. EFL teacher 1 told the researcher that she would like to meet the student's parents to get information about his background in EFL and his general difficulties with studying:

M: He hasn't had any practice so he doesn't remember

T1: Look I don't know when he did these because his mother hasn't come to talk to me. … ok they [parents] know things about their child, he is their child and they have followed his progress so many years. It would be useful if all these people come by and talk to you and tell you how he has reacted generally to the process of studying the rest of the years so that you know with whom you are talking...

Extract 19: Interview with T1

George's parents complained about the lack of provision for George's problem from the school until last year:

M: What has the school offered to you, I mean how satisfied are you? You said before that they are not informed

Mo1: No I can't say, I can't say that the school has helped me, I believe that people that had an immediate relation with the problem, whose child had a problem [helped me].
Extract 20: Interview with George's Parents

The year that the study took place George's parents decided not to go to the school. George asked them not to go to talk to teachers believing that nothing could change (extract 21). He had not had any support and understanding in the previous years, apart from teachers who had children with dyslexia which is what his mother had mentioned (extract 20).

Mo1: this year I haven't gone at all
F1: this year he didn't want anyone [of us] to go, [he wanted to be] alone
Mo1: he doesn't want anyone to go to ask this year, 'don't go to ask' he says, 'come what may,' he says, 'this year' [laughing]...
Extract 21: Interview with George's Parents

Figure 7 shows that EFL teacher 1 (subject) would like to collaborate with George's parents (subject) in order to know his background in studying generally and what he has done in EFL (object). This would help the teacher know how to engage with George and his difficulties. George's parents on the other hand, would like to have information from the school on their child's progress, on what they could have done about his dyslexia the previous years and on the examination process the year that the research took place (object). They did not work with the EFL teacher on this issue but they worked with the researcher and George. The researcher and George are included in the subject position as the researcher worked with George and the EFL teacher on the issue. However, the researcher worked separately with each one of them.

The meeting between George's parents and EFL teacher 1 was not carried out during the study. Hence, there is a contradiction here. The contradiction was probably created by George's parents' work commitments that did not allow them to come to the school or the fact that George asked them not to come to the school.

The finding supported by evidence presented in this section is that both George's parents and EFL teacher 1 wanted to meet in order to exchange information but this meeting did not take place during this study.

On the contrary, Petros' mother from school 2 goes to her son's school twice a week to find all the teachers and be informed about her son's progress:

Mo3: ... I go [to the school] and I go regularly that is in the first trimester I went twice a week in order to go according to every teacher's timetable because if the break is five minutes ... that is the times that you say I will find them all, it takes usually one to one and a half week to go ... to everyone.
Extract 22/Interview with Mo3/11-03-07

In extract 22 Petros' mother mentions the difficulty she faces when she wants to meet her son's teachers regularly. Parents are supposed to meet their children's teachers at lower secondary school once every trimester when they go to take the school report but they can also meet teachers individually in their free time. Petros' mother said she has to go twice in a week or one and a half week to find all the teachers.

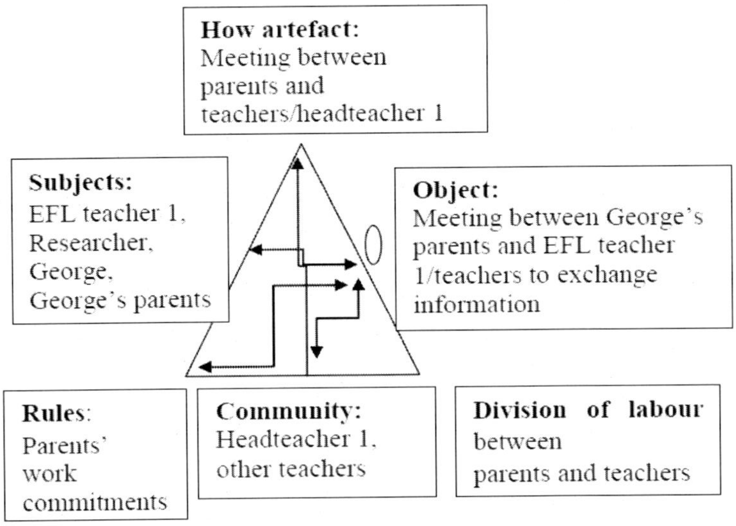

Figure 7. Meeting between parents and EFL Teacher 1.

Thodoris' mother also mentioned the same problem: she said that there are too many teachers in the secondary school to find them all at once:

Mo4: Now there are too many teachers
M: To find them all.
Mo4: You can't find them all.
Extract 23/Interview with Mo4

Therefore, there is a contradiction in the object of Petros' and Thodoris' mother of communicating with teachers created by the timetable which is different for every teacher and the break which is very short (extract 22, Figure 8).

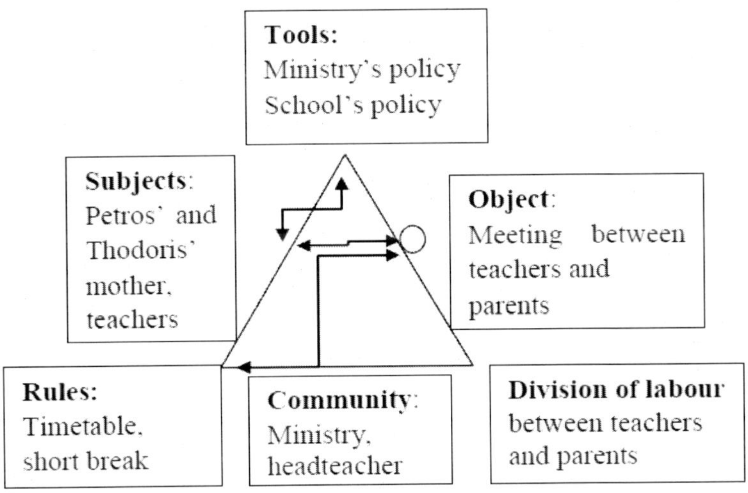

Figure 8. Meeting between parents and teachers in School 2.

Conclusion

Since this is a small-scale study, it could offer insights only for activity systems in secondary schools with similar characteristics to the schools of this study, for example, schools in urban areas of Greece and in other countries with similar policies. This chapter has shown that parents believed that teachers did not have much knowledge on dyslexia or on how to work with learners with dyslexia. Meeting with and exchanging information between parents and teachers on dyslexia issues was an object for all mothers in School 2 as well as in School 1. Parents from School 2 were not informed on their children's difficulties and dyslexia issues by the primary school which their children attended because the lack of training on dyslexia for teachers created a contradiction.

Furthermore, all mothers' object was to have teachers trained on dyslexia issues for their children and teachers who were sensitive, who showed understanding and gave parents information on their children's difficulties and what they could do about them. EFL teacher 2 and some other teachers informed parents on their children's progress and difficulties. However, there was one teacher in the school who disagreed with Stathis' diagnosis and did not show understanding, thus creating a contradiction in the achievement of the parents' object. The study has also shown that parents in School 2 faced difficulties when they attempted to meet teachers. The timetable, parents' work commitments and the unclear Ministry's policy created a contradiction.

The lack of information to parents with seminars has been reported by Constantopoulou (2002), although she has not investigated the specific needs of the parents of students with dyslexia by interviewing parents as in this study. Collaboration with parents in the form of a dialogue, in which teachers offer advice to parents and consult them about effective approaches, is a characteristic of dyslexia-friendly schools according to Mackay (2004). This is the form of collaboration with the teachers that parents in School 1 and 2 would have liked to have. Griffiths et al's (2004) concept of 'extended professionalism' in teachers' collaboration with parents is similar to Mackay's (2004) idea and includes sensitivity to parents' concerns. Parents in School 1 and 2 reported that some teachers did not show 'extended professionalism' which created a contradiction.

Therefore, in order to resolve the contradictions mentioned above and increase teachers' knowledge on dyslexia and their sensitivity to parents' concerns, initial teacher education is needed, which includes reference to Special Educational Needs. In-service training on special needs with specific reference to dyslexia needs to be organized by state services or by the general education or SEN advisers and it needs to be advertised in schools.

Headteachers and teachers also need to work with parents on arranging a time to meet that is convenient for both parts, for example, in the evening. Furthermore, the policy on dyslexia needs to be clearer on what information the headteachers need to give to parents. Finally, seminars and workshops for informing parents on dyslexia issues could be organized by schools or state services.

References

Bedny, G. Z., and Harris, S. R., (2005). The Systemic-structural Theory of Activity: Applications to the Study of Human Work. *Mind, Culture and Activity.* 12 (2), 128-147.

Brewer, J. D., (2000). *Ethnography*. Buckingham: Open University Press.

Cole, M., (1996). *Cultural Psychology: A Once and Future Discipline*. Cambridge: Harvard University Press.

Constantopoulou, X., (2002). *Educational Policy and Practice for Dyslexic Pupils: The Greek Case*. Athens: Educational Issues Publishers.

Cohen, L., Lawrence, M. and Morrison, K., (2007). *Research Methods in Education*. London: Routledge.

Daniels, H., (2004). Activity theory, Discourse and Bernstein. *Educational Review* 56 (2), 121-132.

Davydov, V. V., (1999). The Content and Unsolved Problems of Activity Theory. In *Perspectives on Activity Theory,* edited by Y. Engeström, R. Miettinen, and R L Punamaki, pp. 39-51. Cambridge: Cambridge University Press.

Delamont, S., (2002). *Fieldwork in Educational Settings: Methods, Pitfalls and Perspectives*. London: Routledge.

Denscombe, M., (2003). *The Good Research Guide for Small-scale Social Research Projects* (2nd ed.). Maidenhead: Open University Press.

Engeström, Y., (1999a). Activity Theory and Individual and Social Transformation. In *Perspectives on Activity Theory* edited by Y. Engeström, R. Miettinen, and R. L. Punamaki, pp. 19-38. Cambridge: Cambridge University Press.

Engeström, Y., (1999b). Innovative Learning in Work Teams: Analysing Cycles of Knowledge Creation in Practice. In *Perspectives on Activity Theory,* edited by Y. Engeström, R. Miettinen, and R. L. Punamaki, pp. 377-403. Cambridge: Cambridge University Press.

Engeström, Y., (2001). Expansive Learning at Work: Toward an Activity Theoretical Reconceptualization. *Journal of Education and Work*. 14 (1), 133-156.

Engeström, Y., Engeström, R, and Vahaaho, T., (1999). When the Centre Does not Hold: The Importance of Knotworking. In *Activity Theory and Social Practice,* edited by S. Chaiklin, M. Hedegaard, and U.J. Jensen, pp. 345-374. Aarhus: Aarhus University Press.

Fine, G. A., and Shulman, D., (2009). Lies from the Field: Ethical Issues in Organizational Ethnography. In *Organizational Ethnography: Studying the Complexities of Everyday Life,* edited by S. Ybema, D. Yanow, H. Wells, and F. Kamsteeg, pp. 177-195. London: Sage.

Griffiths, C. B., Norwich, B., and Burden, B., (2004). Parental Agency, Identity and Knowledge: Mothers of Children with Dyslexia. *Oxford Review of Education*. 30 (3), 417-433.

Hunter-Carsch, M., (2009). Learning Support in the Secondary School: Needs Analysis and Provision for Dyslexic Students. In *Dyslexia and Effective Learning in Secondary and Tertiary Education,* edited by M. Hunter-Carsch and M. Herrington, pp. 12-37. London: Whurr Publishers.

Kirby, A., Edwards, L., and Hughes, A., (2008). Parents' Concerns about Children with Specific Learning Difficulties: Insights Gained from an Online Message Centre. *Support for Learning*. 23 (4), 193-200.

Leadbetter, J., (2004). The role of Mediating Artefacts in the Work of Educational Psychologists during Consultative Conversations in Schools. *Educational Review*. 56 (2), 133-145.

Leadbetter, J., (2006). Investigating and Conceptualising the Notion of Consultation to Facilitate Multi-agency Work. *Educational Psychology in Practice.* 22 (1), 19-31.

Leont'ev, A. N., (1978). *Activity, Consciousness, and Personality.* Englewood Cliffs: Prentice-Hall.

Leont'ev, A. N., (1981). *Problems of the Development of the Mind.* Moscow: Progress.

Marshall, C. and Rossman, G. B., (2011). *Designing Qualitative Research* (5th ed.). London: Sage.

Martin, D., (2008). A New Paradigm to Inform Inter-professional Learning for Integrating Speech and Language Provision into Secondary Schools: A Socio-cultural Activity Theory Approach. *Child Language Teaching and Therapy.* 24 (2) 173-192.

MNER., (2006). Examination of Physically Disabled Candidates.

MNER., (2008). Law 3699/2008. Special Education of People with Handicap or Special Educational Needs.

MNER., (2009). Within Schools Exams, Short Time or Hourly Exams for Trimester or Four Month Periods of Secondary School Students with Disability and Special Educational Needs or Specific Learning Difficulties.

Pollock, J., Waller, E. and Politt, R., (2004). *Day-to-day Dyslexia in the Classroom* (2nd ed.). London: Routledge.

Robson, C., (2011). *Real World Research: A Resource for Social Scientists and Practitioner-researchers* (3rd ed.). Oxford: Blackwell.

Vygotsky, L. S., (1978). *Mind in Society: The Development of Higher Psychological Processes.* Cambridge: Harvard University Press.

Vygotsky, L.S., (1987). *Thought and Language.* Cambridge, MA: MIT Press.

BIOGRAPHICAL SKETCH

Dr. Maria Rontou

Affiliation: University of Athens e-learning,
Primary Education of Korinthia

Education:

2004-2010: University of Birmingham.
Doctorate in Education. Strand: Language Studies. Thesis title: Provision for students with dyslexia in EFL: an ethnographic case study
2002-2003: University of Warwick
MA in English Language Studies and Methods
1998-2002: University of Athens
BA with QTS in Greek and English Language and Philology (grade: 8/10)
Direction: literature

Professional Appointments:

2001/2

- teacher of English as a Foreign Language to A, B, D and FCE class at the language school "The Model," Athens.
- private tutor in EFL

2003/4

- EFL teacher at the language school Kerstin Hens, Peristeri, Athens.
- EFL teacher at 28th Primary school of Peristeri, Athens and 26th Primary school of Ilion, Athens.
- EFL teacher at the language school Axon (Egaleo, Athens).
- August 2004: guide in Warwick Castle, UK

2004/5

- English tutor for Midland tutor services and Select tutors.
- supply teacher of Greek in Greek Supplementary schools in Tamworth, Cannock and Stourbridge (5-17 years and adults).
- volunteer learning support assistant in ESOL class of the Adult Education Service in the Cornerstone Family Centre, Coventry.
- 25/7/05-19/8/05: assistant trainer in TEFL certificate in Via Lingua Teacher Training centre in Korinth, Greece.

2005/6

- teaching assistant in primary and secondary schools for Hays Education Coventry and primary school teacher for Select Education
- teacher of Greek in Greek Community school in Stourbridge (ages 4-6 years) and supply teacher of Greek in Greek schools in Tamworth and Birmingham (ages 5-15 years and adults)

2006/7

- administration staff at LEA of Secondary Education of Arkadia, Tripolis
- teacher of EFL at 5th Primary school of Tripolis.
- teacher of English for Nurses at Institute of Vocational Training (IEK) of Tripolis.

2007-08 teacher of EFL at 3rd Senior High School of Petroupolis and 1st and 2nd Technical Vocational Schools of Ilion.

2008-09 teacher of EFL at Night Junior and Senior High schools of Tripolis.

2009-10 teacher of EFL at 2nd Technical Vocational School of Tripolis.

2010-11

- teacher of EFL at 2nd Primary school of Loutraki,
- examiner for the English language for State certificate

2011/12

- Teacher of EFL for Museum Guards and Administrative and Financial Executive at IEK of Corinth-Loutraki
- Teacher of EFL at 2nd primary school of Loutraki
- Reviewer for Journal of Literacy Research
- Examiner for State certificate

2012/13

- Teacher of EFL at 7th Primary school of Egaleo
- Teacher of EFL for specialists in Computerized Accounting at IEK of Egaleo
- Examiner for State certificate

2013/14

- Teacher of EFL at 1st Primary School of Loutraki
- Examiner for State Certificate
- Article editor for Sage Open

2014/2015

- Teacher of EFL at 1st Primary School of Loutraki
- Associate of University of Athens e-learning programme
- Examiner for State certificate
- Reviewer for Professional Journal of primary education teachers of Korinthia and for Learning Disabilities: A Contemporary Journal

2015/2016

- Associate of University of Athens e-learning programme
- Reviewer for Professional Journal of primary education teachers of Korinthia

Honors:
Awards for EdD:

1) All Saints Educational Trust grant towards academic fees for 2006-07
2) Educational Review Progress Scholarship covering academic fees for 2007-09

Publications Last 3 Years:

1) Article titled 'EFL grammatical terminology: how useful is it for teachers and how difficult for students?', Aspects Today, issue 33, January-April 2012
2) Paper titled 'The discourse of disability in Greek policy documents' at Conference titled 'Breaking classroom silences: addressing sensitive issues,' 12/11/13, European University of Cyprus, Nicosia.
3) Article titled 'Contradictions around differentiation for pupils with dyslexia learning English as a Foreign Language at secondary school,' Support for Learning, volume 27, issue 4, 2012.
4) Chapter titled 'Implementation of national policy on dyslexia in EFL provision,' (pp. 115-135) in *Researching dyslexia in multilingual settings: diverse perspectives*, (Ed), D. Martin, (2013), Clevedon: Multilingual Matters.
5) Paper titled 'Differentiation for students with dyslexia,' 16/5/2015, One day seminar by Panhellenic Association of State School Teachers of English, Athens.
6) Chapter titled 'Contradictions around differentiation of homework for students with dyslexia studying EFL' in *Multilingualism, Literacy and Dyslexia: Breaking down barriers for Educators'* Eds Peer, L and Reid, G (2016) Routledge Publishers.
7) Article titled 'The difficulties and needs of students with dyslexia learning EFL: a case study, professional journal of primary education teachers of Korinthia, issue 2, February 2016.

In: Dyslexia: Perspectives, Challenges and Treatment Options ISBN: 978-1-63485-328-6
Editor: Marilyn Frazier

Chapter 5

PARENTS AND TEACHERS OPINION ABOUT LEARNING SKILLS: COMPARISON BETWEEN BRAZILIAN AND ITALIAN DYSLEXIC'S STUDENTS

Simone Aparecida Capellini[1], Catia Giaconi[2] and Giseli Donadon Germano[3]

[1]Investigation Learning Disabilities Laboratory at the Speech and Hearing Sciences Department – São Paulo State University "Júlio de Mesquita Filho," UNESP, Marília, São Paulo, Brazil
[2]Department of Education, Cultural Heritage and Tourism at the University of Macerata, Macerata, Italy
[3]Investigation Learning Disabilities Laboratory at the Speech and Hearing Sciences Department – São Paulo State University "Júlio de Mesquita Filho," UNESP, Marília, São Paulo, Brazil

ABSTRACT

The aim of this chapter is to describe and compare the response of parents and teachers of Brazilian and Italian Dyslexic's students about learning skills. A total of 36 students with dyslexia were assessed by the Learning Skills Checklist (18 Brazilian dyslexic students and 18 Italians's dyslexic students), from both genders, from 3rd to 5th grade of Elementary School. The Learning Skills Checklist included a total of six item, divided into attention skills, visual processing skills, hearing processing skills, math-logical processecing skills, motor skills and behavioral skills. The teacher/parents should response in a scale from 0 to 3 points. The Learning Skills Checklist was distribuited to each parents and teacher students and the response was compared. In the comparison between the responses of teachers and parents of the Italian students, there was a significant difference in the visual processing skills, as teachers showed that the Italian dyslexic's students had greater difficulties in visual processing when compared with the parent response. Regarding the same comparison in Brazilian population, there was no significant diferences in any skill. In comparison between the responses of parents between Brazilian and Italian population there was significant difference between attentional skills, visual processing skills, hearing processing skills, math-logical processing skills. Regarding Brazilian's parents, their children had greater difficulties in these skills when compared to Italian parents. In comparison between the responses of teachers between Brazilian and Italian population, there were significant differences among attention skills, visual processing skills, math-logical processing and behavioral skills. Brazilian teachers indicated that their students had greater difficulties for those skills then Italian teachers, except for behavioral skill, which Italians teachers referred greater difficulties among theirs students. As a conclusion, parents and teachers of Italians students had different points of views of learning skills, indicating that Italian's teachers are more perceptive of the student's deficits. Regarding Brazilian population, there was no difference between parents and teachers response, indicating a lack of knowledge of dyslexics difficulties. However, when compared Italian and Brazilian population, was showed that teachers and parents of Brazilian's students pointed out more difficulties in most of the skills, which can be assumed by the lack of public educational policy support for dyslexic students.

Keywords: dyslexia, checklist, assessment

1. Introduction

Developmental dyslexia, an unexplained difficulty in word reading accuracy and/or fluency, affects 5–12% of children. Also, the manifestations described in Dyslexia's students may be related with others unfavorable outcomes, such as reduced educational attainment and academic self-esteem (Norton, Beach and Gabrieli, 2015).

Researchers had described that reading is a highly complex task, requiring the integration of multiple visual, linguistic, cognitive, and attentional processes. Likewise, reading additionally relies on the integration of visual, orthographic, phonological, and semantic information (Ziegler et al., 2008).

Because of this diversity of manifestations, it is necessary the elaboration of procedures in order to raise the academic potential markers of this population.

Thompson et al. (2015) made a longitudinal study following children at high risk of dyslexia from preschool through the early primary years assessing them from age 3 years and 6 months at approximately annual intervals on tasks tapping cognitive, language, and executive-motor skills. As results, the authors described that at the time of school entry, language skills become significant predictors, and motor skills add a small but significant increase to the prediction probability. They concluded that Dyslexia is the outcome of multiple risk factors and children with language difficulties at school entry are at high risk. Family history of dyslexia is a predictor of literacy outcome from the preschool years.

Also, Dilnot et al. (2016) investigated the role of distal, proximal, and child risk factors as predictors of reading readiness and attention and behavior in children at risk of dyslexia. The parents of a longitudinal sample of 251 preschool children, including children at family risk of dyslexia and children with preschool language difficulties, provided measures of socioeconomic status, home literacy environment, family stresses, and child health via interviews and questionnaires. As results, the authors founded that children at family risk of dyslexia and children with preschool language difficulties experienced more environmental adversities and health risks than controls. The risks associated with family risk of dyslexia and with language status were additive. Both home literacy environment and child health predicted reading readiness while home literacy environment and family stresses predicted attention and behavior.

As described above, the necessity to find ways to assess and predict dyslexia diagnosis is still an obstacle among researches across the worlds. One of the possibilities is the use of checklist or questionnaires addressed to parents or teachers.

Checklists have pointers, which can be very useful in promoting a better self-understanding, and indicate future assessment needs. A rating obtained from the same individual (e.g., the same parent on different occasions) reflects the stability of the child's behavior in a certain environment (e.g., the home), as well as stability in individual characteristics and child interaction characteristics. If ratings on different occasions are obtained from the same type of informant, but from different individuals at different assessments (e.g., different teachers on different occasions), the stability is lower because stability in individual rater characteristics and specific rater-child interaction characteristics are eliminated (Verhulst; Koot and Van der Ende, 1994).

El Nokali, Bachman and Votruba-Drzal (2010) referred that parent involvement is often considered a pathway through which schools enhance the achievement of underperforming children (Berger, 1991). Consequently, it's necessary that parent involvement is encouraged by teachers, childcare providers, policy makers, parents, and researchers (Duch, 2005; Sheldon and Epstein, 2005). Moreover, parent involvement is a key component of early childhood education programs.

The aim of this chapter is to describe and compare the response of parents and teachers of Brazilian and Italian Dyslexic's students about learning skills.

2. METHOD

A total of 36 students with dyslexia were assessed by the Learning Skills Checklist. As part of an international partnership from the Investigation Learning Disabilities Laboratory at the Speech and Hearing Sciences Department – São Paulo State University "Júlio de Mesquita Filho" – UNESP – Marília - São Paulo – Brazil with the Department of Education, Cultural Heritage and Tourism at the University of Macerata, Macerata – Itália, 18 Brazilian dyslexic students and 18 Italians's dyslexic students, from both genders, from 3rd to 5th grade of Elementary School participated of this study.

As a procedure, all students received the Learning Skills Checklist, which was development by Capellini, Giaconi and Germano to this study. As procedure, parents and teachers of each dyslexic student received the questionnaire. They were solicited to complete the questionnaire in relation to the six items assessed in order to make it possible for researchers better characterize the academic problems of students.

The checklist included a total of six items, divided into attention skills (i.e., difficulty maintaining attention during the performance of academic activities), visual processing skills (i.e., Difficult to copy designs, shapes and letters of blackboard or notebook), auditory processing skills (i.e., delay to learn to speak; exhibits changing of similar letters aurally), math-logical processing skills (i.e., Difficult to do mathematical calculations), motor skills (i.e., difficulty with fine motor and global skills) and behavioral skills (i.e., presence of agitated behavior in the classroom and at home).

The teacher/parents should response in a scale from 0 to 3 points (likert scale), with zero referring to no difficulty and 3 great difficulties. All responses were scored according to the scale for comparison of responses.

3. RESULTS AND DISCUSSION

The obtained data were statistically analyzed in order to compare the intragroup and intergroup results. We used the IBM SPSS (Statistical Package for Social Sciences), in its version 22.0, for analysis of results. The results were analyzed statistically with a significance level of 5% (0.050), indicated with an asterisk in the tables on the results.

The Mann-Whitney test was applied in order to verify possible differences between the performance of the variables for the two groups of Brazilian and Italians, regarding parents' opinions (table 1).

Table 1. Mean scores, Standard deviation (SD) and p-value from parents of Italians and Brazilians dyslexic's students in Learning Skills Checklist

	Italians			Brazilian			
	N	Mean	SD	N	Mean	SD	p-value
Attention	18	3,61	2,004	18	7,56	2,749	0,000*
Visual	18	12,00	6,068	18	17,44	6,591	0,011*
Auditory	18	20,39	16,004	18	32,44	15,139	0,015*
Math	18	6,72	4,561	18	10,44	5,447	0,020*
Motor	18	5,72	3,847	18	6,56	3,053	0,498
behavior	18	6,33	4,715	18	6,44	3,399	0,923

At table 1 there was a statistical difference between the opinion of parents regarding attention, visual, auditory, and Math processing skills. The total average score of Brazilian parents was higher than that of Italian parents. This suggests that Brazilian parents showed greater tendency to indicate some academic problems of their children. Parent involvement bridges two key contexts in children's early development, namely the home and school settings (El Nokali; Bachman and Votruba-Drzal, 2010). However, it is important to have attention to these reports because they can raise false interpretations in relation to a diagnosis. Gioia, Andrwes and Isquith (1996) referred that some parents can respond unusually negative manner relative to the clinical manifestation.

Table 2 shows the comparison between groups of Brazilian and Italians, regarding teacher's opinions.

At table 2 there was a statistical difference between the opinion of parents regarding attention, visual, Math and Behavioral processing skills. The total average score of Brazilian teachers was higher than that of Italian parents. This suggests that Brazilian teachers showed greater tendency to indicate some academic problems of their students, with exception of the behavioral process, which the Italians teachers indicated higher score.

Studies with checklist about academic performance still are insufficient for the Brazilian and Italian population. However, Verhulst, Koot, and van der Ende (1994) referred that the comparison of the predictive power of parent and teacher information showed that teacher scores were a stronger predictor of poor outcome than parent scores. Although teachers report fewer problems than parents about the same children, their reports apparently are informative with respect to later functioning. It is therefore important to include teacher information in the diagnostic assessment of children.

Table 2. Mean scores, Standard desviation (SD) and p-value from teachers of Italians and Brazilians dyslexic's students in Learning Skills Checklist

	Italians			Brazilian			
Variables	N	Mean	SD	N	Mean	SD	p-value
Attention	18	3,61	2,004	18	8,00	3,308	0,000*
Visual	18	13,39	5,637	18	18,78	7,811	0,031*
Auditory	18	24,89	9,701	18	33,33	18,746	0,106
Math	18	7,17	1,917	18	10,83	6,290	0,008*
Motor	18	5,28	1,526	18	6,56	3,634	0,183
Behavior	18	5,78	2,533	18	3,83	3,294	0,021*

Thus, the home and school contexts are characterized as autonomous microsystems and parent involvement is conceptualized as a mesosystem, which is made up of interactions between key microsystems. Although each setting can independently influence a child, together the home and school contexts interact to offer a unique influence (El Nokali; Bachman and Votruba-Drzal, 2010). That's one of the reasons that it's important to compare the answers given by parents and teachers.

Table 3 shows the comparison between teachers and parents of the Brazilian students (Wilcoxon Signed Test).

Table 3. Mean scores, Standard deviation (SD) and p-value from teachers and parents of Brazilians dyslexic's students in Learning Skills Checklist

		Brazilian's teachers		Brazilian's parents		p-value
Variables	N	Mean	SD	Mean	SD	
Attention	18	8,00	3,308	7,56	2,749	0,689
Visual	18	18,78	7,811	17,44	6,591	0,316
Auditory	18	33,33	18,746	32,44	1,139	0,794
Math	18	10,83	6,290	10,44	5,447	0,698
Motor	18	6,56	3,634	6,56	3,053	0,875
Behavior	18	3,83	3,294	6,44	3,399	0,004*

Regarding the answers given by teachers and parents of Brazilian's dyslexics students, there was statistical difference between groups only for the behavioral process skills, which had higher score for parents.

Research has supported the negative effects of early problem behaviors, including inattention, problems with social skills, and aggression, on school failure and lower achievement across elementary and secondary schools (Fergusson and Woodward, 2000; Malecki and Elliott, 2002).

Hill et al. (2004) related that parent academic involvement may improve school performance by reducing behavioral problems that may interfere with learning. Aggression, inattention, and social problems are three behavioral issues that have a consistent and negative relation with achievement.

Jellinek et al. (1998) elaborated a Pediatric Symptom Checklist (PSC) that should be completed by parents and designed to help pediatricians in outpatient practice identify school-age children with difficulties in psychosocial functioning. One of the findings of this study highlight that some children who appeared to have "false positive" results on the PSC were actually rated as being just one coding unit away from being considered dysfunctional by the clinicians.

Another finding was that two children classified by the PSC as dysfunctional, one had a PSC score exactly at the cutoff point, and both of these children were living in stressful circumstances, which may have significantly added to their PSC scores. Although the clinicians thought that these children were functioning adequately overall, both had a number of psychosomatic and behavioral symptoms that may have led their mothers to give higher scores when they initially filled out the PSC.

In relation to the Brazilian population, the findings of this study indicate that parents of students with dyslexia related behavioral problems as more impactful than other skills. These results may suggest that there is a shortage about the manifestations present in students with dyslexia.

Table 4 shows the comparison between teachers and parents of the Italians students (Wilcoxon Signed Test).

Table 4. Mean scores, Standard desviation (SD) and p-value from teachers and parentes of Italian's dyslexic's students in Learning Skills Checklist

		Italian's teachers		Italian's parentes		
Variables	N	Mean	SD	Mean	SD	p-value
Attention	18	3,61	2,004	3,61	2,004	1,000
Visual	18	13,39	5,637	12,00	6,068	0,022*
Auditory	18	24,89	9,701	20,39	16,004	0,084
Math	18	7,17	1,917	6,72	4,561	0,511
Motor	18	5,28	1,526	5,72	3,847	0,664
Behavior	18	5,78	2,533	6,33	4,715	1,000

Regarding the answers given by teachers and parents of Italian's dyslexics students, there was statistical difference between groups only for the visual process skills, which had higher score for teachers.

In this study it was possible to observe that Brazilian's parents and teachers showed greater tendency to indicate some academic problems of their children. Also, considering the comparison between parents and teachers' responses, Brazilian's showed a preoccupation regarding the behavioral aspects, while Italian's pointed to visual aspects.

Those results indicate that, besides the socio-economic differences, there are still differences in the way both parents and teachers see and characterize the educational aspects of children, which might be concerning for researchers and impacts the possibilities of the elaboration of educational policy.

Waltenberg (2005) made a review about the PISA 2000 survey (Programme for International Student Assessment), which as aimed to assess the level of cognitive competence of students from different countries (total 32 countries). Specifically, among all surveyed countries, Brazil occupies the last position in terms of average performance in all tests (tests of reading, mathematics and science).

In reading, the Brazilian average is 383 points (31st place last), meanwhile Italy children performance an average of 489 points (21st place). One way to compare the results is to divide students of the results of all the countries in quartiles results and subsequently observed in each country, which is the proportion of students who belong to each quartile performance internationally defined. The proportion of students from each country belonging to the lower hip results is an indicator of the proportion of students who do not reach a level of minimum competence, according to international standards. 72.01% of Brazilian students are in the classification against 25.62% of Italian students.

The justification, pointed by Waltenberg (2005), which emphasizes the socio-economic inequality as explanation presupposes the existence of a causal relationship between socio-economic equality and good average performance on a test of cognitive competencies, which, although it is a plausible hypothesis, further studies that corroborate.

CONCLUSION

As a conclusion, parents and teachers of Italians students had different points of views of learning skills, indicating that Italian's teachers are more perceptive of the students' deficits. Regarding Brazilian population, there was no difference between parents and teachers response, indicating a lack of knowledge of dyslexics difficulties. However, when compared Italian and Brazilian population, was showed that teachers and parents of Brazilian's students pointed out more difficulties in most of the skills, which can be assumed by the lack of public educational policy support for dyslexic students.

REFERENCES

Berger, E.H. (1991). Parent involvement: Yesterday and today. *The Elementary School Journal.* 91, 209– 219.

Dilnot, J.; Hamilton, L.; Maughan, B.; and Snowling, M. J. (2016). Child and environmental risk factors predicting readiness for learning in children at high risk of dyslexia. *Development and psychopathology*, 1-10, http://europepmc.org/abstract/MED/26900040

Duch, H. (2005). Redefining parent involvement in Head Start: A two-generation approach. *Early Child Development and Care,* 175, 23–35.

El Nokali, N. E.; Bachman, H.J.; and Votruba-Drzal, E. (2010). Parent Involvement and Children's Academic and Social Development in Elementary School. *Child Development,* 81(3), 988–1005.

Gioia, G. A., Andrwes, K. and Isquith, P. K. (1996). *Behavior rating inventory of executive function-preschool version (BRIEF-P)*. Psychological Assessment Resources.

Hill, N. E., Castellino, D. R., Lansford, J. E., Nowlin, P., Dodge, K. A., Bates, J. E. and Pettit, G. S. (2004). Parent academic involvement as related to school behavior, achievement, and aspirations: Demographic variations across adolescence. *Child development, 75*(5), 1491-1509.

Jellinek, M.S.; Murphy, J.M.; Robinson, J.; Feins, A.; Lamb, S.; and Fenton, T. (1998). Pediatric Symptom Checklist: Screening school-age children for psychosocial dysfunction, *The Journal of Pediatrics*, 112 (2), 201-209.

Norton, E.S.; Beach, S.D.; and Gabrieli, J.D.E. (2015). Neurobiology of dyslexia. *Current Opinion in Neurobiology,* 30, 73–78.

Sheldon, S.B.; and Epstein, J.L. (2005). Involvement counts: Family and community partnerships and mathematics achievement. *Journal of Educational Research,* 98, 196–206.

Thompson, P.A.; Hulme, C.; Nash, H.M.; Gooch, D.; Hayiou-Thomas, E.; and Snowling, M.J. (2015). Developmental dyslexia: predicting individual risk. *Journal of Child Psychology and Psychiatry*, 56, 9, 976–987.

Verhulst, F.C.; Koot, H.M. and Van der Ende, J. (1994) Differential Predictive Value of Parents' and Teachers' Reports of Children's Problem Behaviors: A Longitudinal Study. *Journal of Abnormal Child Psychology,* 22, 531-546.

Waltenberg, F.D. (2005). Educational inequity in Brazil. A Evaluation with PISA 2000 data. *Economi A,* 6,67–118.

Ziegler, J.C.; Castel, C., Georgel, C.P.; George, F.; Alario, F.X.; and Perry, C.(2008). Developmental dyslexia and the dual route model of reading: Simulating individual differences and subtypes. *Cognition,* 107, 151–178.

In: Dyslexia: Perspectives, Challenges and Treatment Options ISBN: 978-1-63485-328-6
Editor: Marilyn Frazier

Chapter 6

DYSLEXIA AND MULTILINGUAL LEARNERS: ASSESSMENT AND INTERVENTIONS

Mim Hutchings, EdD and Tilly Mortimore, PhD
Bath Spa University, Bath, UK

ABSTRACT

This chapter initially outlines key findings from the Dyslexia and Multilingualism research project (Mortimore et al., 2012) identifying challenges and lessons learnt. This project comprised a literacy intervention for vulnerable learners with English as an additional language (EAL) in English primary schools. The mixed methodology explored the impact of the intervention on learners' skills, incentives and interactions together with the views of children, Teaching Assistants and parents. The second section focuses on lessons relating to screening and assessment processes used for identifying SpLD/Dyslexia within complex multilingual schools and the importance of combining cognitive and psycholinguistic with socio-cultural approaches and understanding of the child's story. It confirms the need for caution in attaching labels too swiftly to children with EAL whose literacy fails to thrive whilst promoting prompt adoption of appropriate interventions, combined with enriched language experience. The third section outlines a staged approach to intervention drawing on our findings. The conclusion indicates ways in which schools and professionals might develop assessment and interventions suitable for complex multilingual contexts.

Keywords: SpLD/Dyslexia, English as an additional language (EAL), literacy intervention, identification of SpLD/Dyslexia

INTRODUCTION

The United Kingdom (UK) Context: Aims and Drivers of the Project

In 2011, the UK Big Lottery funded a research project exploring support needs of learners with English as an Additional Language (EAL), who might also be at risk of

SpLD/Dyslexia. From 1997 to 2013 numbers of students with EAL in English and Welsh schools have increased from 7.6% to 16.2% of all pupils (Strand, and Murphy, 2015) with over 360 languages spoken by 2015 (NALDIC, 2016). Despite population movements driving multi-diversity of language and culture, the English educational systems remains monolingual (Martin, 2016). Minority first language children are expected swiftly to become literate in English.

Levels of achievement across children with EAL are inconsistent (Strand and Murphy, 2015) with concern around how bilingual learners are perceived and catered for in schools, how learning failure can be racialized as learning disability (Ofsted, 2013; Martin, 2016) and how to support bilingualism within a monolingual educational culture. Political policy obviously influences pedagogical decisions but life experiences, social and cultural differences affect EAL and literacy development necessitating a holistic approach to teaching and learning. Transition from junior/primary school to high/secondary school is risky for all vulnerable children (Evangelou et al., 2008). Demands upon reading comprehension, spelling and writing increase and, for children with EAL, the need to move beyond conversational language, (Basic Interpersonal Communicative Skills - BICS) to the increasingly academic language of the secondary curriculum (Cognitive Academic Language Proficiency -CALP) (Cummins, 2000). The added risk of SpLD/Dyslexia increases difficulties mastering rule systems, new phonology and orthography of the second language.

10% of children risk SpLD/Dyslexia (Dyslexia International, 2016). Bilingual learners with EAL are under-represented in SpLD/Dyslexia programmes (Elbeheri and Everatt, 2016). Identifying SpLD/Dyslexia in children acquiring EAL risks misattribution of difficulties to second language acquisition or inappropriate application of SEN labels and expectations (Fawcett, 2016). Difficulties acquiring a second language (L2) can mask signs of SpLD/Dyslexia and levels of skill in oral language affect development or prevention of SpLD/dyslexia (Snowling, 2010). Research (e.g., Ganschow and Sparks, 2000) confirms transfer between languages of strengths and weaknesses in phonology/orthography, syntax and semantics. Learning EAL challenges learners at risk of dyslexia because it necessitates skills compromised in dyslexia - sequencing ability, phonological knowledge and short/long-term memory and listening abilities (Wolf 2008) making acquiring an opaque second language, like English, challenging for dyslexic children (Ziegler and Goswami, 2005).

Pre-2010, little research explored the impact of interventions for this group. Our mixed-methodology project aimed to fill this gap, investigating the potential for identifying dyslexia in children with EAL and successful interventions for those whose literacy was failing to develop. Its combination of expertise from two professional worlds, SpLD/Dyslexia support and the world of those who support bilingual learners was ground-breaking. We aimed to:

- Establish reliable ways of identifying dyslexic type difficulties in EAL children;
- Develop and trial appropriate support strategies and materials;
- Provide training for SENCos and TAs involved in the project.

Dyslexic learners need direct, systematic, multisensory instruction (Brooks, 2008). This also applies to acquiring L2 rule systems (Sparks and Miller, 2000). We therefore explored the literature around dyslexia and working with bilingual learners (e.g., Crombie and McColl, 2001) to devise and trial a daily intervention programme delivered by trained teaching assistants. In UK Government funded schools, a Special Educational Needs Co-ordinator

(SENCo) is responsible for pupils with SEN and for pupils with EAL with an identified SEN. SENCos often do have additional but separate responsibility for EAL although the role of 'SENCo' may be replaced with 'Inclusion leader/ coordinator' covering all vulnerable groups, including EAL. The SENCo co-ordinates varying numbers of staff including teaching assistants according to the school's size and needs. UK schools make extensive use of Teaching Assistants (TAs) whose salaries equate to approximately 30% that of a qualified teacher. They are not qualified teachers so their role is, guided by a teacher, to support teachers in the classroom, prepare resources and equipment, take groups of children who need extra support in, for example literacy or numeracy out of a class and offer work that the teacher cannot always accommodate in class. (Unison, 2016)

The Blatchford Report (2009) questioned the usefulness of teaching assistants. Economic and practical constraints dictated our selection of TAs for this intervention alongside a desire to explore the impact of specific training and support on their effectiveness with vulnerable EAL learners.

The project involved 215 children, aged 9-11, of all social and economic levels, from 55 English rural and urban schools, many containing above average numbers of bilingual learners. All children had attended UK schools for over two years. We developed a screening for the project, described later.

Children were divided into three groups for Phase One of the intervention:

- A - pairs taking the intervention
- B - pairs undertaking a paired reading activity with a trained TA
- C - a waiting control group with no current individual support.

Phase Two enabled groups B and C to undertake the designed intervention and established whether any changes were sustained over time. Children's literacy skills were tested three times - pre and post Phase One and at the end of Phase Two. Data was analysed with SPSS.

To reflect the 'real life' context of the study and provide a rich picture of experience of all involved, our mixed methodology design offered both quantifiable impact of the intervention upon literacy scores alongside the voices of some participants gathered through focus groups and interviews with children, parents and teaching assistants. We feel that mixed methodology enabled the emergence of important issues which might otherwise have remained hidden (Hutchings and Mortimore, 2014).

Section 1: The Intervention Programme and Key Findings

A literature review of research across the fields of SpLD/Dyslexia and EAL informed the design of screening instruments and the intervention (See Mortimore et al., 2012). The organization and structure of the specialist intervention programme was dictated by research into effective teaching for SpLD/Dyslexia and EAL (e.g., Brooks et al., 2008; Geva and Zadeh 2006). It considered precisely targeted ICT packages (Smythe, 2010) and the impact on reading comprehension of vocabulary and repeated reading programmes.

Resources

The funding provided each school with two resources: Rapid reading (RR) (2006) and the ICT programme Nessy (2010). Rapid Reading uses high interest, low reading level, illustrated (fiction and non-fiction) books for 7-11 year old readers, with linked speech recognition software supporting reading practice and worksheets to consolidate word-level work. Nessy was developed specifically for learners with SpLD/dyslexia. It is a computer-based, structured phonics resource for reading and spelling, including letter patterns as well as spelling and reading rules. The material includes humorous visual memory aids, games and activity worksheets. Our intervention highlighted spelling and phonology, with reinforcement through written worksheets.

Both cumulative programmes promote overlearning and reinforcement, essential for dyslexic learners. Furthermore, they offered maximum opportunities for oral language development, explicit vocabulary teaching (including pre-tutoring of key vocabulary), development of comprehension skills (oral and reading) and work with English morphemes.

A similar activity was needed for comparison group B which would not risk wasting the children's time. We therefore adopted a paired reading activity (Boyle and Topping, 2012) which supports reading fluency practice, using interesting texts marginally too difficult for the learner to read independently. This paired reading strategy incorporated oral language development; new vocabulary, ensuring comprehension and retelling the content of texts.

TA and SENCO Training

All project staff received two days of training including pedagogy for dyslexia and bilingual children (for TAs/SENCos); the use of identification screeners and pre-post testing (SENCOs); use of NESSY/Rapid Reading/Paired Reading and record keeping (TAs).

TAs observed demonstrations of paired reading techniques and were issued with detailed handbooks supporting this intervention. They were asked to keep brief daily session records as a fidelity measure and were issued with simple proformas for this. Weekly narrative records were also created to provide the child's view on their reading progress and responses to the material covered.

The TA Handbook explained:

> It helps us to understand the children's preferences and the extent to which the texts have interested or motivated them to read. It also allows you to understand and share with the children their strategies, strengths and weaknesses, and to help them to develop ideas about what critical reading involves and how they can help to improve their understanding. Don't take too long over the review; write it with the child either at the end of a completed book or on a weekly basis – whichever is appropriate.

Findings: Impact on Literacy

Phase One

Statistical analysis of test scores (ANOVA) indicated significant progress in all skills across all three groups except for control group C's progress in single word reading, National Curriculum writing level (NC), number, of words, speed and legibility of writing and of writing speed for groups A and B.

Despite the pre-intervention skills of the control group C being significantly stronger than groups A or B, effect sizes of the changes demonstrated that both intervention groups, A and B, outperformed controls across all skills. Comparing group A with paired reading group B revealed Group A (NESSY, and Rapid Reading) outperforming the paired reading group (B) in spelling, phonological decoding and reading accuracy. However, group B made higher gains in skills associated with reading fluency, silent reading, sentence comprehension and oral receptive language alongside comparative gains in single word reading. It was surprising, however, to see group B outperforming group A in writing speed, word length and in advances in National Curriculum writing standard levels, since the paired reading activities involved no writing tasks.

We concluded that the NESSY/RR intervention had stronger specific impact on spelling and phonological decoding, compared with paired reading. However, paired reading with its added emphasis on comprehension strategies, oral vocabulary and positive feedback from the teaching assistant, produced significant gains in all aspects of literacy skills, with an unexpected trade-off for writing skills. Control group C made some progress in literacy. However, we observed with concern that progress in single word reading skills, number of words written or NC levels over this 15 week period failed to reach significance.

Phase Two

We analysed scores at the end of phase 2 to establish whether the gains from both the NESSY/RR and the paired reading intervention continued over time, particularly in the skills of word reading/decoding and vocabulary which underpin reading comprehension.

Overall, when intervention was not continued, gains from Phase One were sustained across the reading skills but were more fragile in the areas of spelling and writing which tended to level out but did not regress completely.

Once group C completed the Phase two NESSY/RR intervention, they made significant gains with single-word reading and spelling, reading rate and comprehension, vocabulary and non-word reading. However, reading and comprehension gains were only marginally significant and gains in reading accuracy/comprehension and writing speed did not reach significance. The picture here is more mixed.

Summary

This 15 week daily half-hour intervention programme delivered to two children by a trained TA resulted in significant gains in reading and spelling/writing skills. Both the intervention programme and the paired reading activity led to specific improvements and these improvements, particularly in reading skills, were sustained. However, analysis indicated a need for further reinforcement to stabilise spelling gains.

The Participants' Perspectives

Including the voices of children, TAs and families was a crucial trigger for designing future intervention programmes and understanding the importance of connections between communities, family and school. Data was collected through focus groups (children and parents) and interviews (TAs) in six schools at the end of the project. Themes for discussions comprised:

- Pleasure and enjoyment
- The materials used
- Progress and learning
- Being bilingual

Children emphasized how much they enjoyed the time spent with a supportive adult and the importance to them of a close working relationship with a trusted adult. They talked in detail about the materials and books and were clear about their differing interests and preferences for books, aspects of the programme and games. Using materials that speak to children's interests strongly incentivises engagement in learning. Children reported improved vocabulary, reading and spelling, progress was rated mainly in terms of moving through spelling and reading levels.

Children talked enthusiastically about languages and being bilingual. Focus groups stimulated discussion of the range of languages spoken within the group. Main points were:

- Many children were multilingual, sometimes speaking up to 4 languages. Additional languages used were linked to past homes or close relatives. Children made strategic choices about which languages to use in different contexts.
- Children saw the importance of keeping connections to wider family and friends and hence the value of continuing to speak read, and write in home languages.
- Children were comfortable, knowledgeable and interested in language and languages. For example children would discuss differences in spelling in different languages and scripts alongside modes of language use, such as speaking, reading and writing, showing awareness of how good they were in each.
- In some schools, children felt they were 'not allowed' to speak languages other than English unless there was a new non-English speaking child in the school whom they could help.

Overwhelmingly parents showed concern for their children's progress in school. They indicated that the intervention had benefitted their children. However, they showed little precise knowledge of the progress made by individual children throughout the intervention. However, parents reported changes in children's reading behaviors, such as choosing to read more frequently at home and improvements in spelling.

Parents appreciated the value of learning more than one language early in life 'because they never forget' and the importance of children learning English quickly in order to feel socially included. Both parents and children indicated that they speak, read and write more languages at home than schools had recorded.

Overall TAs were positive about their involvement in the project. They enthused about working with the children and how daily sessions had helped build strong relationships with most children. Their knowledge of bilingualism and dyslexia and skills had developed as a result of the training and daily work with children. They did report times when they felt that the school undervalued their increased skills and knowledge or used their time allocated to the project for other unrelated activities.

TAs indicated that, once a routine had been established, materials selected were suitably structured and enabled them to implement the programme confidently. They saw improvements in children's confidence in reading aloud reading comprehension and vocabulary enrichment. The challenging and interesting content motivated children to go beyond decoding to understanding text.

TAs did not discuss detailed aspects of progress in reading, such as phonological awareness, phonics and understanding of morphemes. Comments mainly covered increases in confidence and enjoyment. We had hoped that the daily/weekly and narrative records would provide an evidence base for the kinds of reading and spelling errors occurring plus insights into children's response to the intervention. Patterns of strengths and weaknesses over time can help to determine the reasons for children's difficulties and inform subsequent steps for an intervention programme. In reality many of the records were sparse. TAs concentrated on delivering the intervention and would have benefited from additional training in order to recognize what information could be crucial for future learning.

The more highly qualified and experienced TAs seemed to understand better what was required and how to analyse children's progress, indicating the importance of training and follow up support.

SECTION 2: LESSONS FROM THE PROJECT

Screening and Assessment

Identifying SpLD/Dyslexia

We needed a practical, economical school-based screening protocol for identifying risk of SpLD/Dyslexia, accessible for children with more limited knowledge of English. It should not require one-to-one assessment and should be manageable by teachers with minimal assessment training.

The literature (Mortimore et al., 2012) indicated evaluating the following skills:

- Single word reading
- Single word spelling
- Sentence comprehension
- Processing speed
- Working memory

- Phonological processing – non-word decoding
- Auditory/visual memory
- Verbal and non-verbal reasoning

To cover these skills we selected computer-delivered instruments - The Lucid Assessment System for Schools (LASS) 8-11 and Lucid Ability computer tests (Lucid Research Ltd, 2008) – because they:

- were mainly visual;
- reduced susceptibility to language and cultural differences;
- offered consistent language and format of test instructions.

Lucid Ability offered a Risk of Dyslexia Index and provided information about verbal reasoning, although this might be compromised by limited English. We added the Turner Non –word reading test (1994), the Working Memory Rating Scale Questionnaire (Alloway et al., 2008) and The Dyslexia Checklist - (Ball, 2007) modified slightly for learners with EAL. This checklist explores discrepancies; strengths and weaknesses across literacy attainment; underlying cognitive skills and classroom behaviour.

SENCos were invited to screen children with unexpected literacy difficulties. From a sample of 462 children, the research team selected the 220 who seemed at highest risk. Subsequently, to evaluate screener reliability, 44 of these children underwent a 1-to-1 full assessment for SpLD/Dyslexia undertaken in English by SpLD/Dyslexia qualified professional assessors with working experience of EAL learners. Detailed tests of non-verbal and visual spatial awareness, listening comprehension, short-term working memory, phonological processing, rapid naming and receptive language were added to the battery. Assessor training emphasised culturally appropriate measures and sensitivities and assessors attempted to gather from schools, children and families essential information about the learner's and family's story, culture, current and previous educational experience and reading history.

Unfortunately statistical comparisons of the scores on both the Lucid Dyslexia Index and the Dyslexia Checklist with the full assessment outcomes (risk or no risk of dyslexia) indicated no clear relationship between screener and full assessment identification of risk. Hence, despite all our carefully designed assessment protocols, our screener procedures did not provided reliable indicators of risk of dyslexia.

Some complex lessons emerged. Our analyses suggested:

- children with higher, rather than low, scores in English receptive language were more likely to be labelled as dyslexic;
- children need a certain level of verbal skill before dyslexia is likely to be identified. Poor word knowledge affected reading, spelling and comprehension scores whereas improved word knowledge may have identified more children as 'at risk';
- guard against overlooking those whose vocabulary is less well developed.

EAL children need prompt language enrichment as soon as they are seen to struggle, careful monitoring and follow up both in years 8/9 and before sitting public exams.

The importance of exploring ways to inform parents of their child's development and encouraging liaison between home and school was highlighted. We knew that many parents may not understand the processes and interpretation of full assessment test results, even if translated into L1. Few parents asked to discuss outcomes from full assessments. This did not reflect commitment to the project, more our need to make assessment processes more inclusive. Schools, pupils and parents, however, expressed appreciation of the opportunity to enhance their understanding of why pupils might be 'failing to thrive' in literacy

There may have been cultural bias in terms of subject matter and language across both screening and assessment measures. We should conclude neither was completely reliable. We cannot state that our participants were reliably at risk of SpLD/dyslexia (Hansen and Mortimore, 2013). This offers a strong cautionary lesson. It is challenging to screen this population of 9 to 11 year olds for SpLD/Dyslexia.

Summary

This project showed everyone involved ways to enhance the assessment measures we adopted within the school context to provide a more reliable, informative picture. Evident difficulties in identifying risk of SpLD/Dyslexia prescribe caution in 'diagnosis' but prompt action. The crucial need for speedy intervention suggested that one way forward might be the concept of a staged intervention.

Section 3: The Concept of a Staged Intervention

Evidently, a half hour 15 weeks' daily intervention programme led by trained TAs can boost literacy. Both the paired reading and structured intervention programme suggested that two key elements were significant:

1. Explicit approaches to language development, building confidence in use of language. These should focus on listening and reading comprehension strategies and develop children's metacognitive awareness of their own reading skills and strategies.
2. Any structured programme should involve phonological processing, systematic and explicit teaching of new L2 phonemes supported by carefully structured multi-sensory programmes based on learners' error patterns; explicit teaching of morphology and syllable structure plus strategies for inferring meaning from context and morphology;

However, our difficulties in devising reliable screening and assessment measures suggested the importance of a more dynamic, less static approach to understanding learners' needs. Evidence from parents and children highlighted the necessity of sharing information about the child's story more consistently and accurately between home and school.

Evidence of lack of progress across literacy skills, despite high quality class-based literacy teaching, must trigger intervention. An evidence base involving close communication with families, observing learning over time and evaluating, responses to intervention, can provide important information for disentangling SpLD from issues connected to transferring to a new language. One key area is to distinguish between lack of exposure and difficulty in acquisition.

This dictates a staged approach, focusing on the identification of needs through assessment, intervention, observing and recording learning and review. The process should include child, parents/carers, and school staff collaborating to support a child. Each stage should be followed by a progress review of information involving school staff, children and parents and provide recommendations for next steps. Responses to the intervention should inform decisions about whether to extend the current stage or progress to the next. For example if a child involved in guided reading is progressing in all areas, growing in confidence and generally 'catching up', stage 3 may be inappropriate. If a child at stage 3 continues to show persistent difficulties in language and reading, the review should begin to collate evidence and advice for ways forward.

The following three-stage intervention model incorporates lessons learnt from the project.

Stage 1: Initial identification of children 'at risk' using both school-based assessments of reading levels, assessment of BICS and CALP and checklists such as Ball (2007). Collation of information about child's story.

Stage 2: Initial planned small group intervention programmes, such as, paired reading, which proved successful, or guided reading (Wray, 2004) incorporating language enrichment and discussion to develop critical thinking and metacognitive awareness of strengths and difficulties developing reading fluency and understanding. Systematic documentation should include adult perspective on strengths + weaknesses and child's view of programme and progress. Wherever possible this stage should include working bilingually, using dual language texts and discussion of language/s familiar to the children to enhance literacy.

Stage 3: A more structured multisensory intervention programme linked to language enrichment. Approaches should also incorporate the strategies to develop critical thinking and metacognitive awareness used in stage 2.

B. Observing and recording learning over time

Stage 1: Drawing together of information about the child's story; language/s spoken/reading/writing, prior education, patterns of strengths and weaknesses in learning, reading and writing. Emphasise the importance of L1:

- Explore L1 characteristics to identify areas of need (e.g., phonology) or fluency in English.
- Ascertain oral fluency in L1 with activities such as comparison of Rapid Naming and free writing across L1 and L2. It is possible, without a translator, to sense whether there is fluency in L1. This enriches the holistic profile of the child, even if accuracy cannot be checked. Many project children happily wrote some words in L1, amused by our difficulty pronouncing simple phrases accurately!

Stage 2: Sessions Records, focusing on:

- Reading skills - phonemic awareness and knowledge, word recognition, vocabulary, grammar;

- Reading strategies - predicting from images and surrounding text, comparing differences in similar words and between languages;
- Discussion of texts - comprehension and enjoyment, details of information or story structure, any concepts, words, morphemes, rhymes that were significant;
- Child's response to the text;
- Speed at which child learns new grammar, vocabulary and reading skills;
- Child's growth in understanding of and ability to analyse their strengths and weaknesses in learning (critical thinking and metacognitive awareness).

Stage 3: Records of sessions focusing on:

- Areas included in stage 2;
- Pre and post intervention - assessment of areas identified in the project literature review;
    - Single word reading;
    - Single word spelling;
    - Sentence comprehension;
    - Processing speed;
    - Working memory;
    - Phonological processing – non word decoding;
    - Auditory/visual memory.

The suggestions made above arise from evidence from the Dyslexia and Multilingualism project. They represent a broad outline of the types of programme likely to be beneficial to children with delayed progress and should provide information to disentangle SpLD from problems connected to transferring to a new language.

These suggestions are informed by our recognition of the challenges faced by a school system that is resolutely monolingual resulting in difficulties creating spaces to privilege the emotional and social significance of the culture of learners and their communities(Sternberg 2000). This staged approach also celebrates some of the advantages of being bilingual, such as strengths in cognitive control, problem solving, conceptual transfer and metalinguistic awareness, (Palti, 2016).

SECTION 4: CONCLUSION

These challenges will not disappear; the intention here is to pinpoint how lessons from the project might inform school policy and practices.

Both children and parents highlighted the importance of an additive school environment where being multilingual is seen as a positive resource and where children's knowledge of communication and languages in the classroom is supported. Compiling accurate profiles of children and involving parents more closely would help develop schools' knowledge of children's stories, multi-literacies and cultural contexts to ensure these are celebrated in the classroom. In turn this closer relationship would help in establishing intervention programmes, such as paired reading, in a diversity of languages.

The difficulty of identifying risk of SpLD/dyslexia in children with EAL remains alongside questions about the purpose of identifying this risk. The cognitive and psycholinguistic approaches predominantly used for SpLD/dyslexia assessment under-emphasise socio-cultural issues around cultural differences as well as linguistic difficulties (Rogoff, 2003). Unexpected failure to become literate should instigate prompt intervention, based on exploring a learner's story and developing an appropriate programme.

A cyclical staged approach to intervention has been outlined based on the principles of;

- Developing an evidence base through close communication with families;
- Initiating an intervention programme;
- Observing learning over time;
- Evaluating responses to intervention.

This staged approach includes assessment and intervention - the two key elements of support practice. Aspects from the intervention programmes used in the study have been enhanced to focus more fully on the gathering of evidence to map a child's strengths and weaknesses and support children's linguistic, cognitive and emotional development.

Underpinning these lessons is the importance of staff development. The success of our TA delivered interventions argues for the deployment of trained TAs with small groups of bi/multilingual children for daily support over a relatively short period of time. However the relatively short period of training within the project needs to be followed up with ongoing support especially in relation to introducing metalinguistic awareness and record keeping. Using TAs offers an ideal opportunity for drawing in parents, community members and hence increasing opportunities for understanding children's multi literacies. It was clear, however, that their expertise and potential in this area of SpLD/Dyslexia and EAL was not always recognised by their schools. Evidence from the project suggests that this potential should be supported and exploited if our schools are to offer an inclusive and additive framework for this particular group of children.

REFERENCES

Alloway, T. P., Gathercole, S. E., Kirkwood, H. and Elliott, J. (2008). The working memory rating scale: A classroom-based behavioral assessment of working memory. London: Psychological Corporation.

Ball, S. (2007). The Dyslexia Checklist., Wilts Local Authority.

Blatchford, P., Bassett, P., Brown, P. Koutsoubou, M., Martin, C., Russell, A.,

Webster, R. and with Rubie-Davies, C. (2009). The impact of support staff in schools. Results from the Deployment and Impact of Support Staff project. (Strand 2 Wave 2) (DCSF-RR148). London: Department for Children, Schools and Families.

Boyle, C. and Topping, K. J. (Eds.) (2012). What works in inclusion? New York and Maidenhead: Open University Press.

Brooks, G., Pahl, K., Pollard, A. and Rees, R. (2008). Effective and inclusive practices in family literacy, language and numeracy: a review of programmes and practice in the UK and internationally. Reading: CFBT Trust.

Crombie, M. and McColl, H. (2001). Dyslexia and the teaching of modern foreign languages. In L. Peer, and G. Reid, (Eds.) (2001). Dyslexia-Successful Inclusion in the Secondary School. London: David Fulton.

Cummins, J. (2000). Bilingual education and bilingualism. Clevedon: Multilingual Matters.

Dyslexia International, (2016) www.dyslexia-interntional.org/wp-content/ uploas/2014/10/ DIReport-final-4-29-14..

Elbeheri, G. and Everatt, J. (2016). Principles and Guidelines in Test Construction for Multilingual Children. In L. Peer and G. Reid (Eds.) Multilingualism, Literacy and Dyslexia. Breaking down barriers for educators. 49-61 London: Routledge.

Evangelou, M., Taggart, B., Sylva, K., Melhuish, E. and Sammons, P. (2008). What makes a successful transition from primary to secondary school? (Effective Pre-School, Primary and Secondary Education 3-14 Project) (DCSF research report 019). London: DCSF.

Fawcett, A. (2016). Dyslexia and Learning: Theory and Practice. In L. Peer and G. Reid (Eds.) Multilingualism, Literacy and Dyslexia. Breaking down barriers for educators. 9-21 London: Routledge.

Ganschow, L. and Sparks, R. (2000). Reflections on Foreign Language Study for Students with Language Learning Problems: Research, Issues, and Challenges. *Dyslexia*, *6*, pp. 87-100.

Geva, G. and Zadeh, Z. Y. (2006). Reading efficiency in native English speaking and English-as-a second-language, Children: The role of oral proficiency and underlying cognitive-linguistic processes. *Scientific Studies of Reading*, *10*, 1, 31-57.

Hutchings, M. and Mortimore, T. (2014) Learning from each other. *Special edition of Transylvanian Journal of Psychology*, 147–173.

Martin, D. (2016). Multilingualism and Dyslexia; A critical perspective. In L. Peer and G. Reid (Eds.) *Multilingualism, Literacy and Dyslexia. Breaking down barriers for educators*. 35-49. London: Routledge.

Mortimore, T., Hansen, L., Hutchings, M., Northcote, A., Fernando, J., Horobin, L., Saunders, K. and Everatt, J. (2012). *Dyslexia and Multilingualism: Identifying and Supporting bilingual learners who might be at risk of developing SpLD/Dyslexia*. www.bdadyslexia.org.uk/files/ Big-Lottery-Research- Report.pdf.

Lucid Research, (2008). *Lucid Assessment System for Schools*. Lucid Research Ltd http://www.lucid-research.com.

NALDIC, (2016). *Research and Statistics*. http://www.naldic.org.uk/research-and-information/eal-statistics/.

NESSY, *Learning Programme*, (2010). Net Educational Systems Ltd. http://www.nessy.com/ products.aspx.

Palti, G. (2016) Approaching Dyslexia and Multiple Languages: In L. Peer and G. Reid (eds.) *Multilingualism, Literacy and Dyslexia. Breaking down barriers for educators*. London: Routledge

Rapid Reading for SEN and struggling pupils at KS2 (1st/2nd Level) (2006). www. pearsonschoolsandfecolleges.co.uk/Primary/Literacy/AllLiteracyresources/ RapidReading/RapidReading.aspx.

Rogoff, B. (2003). *The Cultural Nature of Human Development*. Oxford: Oxford University Press.

Smythe, I. (2010). *Dyslexia in the Digital Age: Making IT Work*. London: Continuum.

Snowling, M. J. (2010). Beyond Phonological Deficits: Sources of Individual Differences in Reading Disability. In S. A. Brady, D. Braze and C. A. Fowler (Eds.) *Ex- plaining Individual Differences in Reading: Theory and Evidence*. New Haven, CT: Haskins Laboratories.

Sternberg, R. J. (2000). *Handbook of Human Intelligence*. New York: Cambridge University Press.

Strand, S. and Murphy, V. (2015). *EAL and Educational Achievement in England*. https://v1.educationendowmentfoundation.org.uk/uploads/pdf/EAL_and_Educational_Achievement_-_Executive_Summary.pdf.

Turner, M. (1994). The Non-word Decoding Test. *Dyslexia Review*, *6*, 2, pp. 23-24.

Unison, (2016) http://www.open.ac.uk/choose/unison/develop/my-understanding/role-teaching-assistant.

Wolf, M. (2008). *Proust and the Squid. The story and science of the reading brain*. Cambridge: Icon Books.

Wray, D. (2004). *Teaching Literacy: Using Texts to Enhance Learning*. London: David Fulton.

Ziegler, J. C. and Goswami, U. C. (2005). Reading acquisition, developmental dyslexia and skilled reading across languages: A psycholinguistic grain size theory. *Psychological Bulletin*, *131*(1), 3-29.[pdf].

Biographical Sketch

Dr. Mim (Miriam) Hutchings, EdD

Affiliation: Bath Spa University

Education:
Certificate Education (Nottingham)
BA (Open University)
Diploma in Reading Studies (Open University)
MEd (Bath Spa University)
EdD (Bristol University)
Address: Bath Somerset

Research and Professional Experience:

Mim Hutchings was a senior lecturer in Education and Childhood Studies at Bath Spa University. She specialized in social and educational inclusion within undergraduate and postgraduate programmes. She has taught in mainstream schools, special schools and universities. She has worked in minority ethnic support services and as an advisor for special educational needs.

She was a member of the research team Dyslexia and Multilingualism primarily responsible for the qualitative elements of the project. Other research has focussed on learning experiences of undergraduate students, the transformation and survival of non-traditional entrants to an Education Studies degree. Articles, chapters and conference presentations cover; dyslexia and multilingualism – the voices and experiences of children, parents and support staff and, student learning in higher education.

Professional Appointments:

Senior Lecturer in Education Studies (Inclusion, Special Educational Needs, Language and Literacy) School of Education Bath Spa University

Adviser for Special Educational Needs. Swindon Borough Council

Senior Lecturer in Language and Literacy, Faculty of Arts and Education, University of Plymouth with additional responsibilities for Specialist Teaching Assistant Programme in Devon and Dorset

Advisory Teacher – Special Educational Needs. Avon Section 11 Education Team

Senior Coordinator, Multi-cultural Education Centre, Avon

Teacher, Bath Language Centre, Avon.

Teacher, Featherstone Middle School. Ealing

Teacher, Perivale First School, Ealing

Teacher, Centre Anglo Africain de Langues, Oran, Algeria

Teacher, Ranelagh Junior School, Newham

Publications Last 3 Years:

Hutchings M and Mortimore T (2016) Lessons from the Dyslexia and Multilingualism Project: In L. Peer and G. Reid (eds.) *Multilingualism, Literacy and Dyselxia. Breaking down barriers for educators.* London: Routledge

Hutchings, M. and Mortimore, T. (2014) Learning from each other. *Special edition of Transylvanian Journal of Psychology,* 147–173.

Hutchings M (2013) Arriving in New Place: the ecology of learning: in Ward S A Student's Guide to Education Studies (3rd edition) London Routledge

Mortimore, T., Hutchings, M. and Northcote, A. (2013) Identifying and supporting literacy acquisition in bilingual learners potentially at risk of dyslexia: The Big Lottery Dyslexia and Multilingualism Project. In J. Everatt (Ed.) *Dyslexia, Languages and Multilingualism.* Bracknell: BDA.in

Mortimore, T., Hansen, L., Hutchings, M., Northcote, A., Fernando, J., Horobin, L., Saunders, K. and Everatt, J. (2012) *Dyslexia and Multilingualism: Identifying and Supporting Bilingual Learners Who Might Be at Risk of Developing SpLD/Dyslexia.* www.bdadyslexia.org.uk/ common/ckeditor/filemanager/ userfiles/About_Us/Projects/Big_Lottery_ Research_Report_Final_Version.pdf (accessed 6 June 2015).

Dr. Tilly Mortimore, PhD

Affiliation: Bath Spa University

Education:

BA Reading University

PGCE Goldsmiths College, University of London

Masters in Educational Psychology, Cardiff University

PG Cert Research Methodology Cardiff University
PG Cert Speech and Language Difficulties, Birmingham University
PhD Cardiff University
AMBDA

Address: Bath

Research and Professional Experience:

Following twenty years working with dyslexic learners in a range of educational contexts, running the Hornsby Distance Learning SpLD post-graduate courses and completing her PHD, Dr. Mortimore joined Southampton University to work on the SpLD courses in 2004. She is now senior lecturer in Inclusion and SPLD/ Dyslexia at Bath Spa University where, from 2007 – 2013, she lectured in inclusion and education studies and set up and ran a popular Masters programme in SpLD/dyslexia training teachers in the specialist dyslexia skills leading to AMBDA. Having completed a large scale research project exploring dyslexia in learners with English as an additional language, she currently researches dyslexia, inclusion and vulnerable learners, acts as consultant to international specialist dyslexia course providers and lectures in a range of international educational and training contexts. Her recent publications include chapters and articles on varying aspects of SpLD/dyslexia and inclusion, subsequent to the 2008 books, a second edition of Dyslexia and Learning Style and, with Jane Dupree, Supporting Learners with SpLD/dyslexia in the Secondary Classroom.

Professional Appointments:

Senior Lecturer in SpLD/Inclusion and Education Studies: School of Education; Bath Spa University

Lecturer in SpLD/Dyslexia: Southampton University
Head of PG Distance Learning Hornsby International Dyslexia Centre, London
Head of English: Mark College, Somerset, England
Head of English: Shapwick School, Somerset, England
Deputy Head, English Department, Kings of Wessex Secondary School, Somerset
External Examiner for Birmingham and Kingston Universities
Accreditation Board: British Dyslexia Association UK
Associate Editor Patoss Bulletin

Publications Last 3 Years:

Mortimore, T. (2012) Dyslexia in higher education: creating a fully inclusive institution *Journal of Research in Special Educational Needs*. 1-10

Mortimore, T. (2013) Learning Disability/Dyslexia and Higher Education. Creating an inclusive institution in Higher Education: In L. Smith (Ed.) Recent *Trends, Emerging Issues and Future Outlook*. New York: Nova Science Publishers, Inc

Hutchings, M. and Mortimore, T. (2014) Learning from each other. Special edition of *Transylvanian Journal of Psychology*

Hutchings, M. and Mortimore, T. (2016) Lessons from the Dyslexia and Multilingualism Project: in L. Peer and G. Reid (eds) *Multilingualism, Literacy and Dyslexia. Breaking down barriers for educators*. London: Routledge

Mortimore, T., Hansen, L., Hutchings, M., Northcote, A., Fernando, J., Horobin, L. Saunders, K. and Everatt, J. (2012) Dyslexia and Multilingualism: Identifying and Supporting bilingual learners who might be at risk of developing SpLD/dyslexia. www.bdadyslexia.org.uk/files/Big-Lottery-Research-Report.pdf

Mortimore, T, Heale, C and Ullyatt. P. (2013) Assessment *Reports, Making Real Life recommendations*: Patoss Winter Bulletin

Mortimore, T., Hutchings, M. and Northcote, A. (2013) Identifying and supporting literacy acquisition in bilingual learners potentially at risk of dyslexia: The Big Lottery Dyslexia and Multilingualism Project: in J. Everatt (Ed.) *Dyslexia, Languages and Multilingualism*. Bracknell; BDA

Mortimore, T and Zholnai, A. (2014) *Inclusive education and social competence development*. HERJ (Hungarian Educational Research Journal)"

In: Dyslexia: Perspectives, Challenges and Treatment Options ISBN: 978-1-63485-328-6
Editor: Marilyn Frazier

Chapter 7

INVESTIGATION OF THE SUBTYPES OF DEVELOPMENTAL DYSLEXIA IN BRAZILIAN'S CHILDREN

Giseli Donadon Germano,
Gabriela Franco dos Santos Liporaci
and Simone Aparecida Capellini
Investigation Learning Disabilities Laboratory at the
Speech and Hearing Sciences Department,
São Paulo State University "Júlio de Mesquita Filho,"
UNESP, Marília, São Paulo, Brazil

ABSTRACT

Dyslexia refers to individual differences in processing, often characterized by difficulties in early literacy, affecting the acquisition of reading, writing and spelling. They can also occur in cognitive failure, phonological and / or visual processes. Dyslexia can be classified into three subtypes: Phonological Dyslexia, Visual Dyslexia and Mixed dyslexia. The aim of this chapter was to investigate whether Brazilian's students with developmental dyslexia could be classified according with subtypes. Sixty-six children with developmental dyslexia and normal Brazilian Portuguese children participated in this study. Were administered three tasks of phonological skills (phoneme identification, phoneme, and syllable blending) and three visual tasks (a letter global report task and two non-verbal tasks of visual closure and visual constancy). The results indicated that students with dyslexia presented lower performance when compared to students from the control group and to reading processes (identifying letters, same-different, lexical decision, understanding phrases, reading comprehension, reading words and reading nonwords), the phonological tests (phonemic identification phonemic combination, syllabic combination) and visual (constancy, visual closure and global print report). Two subgroups of children with developmental dyslexia were identified a single cognitive impairment, phonological or visual having another group presented a double deficit and some children showed no disorder. In this study, the results indicated the predominance of visual and mixed subtypes. Also, this study brings a contribution to heterogeneity of the dyslexic subtypes in Brazilian Portuguese.

Keywords: developmental dyslexia, phonological processing, visual processing, subtypes, visual attention span

1. INTRODUCTION

Developmental dyslexia is a specific disorder of learning, of neurological origin, characterized by difficulty with the correct fluency in reading and difficulty in decoding and spelling skills, resulting in a deficit in the phonological component of language (Lyon; Shaywitz and Shaywitz, 2003).

However, recent studies (Germano and Capellini, 2011, 2015; Germano et al., 2014; Peyrin et al., 2012; Valdois, Bosse and Tainturier, 2004; Valdois et al., 2003, 2012, 2014) reported that there is no single pattern of expression that affects the individual with dyslexia. Therefore, to attribute the cognitive-linguistic manifestations of dyslexics to a single theory would be a reductionist view, which does not favor the understanding of the variety of manifestations of each subtype of dyslexia.

In this way, in the international literature (Germano and Capellini, 2011; Germano et al., 2014; Lyon; Shaywitz and Shaywitz, 2003; Peyrin et al., 2012; Valdois, Bosse and Tainturier, 2007) it is clear the concern of researchers regarding the classification of the developmental dyslexia subtypes. Peyrin et al. (2012) highlighted that the heterogeneity of the dyslexic population is widely recognized it should allow the identification of distinct subgroups characterized by different cognitive disorders and different neurobiological dysfunctions.

Still, despite recent research has been conducted, Galaburda and Cestnick (2003) had described three subtypes of developmental dyslexia, as follows phonological and surface dyslexia, respectively reflecting dissociations between irregular word and pseudo-word reading and mixed dyslexia that is characterized by readers who have problems of both subtypes.

Ramus et al. (2003) referred that several researches had attributed single or several deficits to explain the dyslexic's manifestations or to formulate some of the most known theories. The phonological theory postulates that dyslexics have a specific impairment in the representation, storage and/or retrieval of speech sounds, explaining the reading impairment by the deficit in acquiring the grapheme-phoneme correspondence (Bradley and Bryant, 1978; Vellutino, 1979; Brady and Shankweiler, 1991).

Ramus et al. (2003) also referred the rapid auditory processing theory, which specifies that the deficit lies in the perception of short or rapidly varying sounds (Tallal, 1980; Tallal et al., 1993). Because of this deficit, the student with dyslexia might hav difficulties in performance tasks such as auditory tasks and temporal order judgement. Another theory is the visual theory (Lovegrove et al., 1980; Livingstone et al., 1991; Stein and Walsh, 1997) that of considers a visual impairment was due difficulties with the processing of letters and words on a page of text.

Additional view such as the cerebellar theory (Nicolson and Fawcett, 1990) regarding the automatization processes, which might affect the capacity of learning of grapheme-phoneme correspondences.

Finally, Ramus et al. (2003) described a unifying theory that attempted to integrate all the findings mentioned above. A generalization of the visual theory, the magnocellular theory (Stein and Walsh, 1997) postulates that the magnocellular dysfunction is not restricted to the visual pathways but is generalized to all modalities (visual and auditory as well as tactile).

Despite these studies, most reading theories do not specify the attentional processes involved in the visual analysis of letter strings. The VA span deficit hypothesis is theoretically grounded in the connectionist multi-trace memory model of polysyllabic word reading proposed by Ans, Carbonnel, and Valdois (1998). A visual attention (VA) span disorder, namely a limitation in the number of distinct visual elements that can be processed simultaneously in a visual display. The VA span is expected to play an important role in reading acquisition, as it delineates the amount of orthographic information that can be processed at each step of the reading process (Bosse et al., 2007).

Although several studies have been conducted internationally, studies with the Brazilian population are rare. Thus, the aim of this chapter was to investigate whether Brazilian's students with developmental dyslexia could be classified according with subtypes.

2. METHOD

Sixty-six Brazilian Portuguese children took part in this experiment. All were monolingual native speakers of Portuguese who lived in the São-Paulo state (Brazil). All the participants of the students signed the Term of Free and Informed Consent (TFIC).

The 33 participants of the control group were typically developing children with no history of learning disability. The control participants had normal visual acuity and hearing and were identified by their teachers as being average or good readers.

The developmental dyslexia group consisted of 33 children (24 males). The diagnosis of dyslexia was done by an interdisciplinary team of pediatric neurologists, neuropsychologists, educational psychologists and Speech Language Therapists from the Laboratory of Investigation of Learning Deviations of the Center for the Study of Education and the Faculty of Health Sciences - São Paulo State University "Júlio de Mesquita Filho" – UNESP – Marília – São Paulo – Brazil.

2.1. Procedures

For the characterization of subtypes, phonological and visual tests were used. As procedure, all students were submitted to the follows tasks:

2.1.1. Metalinguistic Skills Evaluation Battery (PROHFON Battery, Germano and Capellini, 2011, 2015)

This is a standardized test, was used for the assessment of phonological skills. The test was designed for the Brazilian population of children from 8 to 13. The three subtests of Phonemic Identification, Combination of syllables and combination of phonemes were administered, as processing similarly develops for the syllable and phoneme units in Portuguese. Each subtest consisted in the presentation of 5 cards with six pictures each. The child was first asked to name the six pictures successively. When a picture was erroneously named, the experimenter provided the corresponding name. Then the child was asked to perform a phonological task and provide his/her response by pointing to one of the pictures. Each card was used for three successive trials, so that 3 pictures out of 6 had to be successively pointed at to provide the answer. For each task, the experiment began with three training trials (on one card of six pictures, only used for training), for which the child received corrective feedback. No feedback was provided during the experimental trials. There was no time pressure for providing the answer. Each correct pointing received one point, for a maximal score of 15 on each of the three tasks.

Phoneme Identification (PhoId)

The experimenter said a single phoneme and the child had to point at the picture of the object whose name included the target phoneme. For example, the child was asked to point at the picture depicting the word that included the phoneme /b/ among *"balde," "galinha," "sapo," "noz," "pato" and "cola"* (bucket, chicken, frog, nut, duck, glue). The task was designed to include one close distractor for each target phoneme (the /p/ of *"pato"* in the example). Three phonemes were successively provided so that three different pictures had to be successively pointed at on each card of 6 pictures. On each card, a single picture included each target phoneme. The child was instructed that the target phoneme could occur randomly at the beginning, in the middle or at the end of the phonological word.

Syllable Blending (SyBl)

At each trial, two or three syllables were successively pronounced by the experimenter. The child was asked to blend them to form a word and then point to the corresponding picture. For example, a card was presented with the following pictures: *"sapo," "chuva," "coração," "girafa," "casa"* and *"pé"* (frog, rain, heart, giraffe, house and foot). The experimenter said "Take the first syllable of the word "cara" /ka/ and blend it with the last syllable of the word "mesa" /za/ which word do you get? The child had to point to the picture of the word "*casa,*" among the 6 distractors. All target syllables were stressed syllables that could be located in initial, medial or final position within the phonological word.

Phoneme Blending (PhoBl)

The instruction was very similar as for the syllable blending task except that two phonemes had to be blended to form a word. For example, the child was asked to blend the initial sound/phoneme of *"chapéu" /ʃ/* with the last sound/phoneme of "mesa" /a/ and then point at the corresponding picture "chá." The distractors for this trial were *"sol," "pente," "girafa," "oca"* and *"ovo"* (tea, sun, comb, giraffe, teepee, egg). "*Chá," "ovo,"* and "*oca"* were target drawings for the three successive trials using the same set of 6 drawings.

2.1.2. Test of Visual Perception Skills – TVPS (Martin, 2006) and Whole Letter Report Task (Bosse et al.*, 2007)*

Three different visual tasks were administered, two were taken from the Test of Visual Perception Skills – TVPS (Martin, 2006); the third one was the whole letter report task typically used to assess visual attention span abilities (Bosse et al., 2007).

2.1.2.1. Test Visual Perception Skills – TVPS (Martin, 2006)

The two subtests of visual closure and visual form constancy of the Test Visual Perception Skills – TVPS (Martin, 2006) utilize black and white designs as stimuli and a forced choice paradigm. Each subtest starts with two training trials (not scored and with feedback) that are followed by 16 experimental items arranged in order of difficulty. The children can answer either verbally or by pointing at the target drawing. For each trial, a maximum of 20 sec was provided for the response. Maximum score for each test is 16. Raw scores were recorded at the end of each subtest. The tests were applied individually, in a quiet room (without auditory or visual distraction).

Visual Form Constancy Subtest (VFC)

A visual shape (the target) was presented at the top of a card. The child was asked to retrieve the top shape among five alternatives. The alternatives were either similar to the top shape while differing in size or orientation or were complex configurations, one of which included the target after transformation (rotation or size change). There was 1 practice trial and there were 16 test trials for a maximal score of 16. Each participant progressed on the subtest until he or she failed four out of five consecutive items.

Visual Closure Subtest (VC)

The black outline drawing of a complex geometrical shape was presented at the top of the sheet and the participant was asked to match it with one out of 4 fragmented shapes displayed below. The fragmented visual shapes of the distractors included similar features as the target but the orientation, the size or the position of some features had been changed. The target was a fragmented shape derived from the outline drawing. There was 1 training trial followed by 16 test trials.

2.1.2.2. Letter Global Report Task (LGR) (Bosse et al., 2007)

On each trial, a five-consonant string was displayed for 200msec at the centre of the computer screen. The strings built-up from 10 consonants (BPTFLMDSRH) contained no repeated item. To prevent lexical activations, they never matched the skeleton of a real word. Each letter was used 10 times and appeared twice in each position. Letters were presented in upper case (Geneva 24) in black on a white background; each letter subtended a visual angle of 0.7°. To minimize crowding, the distance between adjacent letters was increased (inter-letter space of 0.57cm). The whole array subtended an angle of approximately 5.4°. The task began with 10 training trials, for which children received feedback. No feedback was provided on the experimental trials.

At the beginning of each trial, a central fixation point was presented for 1000ms followed by a blank screen for 50ms. Then, the consonant string was presented at the centre of the display for 200msec. Twenty experimental trials were displayed. The child had to report verbally (identification not location) the name of the letters he had identified. We measured the number of items accurately reported, irrespective of location, across the 20 experimental trials (maximum score = 100).

3. Results and Discussion

For the results, it was used t-tests (one tailed) to compare performance of the two groups (children with developmental dyslexia and typical readers on the reading), phonological awareness and visual attention tasks (Table 1).

In Table 1 shows that there was significant difference in all variables in the comparison between the two groups, and the performance of students with dyslexia was lower.

Regarding the phonological awareness tasks, Peterson and Pennington (2012) referred that the ability to attend to and to manipulate linguistic sounds is crucial for the establishment and automatization of letter–sound correspondences, which in turn underlie accurate and fluent word recognition through the process of phonological coding. The general consensus is that the phonological deficits of dyslexia result from faulty development of phonological representations, which are characterized as poorly segmented, imprecise, or otherwise degraded. However, still, it's not a total agreement among the researchers.

Table 1. Mean scores (and SD) of the control and children with developmental dyslexia for text reading, phonological awareness and visual processing

Tasks	Developmental dyslexia group	Control group	t-test, p
Phonological awareness			
Phoneme identification (/15)	9,15 (3,37)	11,70 (2,68)	t=-3,39, p<.00001
Phoneme blending (/15)	5,87 (4,51)	13,84 (2,64)	t= -6,79, p<.00001
Syllable blending (/15)	8,70 (4,74)	13,84 (1,46)	t= -5,95, p<.00001
Visual processing			
Form constancy (/16)	5,15 (2,95)	10,45 (2,03)	t= -8,50, p<.00001
Visual closure (/16)	5,00 (3,13)	10,81 (2,43)	t= -8,43, p<.00001
Letter global report (/100)	50,88 (14,10)	65,21 (11,46)	t= -4,53, p<.00001

Phonological deficits is also linked with the retrieval of speech sounds. It explains dyslexics' reading impairment by appealing to the fact that learning to read an alphabetic system requires learning the grapheme-phoneme correspondence, i.e., the correspondence between letters and constituent sounds of speech. If these sounds are poorly represented, stored or retrieved, the learning of grapheme- phoneme correspondences (Bradley and Bryant, 1978; Vellutino, 1979; Brady and Shankweiler, 1991).

These findings related performance difficulties of students with dyslexia in phonological awareness tests have been described in studies with the Brazilian population (Germano et al, 2008, 2009; Germano and Capellini, 2008, 2011, 2015).

The results of Table 1 also showed that dyslexic students had lower performance when compared with control group. A recent Brazilian study had been conducted to verify the efficacy of a perceptual and visual-motor skill intervention program for students with dyslexia and control group (Fusco, Germano and Capellini, 2015). In pre- and post-testing situations, both groups were submitted to the Test of Visual-Perceptual Skills (TVPS-3). Comparing the means between the pre- and post-testing situations of students from dyslexic group, differences were observed in visual discrimination skills, visual memory, visual-spatial relationship form constancy, visual sequential memory, visual figure-ground and visual closure, as the dyslexic group had inferior performance in all those subtests.

Also, regarding the VA span, there was significant difference comparison between the two groups in letter global report task, and the performance of students with dyslexia was lower. According with Lobier, Zoubrinetzky and Valdois (2012) dyslexic children cannot process as many visual elements as their normal reading peers, regardless of element type. Impaired performance on these tasks was interpreted as evidence for a deficit in the number of individual visual elements that can be processed simultaneously.

Subsequently, others statistical analysis had been made. A principal components analysis with *varimax* rotation had been executed in the performance for the three phonological tasks and the three visual processing tasks. The analysis revealed a two-factor solution. The first factor (called the visual factor hereafter) accounted for 36.82% of the variance and received high loading from the shape constancy, visual closure and global report tasks. The second "phonological" factor that received high loadings from the three phonological tasks accounted for a further 36.28% of variance.

Figure 1 shows the scatterplot of the participants based on their phonological and visual coefficients.

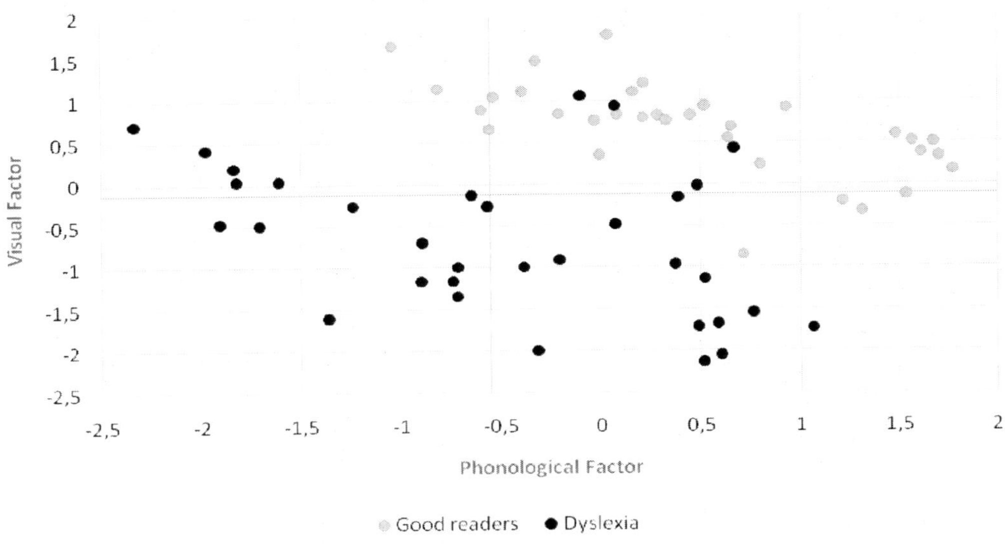

Figure 1. Scatterplot´s graphic of the distribution of children with developmental dyslexia and control group based on their phonological and visual coefficients.

The results of this study show the existence of different developmental dyslexia profiles in speaking population of Brazilian Portuguese. It was possible to verify that they exhibited a visual and phonological processing.

The results indicated that only 5 children (15.1%) showed poor phonological skills but normal visual processing, thus defining a group with a selective phonological disorder. In contrast, a high proportion of children (72.7%) exhibited a visual processing disorder. This group of children split into a first subgroup of 13 children (39.4%) who showed a selective visual disorder (in the absence of phonological problems) and a second subset of 11 children

(33.3%) with both visual and phonological disorders. Only 4 children with developmental dyslexia (12.1%) showed no phonological or visual disorder.

Although the phonological deficit be considered as the basis of the manifestations of developmental dyslexia and being widely researched and accepted in national and international literature (Fusco, Germano and Capellini, 2015; Galaburda and Cestnick, 2003; Germano et al, 2008, 2009; Germano and Capellini, 2008, 2011, 2012; Peyrin et al, 2012), the results of this study reveled that the phonological dyslexia subtype was not as frequent as the other subtypes.

The viso-perceptual skills are related to learning of reading and writing, as they allow the students use the breakdown between breakdown of letters and general configuration of words (a - f - t, n - u) form a visual image of the words; in writing, enables the correct use of spelling, notice the position of objects relative to the body itself or in relation to another object and recognize visual cues and / or fragments and then determine the appearance of the final product without the details are present (Martin, 2006).

Thus, difficulties in visual skills can have a negative impact on school activities, such as reading, spelling, text production, copy, dictation and math. In addition, visual perception dysfunction can negatively affect the ability of school children succeed to complete their activities of daily living, participate in leisure activities, and complete school work (Brown and Rodger, 2009).

Regarding the phonological tasks, the ability to identify phonemes at the beginning, middle and end and target phoneme, favors the perception that these phonemes can be either deleted the words forming a new word, as combined to form another word. Also, The perception of the phoneme enables the student to make the grapheme-phoneme association, and realize that phonemes can be combined to form another word, contributing thus to the generative mechanism of memory, which converts the phonology in spelling (Chappell et al., 2009; Germano and Capellini, 2011, 2015).

Also, visual perception had an important role in dyslexic's performance. The students had difficulties complex processes, such as figure-ground and visual closura. The ability to visually closure refers to the ability to determine one of four incomplete shapes similar to the original stimulus (Gardner, 1996).

Conclusion

The results of this study suggest the heterogeneity of developmental dyslexia, since the demonstrations dissociate in terms of cognitive-linguistic characteristics.

The above findings show that, regardless of phonological or visual impairment, difficulties in reading and writing expressed by dyslexics may result from only one deficit or from a combination of deficits. However, we emphasize that the continuation of this study may contribute to a greater understanding of cognitive-linguistic manifestations caused these deficits.

Moreover, we point out that for health professionals and education, the results of this study indicate the need for better research of students with developmental dyslexia to establishing an accurate and differential diagnosis, which will facilitate the planning strategies interventional clinical and educational.

REFERENCES

Ans, B., Carbonnel, S. and Valdois, S. (1998). A connectionist multi-trace memory model of polysyllabic word reading. *Psychological Review*, 105, 678–723.

Bradley, L. and Bryant, P.E. (1978). Difficulties in auditory organisation as a possible cause of reading backwardness. *Nature*, 271, 746-7.

Brady, S.A. and Shankweiler, D.P. (1991). Phonological processes in literacy. Hillsdale, NJ: Lawrence Erlbaum.

Brown, T. and Rodge, S. (2009). An Evaluation of the Validity of the Test of Visual Perceptual Skills – Revised (TVPS-R) using the Rasch Measurement Model. *British Journal of Occupational Therapy*. February, 72, 66-78.

Chappell, J., Stephens, T., Kinnison, L. and Pettigrew, J. (2009). Educational diagnosticians' understanding of pho- nological awareness, phonemic awareness, and reading fluency. Assessment for effective intervention, 35(1), 24-33.

Ramus, F., Rosen, T., Dakin, S.D., Day, B.L, Castellote, J.M., White, S, and Frith, U. (2003). Theories of developmental dyslexia: insights from a multiple case study of dyslexic adults. *Brain*, 126, 841-865.

Fusco, N., Germano, G.D. and Capellini, S.A. (2015). Eficacy of a perceptual and visual-motor skill intervention program for students with dyslexia. CoDAS, 27(2),128-34.

Gardner MF (1996) Test of Visual Perceptual Skills (Non-Motor) – Revised. San Francisco, CA: Psychological and Educational Publications.

Galaburda, A.M. and Cestnick, L. (2003). Dislexia del desarollo. Revista de Neurología, 36, supl.1, 13-23.

Germano, G. D et al. (2009). Relationship between neuroimaging findings and auditory and metaphonological abilities in students with developmental dyslexia. Rev. soc. bras. fonoaudiol., 14, 315-322.

Germano, G. D., Pinheiro, F. H., and Capellini, S. A. (2008). Performance of students with developmental dyslexia in phonological and syllabic tasks. Rev. CEFAC. 11, 213-220.

Germano, G. D. and Capellini, S.A. (2008). Efficacy of an audio-visual computerized remediation program in students with dyslexia. *Pró-Fono R. Atual. Cient.*, 20, 237-242.

Germano, G. D. and Capellini, S.A. (2011). Performance of students with dyslexia, learning disabilities and learning difficulties in metaphonological abilities tests (PROHFON). *J. Soc. Bras. Fonoaudiol.* 23, 135-141.

Germano, G.D. and Capellini, S.A. (2015). Metalinguistic Skills Evaluation (PROHFON): Characterization and Comparison of Students' Performance. 28(2), 213-222. 28(2), 213-222.

Livingstone, M.S., Rosen, G.D., Drislane, F.W. and Galaburda, A.M. (1991). Physiological and anatomical evidence for a magnocellular defect in developmental dyslexia. *Proc Natl Acad Sci USA*, 88, 7943-7.

Lobier, M., Zoubrinetzky, R. and Valdois, S. (2012). The visual attention span deficit in dyslexia is visual and not verbal. *Cortex,* 48, 768-773.

Lovegrove, W.J., Bowling, A., Badcock, B. and Blackwood, M. (1980). Specific reading disability: differences in contrast sensitivity as a function of spatial frequency. *Science,* 210, 439-40.

Lyon, R.; Shaywitz, S.; and Shaywitz, B. (2003). Defining dyslexia, comorbidity, teachers' knowledge of language and reading. *Annals of dyslexia*, 53.

Nicolson, R.I. and Fawcett, A.J. (1990). Automaticity: a new framework for dyslexia research? *Cognition*, 35, 159-82.

Peterson, L.R., Pennington, B.F. (2012). Developmental dyslexia. *Lancet,* 379, 1997–2007.

Peyrin, C., Lallier, M., Démonet, J. F., Baciu, M., Le Bas, J. F. and Valdois, S. (2012). Neural dissociation of phonological and visual attentional span disorders in developmental dyslexia: fMRI evidence from two case reports. *Brain Lang*. 120, 381-394.

Martin, N. A. (2006). Test of Visual Perceptual Skills. Third Edition (TVPS-3). Flórida: PAR.

Ramus, F., Rosen S., Dakin, S.C., Day, B.L., Castellote, J.M., White, S. and Frith, U. (2003). Theories of developmental dyslexia: insights from a multiple case study of dyslexic adults. *Brain*, 126, 841-865.

Stein, J. and Walsh, V. (1997). To see but not to read; the magnocellular theory of dyslexia. *Trends Neurosci,* 20, 147-52.

Tallal, P., Miller, S., Fitch, R.H. (1993). Neurobiological basis of speech: a case for the preeminence of temporal processing. [Review]. *Ann NY Acad Sci,* 682, 27-47.

Tallal P. (1980). Auditory temporal perception, phonics, and reading disabilities in children. Brain Lang, 9, 182-98.

Valdois, S., Bosse, M. L., Ans, B., Carbonnel, S., Zorman, M., David, D., et al. (2003). Phonological and visual processing deficits can dissociate in developmental dyslexia: Evidence from two case studies. *Read Writ.* 16, 541-572.

Valdois, S., Bosse, M.L., and Tainturier, M.J. (2004). Cognitive correlates of developmental dyslexia: Review of evidence for a selective visual attentional deficit. Dyslexia. 10, 1-25.

Valdois, S., Lassus-Sangosse, D., and Lobier, M. (2012). Poor letter string processing in developmental dyslexia: What visual-to-phonological code mapping disorder. *Dyslexia,* 18, 77-93.

Valdois, S., Peyrin, C., Lassus-Sangosse, D., Lallier, M., Démonet, J. F., and Kandel, S. (2014). Dyslexia in a French Spanish bilingual child: Behavioural and neural modulation following a specific VA span intervention program. *Cortex.* 53, 120-145.

Vellutino, F.R. (1979). Dyslexia: research and theory. Cambridge (MA): MIT Press.

In: Dyslexia: Perspectives, Challenges and Treatment Options ISBN: 978-1-63485-328-6
Editor: Marilyn Frazier

Chapter 8

DYSLEXIA: NEW ASSESSMENT TRENDS AND CHALLENGES FOR THE FUTURE

Débora Areces[1,*], Trinidad García[1], Stephen Loew[2], Marisol Cueli[1], Paloma González-Castro[1] and Celestino Rodríguez[1]
[1]University of Oviedo, Oviedo, Spain
[2]University of New England, Armidale NSW, Australia

ABSTRACT

Dyslexia is one of the most common problems in childhood, even affecting adult population, and its prevalence situates between 5% to 17% of school-age children, according to different studies (Katusic, Colligan, Barbaresi, Schaid, and Jacobsen, 2001; Shaywitz and Shaywitz, 2003). This is important since reading disabilities have shown to be an important determining factor in children and adolescent academic performance (Ewing and Parvez, 2012). Dyslexia has been traditionally attributed to different factors, from defects in the visual system to language or phonological coding deficits (Vellutino, Fletcher, Snowling, and Scanlon, 2004), without reaching an agreement on its specific cause. This may explain the fact that diagnosis of dyslexia sometimes lacks objective criteria, which makes it difficult to make an early detection and intervention. Within this context, in the present chapter, a comprehensive revision of previous literature on this disorder will be conducted, paying special attention to new assessment tendencies and the challenges that the need for objective and reliable measures of reading disabilities supposes for future research and practice. Specifically, a special emphasis will be made in those factors related to visual and perceptual skills (i.e., saccadic movements, fixation, visual fusion), and fluency (i.e., naming speed variables), and how to evaluate them, in concordance with previous theories that support these assessment methods. By means of this analysis, we will intend to make readers familiar with some innovative techniques that are being used nowadays, their main characteristics and potential usefulness for the assessment of reading disabilities in childhood and adolescence; inviting researchers and professionals to consider these techniques in their daily practice. Some implications of the use of these measures will also be outlined.

* Corresponding author: Débora Areces. Department of Psychology. University of Oviedo. Plaza Feijoo s/n. 33003 Oviedo (Spain). Email: arecesdebora@uniovi.es.

Keywords: dyslexia, assessment, visual-perceptual skills, fluency, childhood and adolescence

INTRODUCTION

Learning to read properly is one of the most important skills that children are supposed to acquire at the beginning of their education process. However, in many cases, this activity is far from being easy for students. This difficulty is even more pronounced when specific impairments, such as dyslexia, are present.

Dyslexia is defined by the presence of reading and spelling impairments. Dyslexic readers show difficulties with word-level reading and spelling, and frequently reverse the orientation of letters when writing, despite of having adequate intelligence and opportunities to learn (Lyon, Shaywitz, and Shaywitz, 2003; Snowling, 2000). Prevalence rates for dyslexia are very high, ranging between 5% and 15% of school age children (Shaywitz and Shaywitz, 2008; Snowling and Hayiou-Thomas, 2006; Vellutino, Fletcher, Snowling, and Scanlon, 2004).

EFFECTS OF DYSLEXIA ON ACADEMIC PERFORMANCE

Reading skills have import implications for every child's school performance. In fact, both oral and written language skills have a key role in the acquisition of basic skills and knowledge during childhood. However, many students struggle with reading from the early beginning of their schooling. This problem becomes even more relevant as students progress throughout elementary school, where reading proficiency is essential for learning more complex academic concepts and developing multiple cognitive skills. This predisposes students with reading difficulties to a serious risk of academic failure, and subsequent related issues (Bellocchi, Muneaux, Bastien-Toniazzo, and Ducrot, 2013; Savage, Carless, and Ferrero, 2007). For instance, implicit learning seems to be impaired in dyslexic children, as previous research has indicated (Stoodley et al., 2006b, 2008), while it has also been shown that dyslexic students have a lower academic self-perception of their scholastic competence and negative views of their self-worth (Baker and Zigmond, 1990). Similarly, Borkowski, Weyhing, and Carr (1988) showed that children who are affected by a specific learning disability usually make more uncontrollable attributions for their academic performance than their peers, which may possibly lead to further negative consequences at the emotional level.

CAUSES OF DYSLEXIA

Different causes have been proposed as the basis for dyslexia, with the *phonological theory* being the most widely studied. According to this theory, dyslexia is primarily related to poor phonemic awareness (Vellutino et al., 2004), which then translates to difficulties in consolidating and accessing phonological representations of the words (Elbro, 1996; Snowling, 2000).

Within this same concept, different studies maintain that some reading impairments are related to low-level auditory perceptual dysfunction that negatively influence the ability to use phonics skills adequately (Tallal, 1980). Children with reading difficulties exhibit deficits in phoneme perception (Mody, Studdert Kennedy, and Brady, 1996), which may also play a role in the difficulties they have in acquiring phonological processing skills (McBride-Chang et al., 2008).

Other investigations suggest that dyslexic people are considerably slower than their peers in *naming tasks* (Wolf, 2007). The causes of these findings are, however, controversial. In this sense, while for some authors believe it is due to a problem of phonological labels recovery (Breznitz, 2003; Wolf and Bowers, 1999), others suggest that it could be caused by a *processing speed deficit* (Geiger Lettvin, and Zegarra-Moran, 1992). Previous research indicates that the longer inter-stimulus pauses shown by dyslexic readers while performing these tasks could be related to difficulties in disengaging from an already-named stimulus in order to focus on processing the current stimulus (Wolf and Bowers, 1999). Alternatively, Hari and Renvall (2001) proposed that dyslexic children exhibit a 'Sluggish Attentional Shifting' (SAS), which impairs their ability to disengage from processing one item in order to engage to the following item. According to this evidence, although dyslexic readers may not have problems recognizing letters when presented isolated, their attention processes seem to be affected when the target item is presented within a set of stimulus.

This would be coherent with the evidence of a visual attentional deficit in dyslexia (Hari and Renvall, 2001; Bosse, Tainturier, and Valdois, 2007). As some authors suggest, low processing speed could be related to impaired *attention mechanisms* in dyslexic people (Bellochi et al., 2013; Stenneken et al., 2011; Whitney and Cornelissen, 2005). Specifically, the presence of attentional deficits can have detrimental effects on orthographic processing, and the segmentation of strings of letters into graphemes. Similarly, Facoetti, Lorusso, Paganoni, Umiltra and Mascetti (2003) found auditory and visual selective-attention deficits in dyslexic children, while Facoetti et al. (2000) highlighted the existence of an asymmetrical allocation of attention to the right visual field in this population, which they interpreted as a sort of left neglect phenomenon. In the same light, a more recent study conducted by this group found impairments in visual-spatial attention and syllabic segmentation tasks in students at familial risk for developmental dyslexia, indicating that using measures of both phonological skills (i.e., syllabic segmentation and attention), are more reliable than using a single measure to identify students with dyslexia (Facoetti, Corradi, Ruffino, Gori, and Zorzi, 2010).

Among other possible explanations for dyslexia, some research has focused on the role of word processing functions, such as *word prediction*. The prediction of an upcoming word and its alignment with the parafoveal visual perception of the word must be well synchronized to prevent "an overabundance of prediction errors," which would hinder reading more than it would accelerate the process. Such investigations (Kintsch, 1998; Staub, 2015) affirm that, for students with high reading skills, this is related to automatic access to context-based inferences, whereas those with poorer reading skills do so in a more restricted manner, which impairs their reading efficiency. Despite the feasibility of this approach, the fact is that phonological theories and, more recently, those focused on processing speed and attention deficits, are the most prevailing concepts today. New assessment tools and methods have emerged from the latter perspective, as it is also the case for naming speed tasks such as

RAN/RAS (Denckla and Rudel, 1974; Zoccolotti et al., 2013), as well as multiple eye-movements paradigms, both of which will be extensively described in the present chapter.

NEUROLOGICAL BASIS FOR DYSLEXIA

Different studies have tried to identify the brain areas affected in dyslexia. In the last few years, many authors have found that the cerebellum is involved in the performance of a broad range of reading tasks.

This area of the brain has traditionally been associated with the coordination of smooth movements, the maintenance of balance and/or posture, visually guided movements, and other motor-controlled neurological learning. However, some current research is now linking the cerebellum with other capacities without a motor output; such as executive function, linguistic abilities, as well as emotional and affective regulation (Molinari, Petrosini, Misciagna, and Leggio, 2004; Schmahmann, Weilburg, and Sherman, 2007; Stoodley and Stein, 2011).

Most previous research has focused upon the study of reading difficulties after cerebellar damage (Carreiras, Mechelli, Estevez, and Price, 2007). In this line, Scott et al. (2001) found that right cerebellar damage in children impaired the development of verbal and/or literacy skills. Likewise, Karaci, Ozturk, Ozbakir, and Cansaran (2008) found a relationship between the presence of right-sided cerebellar infarcts in patients and impairments in reading and language tasks. Furthermore, using neuro-imaging techniques, Aylward et al. (2003) and Eden et al. (2004) found alterations in cerebellar activity during phonological tasks in both children and adults with dyslexia. But, what is the actual relationship between the cerebellum and reading? Stoodney and Stein (2009) argue that this relationship is due to the involvement of the cerebellum in sensory and language processing, as well as in eye-movement control. These authors also highlight the importance of this specific brain-region in relation to: attention; word-error detection; and timing/sequencing mechanisms. The cerebellum has also been associated with implicit learning, which affects literacy development (Peng et al., 2003; Ruz, Wolmetz, Tudela, and McCandliss, 2005).

If we take into consideration neuro-imaging studies, the major prime findings on the relationship between the cerebellum and dyslexia suggest that: a) both motor and non-motor cerebellar regions are activated for reading tasks, and the differential activation of these areas depends upon task demands; b) the cerebellum is activated by tasks involving lexical, sub-lexical and semantic processing; c) the right posterolateral cerebellum is especially important for reading tasks. These areas are also activated during language tasks (Stoodney and Stein, 2009).

Obviously, additional research has also been conducted in order to explore the relationship between dyslexia and other brain areas (McCrory, Mechelli, Frith, and Price, 2005). These authors highlighted three left hemisphere regions: the left frontal regions, largely centered on the inferior frontal gyrus; the left temporal-parietal region; and the left posterior inferior temporal lobe, commonly referred to as the occipital-temporal region. Within this context, the most robust differences between dyslexic and normal readers would arise in the left occipital-temporal area (Shaywitz et al., 2002), which has been previously associated with impairments in phonological processing in cases of dyslexia (Shaywitz et al.,

2002). Despite these findings, however, evidence from both dyslexic and normal readers suggests that the cerebellum may play a more important role as a part of the reading network than other brain areas.

Some of the functions attributed to the cerebellum are in fact present in current assessment tools and methods. In the present chapter, a special emphasis will be placed on two of these methods: 1) *naming tasks,* as a measure of fluency and processing speed; and 2) *eye-movement paradigms*, as a strategy to evaluate visual-attentional networks involved in reading.

Assessment of Dyslexia: Processing Speed and Visual Attention

Undoubtedly, as mentioned in the previous paragraphs, there are many causal-factors that have been explored in relation to dyslexia, which may explain the extent of heterogeneity that exists among the different subtypes of dyslexia, as well as the variety of symptoms reported. In this respect, the assessment of dyslexia is extremely complicated, as it is quite possible to confuse it with other disorders, such as attentional problems, visual-perceptual deficits, or even a lack of school adaptation.

For this reason, it is important to be familiar with recent innovative assessment techniques, the main objectives of which, are to enhance the likelihood of early assessment, in order to provide timely intervention for children, and thus prevent the development of further (and less treatable) difficulties in the future.

RAN/RAS Tests

RAN/RAS (Rapid Automatized Naming/Rapid Alternating Stimulus) are tests which involve the rapid naming of visual symbols, such as letters, digits, colors, and objects (Denckla and Rudel, 1974). These stimuli consist of five items repeated 10 times in random sequences, and the child is asked to name each stimulus as quickly as possible.

Despite the simplicity of its administration, RAN/RAS test performance has been shown to strongly correlate with early reading development (Manis, Doi, and Bhadha, 2000; Jones, Branigan, and Kelly, 2009). RAN and reading might be related because several items are visible at once in both tasks, and the reader needs to pre-process some stimuli in the parafovea (Sereno and Rayner, 2000). As a consequence, the parafoveal information could act as a source of interference for children with reading disabilities, in both reading (Pernet, Valdois, Celsis, and Démonet, 2006), and in RAN tasks (Jones et al., 2009). Interestingly, Wolf and Bowers' (1999) interpreted the relationship between RAN and orthographic knowledge as being linked to both, the speed of visual activation of letters, and the likelihood of co-activations of adjacent letters.

The evidence shown in several investigations has led to different points of view about the relationship between naming speed and reading abilities. For some authors, naming speed could be considered as a phonological skill (Torgesen and Burgess, 1998). According to this hypothesis, naming speed can predict reading performance at early ages, as this measure is closely related to the ability to access phonologically-based codes (Torgesen and Burgess, 1998).

However, other researchers (Wolf, Bowers, and Biddle, 2000) have reported that rapid naming tasks set-off attentional, visual, lexical, temporal, and recognition sub-processes, and all of these are implied on all of which have an influence on naming speed performance. From this perspective, to classify these sub-processes under the category of phonological awareness would be a reductionism simplification that would not specifically explain the underlying complexity involved in naming speed tasks. For this reason, Wolf and Bowers (1999) argue that the processes involved in naming tasks are independent of phonological skills, and they therefore propose a "double deficit" theory, and base this upon the hypothesis that three subtypes of dyslexia exist: 1) Phonological deficit, based on poor phonological awareness and intact naming speed; 2) Rate deficit-naming, characterized by naming speed deficits, but intact phonological awareness skills; and 3) Double deficit, based on comorbidity of impaired naming speed and phonological skills.

On the other hand, some researchers have aimed to analyze the predictive power of the naming tasks according to the nature of the stimuli utilized [e.g., alphanumeric (letters and digits), and non-alphanumeric (colors and objects)]. The results showed different patterns of performance, wherein it was observed that both alphanumeric and non-alphanumeric RAN tasks related well to reading measures in kindergarten, but only alphanumeric RAN related strongly to reading measures in the first and second grades (Meyer, Wood, Hart, and Felton, 1998). One explanation for these findings may be that, while the alphanumeric naming tasks only have a single name for each stimulus, the non-alphanumeric naming tasks may have more than one name for each stimulus (Narhi et al., 2005).

However, despite the different findings provided by several studies, all of these studies are consistent in reporting that naming tasks were found to be effective in the early diagnosis of reading difficulties. This also means that naming speed tests are likely to be good early indicators of children at risk for reading problems, which would thus allow far earlier interventions, perhaps even before children can read.

EYE-MOVEMENT PARADIGMS

Eye movements are commonly evaluated by means of eye-tracking methods (Bartl-Pokorny et al., 2013). This is a non-invasive technique based on infrared video technology, which easily provides insights into perceptual and cognitive capacities. Eye-movements are studied within many different contexts, from experimental and clinical psychology, and psychiatry, to the fields of ophthalmology, neurology, and neuropsychology.

In the context of dyslexia, evidence from previous research suggests that dyslexics commonly show more frequent and longer fixations, an increased amount of loss of fixation, smaller saccades, and more regressions in comparison to normal readers (Bartl-Pokorny et al., 2011, 2013; Berget and Sandnes, 2015; Kraljevic and Palmovic, 2011; Vagge, Cavanna, Traverso, and Iester, 2015). Berget et al. (2015) also found that people with dyslexia performed significantly slower on textual tasks than controls, and that this was related to longer saccade-fixation durations. These sorts of studies have also revealed specific aspects of reading that dyslexic students may struggle with. For example, Kunert and Scheepers (2014) found that dyslexics (but not controls) had significant problems recognizing rhyme-inconsistent words, which suggests a representational deficit for such words in this group.

Eye-movement behavior is also being currently used to examine individual differences in the size of readers' perceptual span. The so-called "gaze-contingent moving window" technique is an example of this. Choi, Lowder, Ferreira, and Henderson (2015) used this technique with a sample of normal readers, who were asked to read different paragraphs while the size of the rightward window of visible text was systematically manipulated across trials. These authors found a relationship between language proficiency and visual span, in the sense that greater proficiency was associated with better performance extracting linguistic information beyond the fixated word.

The applicability of eye-movement measurements is not only related to its potential usefulness in the identification of visual-perceptual networks related to reading. Current research suggests its usefulness as a complementary means of monitoring the effects of intervention strategies aimed at improving reading in dyslexic patients. This was the case in a study conducted by Ablinger, Huber, and Radach (2014). These authors analyzed the time and course of recovery in a sample of five readers with acquired dyslexia, using eye tracking methodology to examine word processing in real time. They found differences in the distributions of fixation positions during word processing throughout the intervention process, and these differences were related to changes from predominantly lexical to more segmental word processing and improved reading performance in three of the five patients.

Despite of the advantages that this measure may offer compared to traditional methodologies, it is worth noticing at this point that eye movements have been traditionally used to investigate how skilled adult readers process written language. However, relatively little research has been conducted with children (Blythe, 2014; Joseph, Nation, and Liversedge, 2013). Nevertheless, one of the few studies conducted with young samples indicated that reading ability is better predicted by fixation-duration and fixation-count measurements of eye movements than by general verbal ability, which supports the relevance of visual-perceptual mechanisms in reading (Orlovska, Bluss, and Rascevska, 2014). However, references to studies of this kind that were conducted with children still remain scant to date. This is important, since by recording eye-movement behavior in children, researchers and clinicians will be able to better understand how children progress to skilled adult reading, which would open the pathway to more adaptive interventions. Additional research on this issue would not only allow us to better understand the relationship between changes in both cognitive processing and eye-movement behavior, but it would also lead to increased understanding of how developmental changes can affect these processes. As Al-Wabil and Al-Sheaha (2010) pointed out, the application of eye movement technologies in investigating the nature of the reading problems, and the tailoring of interventions to the particular needs of individuals with dyslexia, is more than necessary if we wish to achieve major advancements in both of these areas.

Conclusion and Future Lines of Research

Reading skills have a great relevance today, not only regarding academic performance and literacy, but also in relation to social and affective-motivational development and regulation. The high prevalence rates for dyslexia, together with the heterogeneity that characterizes the disorder, makes it necessary to design and implement reliable, valid and economic assessment measures, aimed at obtaining an adjusted and early diagnosis.

There are some theories that have tried to uncover the causes behind dyslexia. While the phonological theory is one of the most widely extended models, more recent theories highlight the relevance of processing speed and visual attentional mechanisms as key points for diagnosis. In the context of these theories, some assessment measures have emerged in the last decades, such as naming tasks and eye-movement paradigms.

These measures were extensively described in the present chapter. Although they have some differential characteristics, both provide interesting insights into the mechanisms involved in reading, beyond the information that may be obtained from traditional measures or laboratory batteries, commonly based on performance.

In the case of naming tasks, it also supposes an economic measure, as it is easily administered and lasts for a few minutes. This measure has demonstrated to be predictive of verbal fluency, reading speed and also comprehension in both adults and children. Within the context of dyslexia, there is a good deal of evidence on the diagnostic usefulness of these tasks, which lies in the fact that naming tasks allow to identify students at risk of dyslexia at very early stages, even before formal reading instruction starts.

Concerning eye-movement measures, previous research suggests that there are different oculomotor patterns in dyslexia and normative readers. Number, speed, duration and accuracy of saccadic movements and fixations are some of the most widely used indicators in this sense. As naming tasks, eye-movement measures provide objective information, which can be interpretable in terms of visual and attentional mechanisms functioning. These measures have demonstrated its usefulness in the diagnosis of dyslexia. In addition, there are important lines of research that use these measures a complement to examine the influence of certain characteristics of the word (familiarity, length, homophony, etc.) on reading performance, as well as in the treatment of reading difficulties. Eye-movement behavior is in fact one of the areas where more progress is being made today. Obviously, different factors such as the difficulty that analyzing and interpreting data from eye-movements implies, or the high cost of the systems and equipment commonly used, pose some barriers to a more widespread use of this technique. However, increasingly more economical and intuitive systems are appearing today, which will make easier carry out studies within this perspective.

Our recommendation in this sense is that researchers and clinicians will gradually incorporate these techniques as a complement to traditional batteries and measures based on performance. The use of both sort of measures should not be exclusive in any case, and, in turn, may provide privileged information about the mechanisms impaired in dyslexia.

Acknowledgments

This work has been supported by a project of the Principality of Asturias (FC-15-GRUPIN14-053) and a predoctoral grant from Severo Ochoa Program-FICYT (BP14-030).

REFERENCES

Ablinger, I., Huber, W., and Radach, R. (2014). Eye movement analyses indicate the underlying reading strategy in the recovery of lexical readers. *Aphasiology*, 28(6), 640-657. doi: 10.1080/02687038.2014.894960.

Al-Wabil, A., and Al-Sheaha, M. (2010). Towards an Interactive Screening Program for Developmental Dyslexia: Eye Movement Analysis in Reading Arabic Texts. *Computers Helping People with Special Needs, Proceedings, PT2. Lecture Notes in Computer Science*, 6180, 25-32.

Aylward, E.H., Richards, T.L., Berninger, V.W., Nagy, W.E., Field, K.M., Grimme, A.C.,… and Cramer, S.C. (2003). Instructional treatment associated with changes in brain activation in children with dyslexia. *Neurology*, 61, 212-219. doi: 10.1212/01.WNL.0000 068363.05974.64.

Baker, J.M. and Zigmond, N. (1990). Are regular classes equipped to accommodate students with learning disabilities? *Exceptional Children*, 56, 515-528. doi: 10.1177/001440299 005600603.

Bartl-Pokorny, K. D., Pokorny, F., Boelte, S., Langmann, A., Falck-Ytter, T., Wolin, T., … and Marschik, P. B. (2013). Eye Tracking in Basic Research and Clinical Practice. *Klinische Neurophysiologie*, 44(3), 193-198. doi: 10.1055/s-0033-1343458.

Bellocchi, S., Muneaux, M., Bastien-Toniazzo, M., and Ducrot, S. (2013). I can read it in your eyes: What eye movements tells us about visuo-attentional processes in developmental dyslexia. *Research in Developmental Disabilities*, 34(1), 452-460. doi: 10.1016/j.ridd.2012.09.002.

Berget. G., and Sandnes, F. E. (2015). *The Effect of Dyslexia on Searching Visual and Textual Content: Are Icons Really Useful?* 9th International Conference on Universal Access in Human-Computer Interaction (UAHCI) Held as Part of 17th International Conference on Human-Computer Interaction (HCI). Los Angeles, CA. AUG 02-07, 2015.

Blythe, H. (2014). Developmental Changes in Eye Movements and Visual Information Encoding Associated With Learning to Read. *Current Directions in Psychological Science*, 23(3), 201-207. doi: 10.1177/0963721414530145.

Borkowski, J.G., Weyhing, R.S., and Carr, M. (1988). Effects of attributional retraining on strategy based reading comprehension in learning disabled students. *Journal of Educational Psychology*, 80, 46-53. doi: 10.1037/0022-0663.80.1.46.

Bosse, M.L., Tainturier, M.J., and Valdois, S. (2007). Developmental dyslexia: The visual attention span hypothesis. *Cognition*, 104, 198-230. doi:10.1016/j.cognition.2006.05.009.

Breznitz, Z. (2003). Speed of phonological and orthographic processing as factors in dyslexia: Electrophysiological evidenc. *Genetic, Social, and General Psychology Monographs*, 129(2), 183-206.

Carreiras, M., Mechelli, A., Estevez, A., and Price C.J. (2007). Brain activation for lexical decision and reading aloud: Two sides of the same coin? *Journal of Cognitive Neuroscience*, 19, 433-444. doi: 10.1162/jocn.2007.19.3.433.

Choi, W., Lowder, M. W., Ferreira, F., Henderson, J. M. (2015). Individual differences in the perceptual span during reading: Evidence from the moving window technique. *Attention, Perception and Psychology*, 77(7), 2463-2475. doi: 10.3758/s13414-015-0942-1.

Denckla, M. B., and Rudel, R. (1974). «Rapid automatized» naming of pictured objects, colors, letters, and numbers by normal children. *Cortex*, 10, 186-202. doi:10.1007/s11 881-999-0018-9.

Eden, G. F., Jones, K. M., Cappell, K., Gareau, L., Wood, F. B., Zeffiro, T. A., ... and Flowers, D. L. (2004). Neural changes following remediation in adult developmental dyslexia. *Neuron*, 44(3), 411-422. doi:10.1016/j.neuron.2004.10.019.

Elbro, C. (1996). Early linguistic abilities and reading development: A review and a hypothesis. *Reading and Writing*, 8(6), 453-485. doi:10.1007/BF00577023.

Geiger, G., Lettvin, J. Y., and Zegarra-Moran, O. (1992). Task-determined strategies of visual process. *Cognitive Brain Research*, 1(1), 39-52. doi:10.1016/0926-6410(92)90004-B.

Hari, R., and Renvall, H. (2001). Impaired processing of rapid stimulus sequences in dyslexia. *Trends in Cognitive Sciences*, 5(12), 525-532. doi:10.1016/S1364-6613(00)01801-5.

Joseph, H. S. S. L., Nation, K., and Liversedge, S. P. (2013). Using Eye Movements to Investigate Word Frequency Effects in Children's Sentence Reading. *School Psychology Review*, 42(2), 207-222. doi: 10.1371/journal.pone.0054141.

Karaci R, Ozturk S, Ozbakir S, and Cansaran N. (2008). Evaluation of language functions in acute cerebellar vascular diseases. *Journal of Stroke and Cerebrovascular Diseases*, 17, 251-256. doi:10.1016/j.jstrokecerebrovasdis.2008.02.009.

Kintsch, W. (1998). *Comprehension: A paradigm for cognition*. Cambridge, England: Cambridge University Press.

Kraljevic, J. K., and Marijan, P. (2011). Spatial and Temporal Measurements of Eye Movement in Children with Dyslexia. *Collegium Antropologicum*, 35(1), 191-198.

Kunert, R., and Scheepers, C. (2014). Speed and accuracy of dyslexic versus typical word recognition: an eye-movement investigation. *Frontiers in Psychology*, 5, 1129. doi: 10.33 89/fpsyg.2014.01129.

Jones, M.W., Branigan, H.P., and Kelly, M.L. (2009). Dyslexic and non dyslexic reading fluency: rapid automatized naming and the importance of continuous lists. *Psychonomic Bulletin and Review*. 16, 567-572 doi:10.3758/pbr.16.3.567.

Lyon, G. R., Shaywitz, S. E., and Shaywitz, B. A. (2003). A definition of dyslexia. *Annals of Dyslexia*, 53(1), 1-14. doi:10.1007/s11881-003-0001-9.

Manis, F. R., Doi, L. M., and Bhadha, B. (2000). Naming speed, phonological awareness, and orthographic knowledge in second graders. *Journal of Learning Disabilities*, 33, 325-333. doi:10.1177/002221940003300405.

McBride-Chang, C., Lam, F., Lam, C., Doo, S., Wong, S.W. and Chow, Y.Y. (2008). Word recognition and cognitive profiles of Chinese pre-school children at risk for dyslexia through language delay or familial history of dyslexia. *Journal of Child Psychology and Psychiatry*, 49(2), 211-218. doi:10.1111/j.1469-7610.2007.01837.x.

McCrory, E. J., Mechelli, A., Frith, U., and Price, C. J. (2005). More than words: a common neural basis for reading and naming deficits in developmental dyslexia? *Brain*, 128(2), 261-267. doi: 10.1093/brain/awh340.

Meyer, M. S., Wood, F. B., Hart, L. A., and Felton, R. H. (1998). Longitudinal course of rapid naming in disabled and nondisabled readers. *Annals of Dyslexia*, 48, 91-114. doi: 10.1007/s11881-998-0005-6.

Mody, M., Studdert-Kennedy, M., and Brady, S. (1996). Speech perception deficits in poor readers: auditory processing or phonological coding? *Journal of experimental child psychology*, 64(2), 199-231. doi:10.1006/jecp.1996.2343.

Molinary, M., Petrosini, L., Misciagna, S., and Leggio, M. (2004). Visuospatial abilities in cerebellar disorders. *Journal of Neurology, Neurosurgery and Psychiatry*, 75, 235-240. doi:10.1136/jnnp.2003.015453.

Narhi, V., Ahonen, T., Aro, M., Leppäsaari, T., Korhonen, T. T., Tolvanen, A., and Lyytinen, H. (2005). Rapid serial naming: Relations between different stimuli and neuropsychological factors. *Brain and Language*, 92(1), 45-57. doi:10.1016/j. bandl. 2004.05.004.

Orlovska, M., Bluss, K., and Rascevska, M. (2014). The relationship between children's reading ability, verbal and fluid intelligence and measurements of eye movements during reading. *4th International Interdisciplinary Scientific Conference on Society, Health, Welfare. SHS Web of Conferences*, 10, paper 0030.

Paulesu, E., Démonet, J. F., Fazio, F., McCrory, E., Chanoine, V., Brunswick, N., ... and Frith, U. (2001). Dyslexia: cultural diversity and biological unity. *Science*, 291(5511), 2165-2167. doi: 10.1126/science.1057179.

Peng, D. L., Xu, J. Z., Luo, Q., Ding, G. S., Perry, C., Zhang, L., and Liu, Y. (2003). Neural basis of the non-attentional processing of briefly presented words. *Human Brain Mapping*, 18, 215-221. doi: 10.1016/j.neuropsychologia.2008.03.024.

Pernet, C., Valdois, S., Celsis, P., and Démonet, J.F. (2006). Latera lmasking Levels of processing and stimulus category: a comparative study between normal and dyslexic readers. *Neuropsychologia*, 44, 2374-2385. doi:10.1016/j.neuropsychologia.2006.05.003.

Ruz, M., Wolmetz, M. E., Tudela, P., and McCandliss, B. D. (2005). Two brain pathways for attended and ignored words. *Neuroimage*, 27, 852-861. doi:10.1016/j.neuroimage. 2005.05.031.

Savage, R. S., Carless, S., and Ferrero. (2007). Predicting curriculum and test performance from pupil background, baseline skills and phonological awareness at age 5: A six-year follow-up at the end of Kay Stage 2. *Journal of Child Psychiatry*, 48(7), 732-739. doi: 10.1111/j.1469-7610.2007.01746.x.

Sereno, S.C. and Rayner, K. (2000). Spelling-sound regularity effects on eye-fixations in reading. *Perception and Psychophysics*, 62, 402-409.doi:10.3758/bf03205559.

Schmahmann, J. D., Weilburg, J., and Sherman, J. (2007). The neuropshychiatry of the cerebellum-insights form the clinic. *Cerebellum*, 6, 254-267. doi:10.1080/147342207014 90995.

Shaywitz, S. E., and Shaywitz, B. A. (2008). Paying attention to reading: The neurobiology of reading and dyslexia. *Development and Psychopathology*, 20(4), 1329-1349. doi: 10.1017 /S0954579408000631.

Shaywitz, B. A., Shaywitz, S. E., Pugh, K. R., Mencl, W. E., Fulbright, R. K., Skudlarski, P., ... and Gore, J. C. (2002). Disruption of posterior brain systems for reading in children with developmental dyslexia. *Biological Psychiatry*, 52(2), 101-110. doi:10.1016/S1053-8119(00)91048-6.

Snowling, M. J. (2000). *Dyslexia*. Oxford: Blackwell Publishing.

Snowling, M. J., and Hayiou-Thomas, M. (2006). The Dyslexia spectrum: Continuities between reading, speech, and language impairments. *Topics in Language Disorders*, 26(2), 110-126. doi:10.1097/00011363-200604000-00004.

Staub, A. (2015). The effect of lexical predictability on eye movements in reading: Critical review and theoretical interpretation. *Language and Linguistics Compass*, 9(8), 311-327. doi:10.1111/lnc3.12151.

Stenneken, P., Egetemeir, J., Schulte-Koerne, G., Müller, H. J., Schneider, W. X., and Finke, K. (2011). Slow perceptual processing at the core of developmental dyslexia: A parameter-based assessment of visual attention. *Neuropsychologica*, 49(12), 3454-3465. doi:10.1016/j.neuropsychologia.2011.08.021,

Stoodley, C. J., Harrison, E. P., and Stein, J. F. (2006). Implicit motor learning deficits in dyslexic adults. *Neuropsychologia*, 44, 795-798. doi: 10.1080/00207594.2010.509800.

Stoodley, C. J., Ray, N. J., and Stein, J. F. (2006). Implicit learning in control, dyslexic, and garden-variety poor readers. *Annals of the New York Academy of Sciences*, 1145, 173-183. doi: 10.1196/annals.1416.003.

Stoodley, C. J., and Stein, J. F. (2011). The cerebellum and dyslexia. *Cortex*, 47(1), 101-116. doi: 10.1016/j.cortex.2009.10.005.

Tallal, P. (1980). Auditory temporal perception, phonetic, and reading disabilities in children. *Brain and Language*, 9, 182-198. doi: 10.1016/0093-934X(80)90139-X.

Torgesen, J. K., and Burgess, S. R. (1998). Consistency of reading-related phonological processes throughout early childhood: Evidence from longitudinal-correlational and instructional studies. *Word recognition in beginning literacy*, 161-188.

Vagge, A., Cavanna, M., Traverso, C. E., and Iester, M. (2015). Evaluation of ocular movements in patients with dyslexia. *Annals of Dyslexia*, 65(1), 24-32. doi: 10.1007/s 11881-015-0098-7.

Vellutino, F. R., Fletcher, J. M., Snowling, M. J., and Scanlon, D. M. (2004). Specific reading disability (dyslexia): What have we learned in the past four decades? *Journal of Child Psychology and Psychiatry*, 45(1), 2-40 . doi:10.1046/j.0021-9630.2003.00305.x.

Whitney, C., and Cornelissen, P. (2005). Letter position and dyslexia. *Journal of Research in Reading*, 28(3), 274-301. doi: 10.1080/02643290143000051.

Wolf, M. (2007). *Proust and the squid: The story and science of the reading brain.* New York: Harper Collins.

Wolf, M., and Bowers, P. G. (1999). The double-deficit hypothesis for the developmental dyslexias. *Journal of Educational Psychology*, 91(3), 415-438. doi:10.1037/0022-0663.91.3.415.

Wolf, M., Bowers, P. G., and Biddle, K. (2000). Naming-speed processes, timing, and reading A conceptual review. *Journal of Learning Disabilities*, 33(4), 387-407.

Zoccolotti, P., De Luca, M., Lami, L., Pizzoli, C., Pontillo, M., and Spinelli, D. (2013). Multiple stimulus presentation yields larger deficits in children with developmental dyslexia: A study with reading and RAN-type tasks. *Child Neuropsychology*, 19(6), 639-647.

Biographical Sketch

Débora Areces

Affiliation: Department of Psychology, University of Oviedo
Date of Birth: 04-August-1990
Education: PhD student in Psychology

Address: Department of Psychology, University of Oviedo. Plaza Feijoo s/n, 33003, Oviedo, Spain.

Research and Professional Experience: PhD student at the University of Oviedo

Publications Last 3 Years:

Cueli, M., Rodríguez, C., García, T., Areces, D. and González-Castro, P. (2015). Estudio experimental sobre el Neurobiofeedback: una mejora de la concentración en el TDAH a través del nirHEG y la fluidez sanguínea. *Revista de Psicología Clínica con Niños y Adolescentes.* 2(2), 9-21.

Fernández, T. G., Castro, P. G., Areces, D., Cueli, M. S. F. and Pérez, C. R. (2014). Funciones ejecutivas en niños y adolescentes: implicaciones del tipo de medidas de evaluación empleadas para su validez en contextos clínicos y educativos. *Papeles del psicólogo*, *35*(3), 215-223.

Fernández, T. G., Pérez, C. R., González-Castro, P. and Areces, D. (2014). Executive Functions and their assessment in Children and Adolescents. *Cognitive Sciences*, *9*(2),102-116.

Rodríguez, C., Areces, D., García, T., Cueli, M., Loew, S.J. and González-Castro, P. (2015). ADHD and writing learning disabilities, overlapping and educational implications. *Insights on Learning Disabilities*, *12*(2), 121-146

Areces, D., Rodríguez, C., García, T., Cueli, M., González-Castro, P. (In press, 2016). Efficacy of a Continuous Performance Test based on Virtual Reality in the Diagnosis of ADHD and Its Clinical Presentations. *Journal of Attentional Disorders.* doi:10.1177/1087054716629711

Trinidad García, PhD

Affiliation: Department of Psychology, University of Oviedo
Date of Birth: 12-March-1968
Education: PhD in Psychology
Address: Department of Psychology, University of Oviedo. Plaza Feijoo s/n, 33003, Oviedo, Spain.

Research and Professional Experience: Lecture at the University of Oviedo

Publications Last 3 Years:

García, T., Rodríguez, C., González-Castro, P., González-Pienda, J. A. and Torrance, M. (In Press). Elementary students' metacognitive processes and post-performance calibration on mathematical problem-solving tasks. *Metacognition and Learning*, *10*, 2.

García, T., Rodríguez, C., González-Castro, P., Álvarez-García, D. and González-Pienda, J. A. (In Press). Metacognition and executive functions in Primary School. *Annals of Psychoology.*

García, T., González-Castro, P., Rodriguez, C., Cueli, M., Álvarez-García, D. and Álvarez, L. (2014). Executive Functions impairments in ADHD and its subtypes. *Psicología Educativa*, *20*, 23 - 32.

García, T., Álvarez-Garcia, D., González-Castro, P., Álvarez, L. and Segurola, L. A. (2014). Psychometric Properties of the Executive Functioning Scale for Teachers (EFS-T). *Revista de Psicología y Educación*, *9*(1), 49 – 69

García, T., Rodríguez, C., González-Castro, P., Álvarez, D., Cueli, M. and González-Pienda, J. A. (2013). Executive Functions in children and adolescent with Attention Deficit Hyperactivity Disorder and Reading Difficulties. *International Journal of Psychology and Psychological Therapy*, *13*(2), 179 - 194.

Stephen John Loew, PhD

Affiliation: University of New England, Armidale, Australia
Date of Birth: 18/4/57
Education: PhD, BSc(Hons)
Address: 16 Clemenceau Crescent, Tanilba Bay, NSW 2319, Australia

Research and Professional Experience:

2014: Visiting Researcher - International joint-research study (Fluorescent lighting, ultra-white paper: effects on reading discomfort in 1st-year nursing students)Sunway University, Malaysia.
2010 – 2014: PhD Research Project
School of Science and Technology, University of New England, Armidale, Australia
2014: Visiting Researcher - International Collaborative Research Project (Levels of visual stress in expert readers; Effects of spectral-filtering), Sunway University, Selangor, Malaysia.
2013: Visiting Researcher - International Collaborative Research Project (Levels of visual stress in expert readers; Effects of spectral-filtering), Sunway University, Selangor, Malaysia.
2013: Short-Term Research Attachment (3 months)
Faculty of Psychology, University of Oviedo, Asturias, Spain.
2008 – 2009: BSc Honours Research Project
School of Science and Technology, University of New England, Armidale, Australia

Professional Appointments: 2006 – 2007: Chief-Investigator / Research Asst. to Head of School of Science and Technology, Centre for Bioactive Discovery in Health and Ageing, University of New England, Australia

Honors:

Golden Key International Honour Society - (Life-time membership "In Recognition of: Outstanding Scholastic Achievement and Excellence", September, 2005).

Publications Last 3 Years:

Loew, S.J., Rodríguez, C., Marsh, N.V., Jones, G.L., Núñez, J.C. and Watson, K. (2015).Levels of visual stress in proficient readers: effects of spectral filtering of fluorescent lighting on reading discomfort. *Spanish Journal of Psychology*, *18*, 1-11.

Loew, S.J., Jones, G.L. and Watson, K. (2014).Meares-Irlen/visual stress syndrome, classroom fluorescent lighting and reading difficulties: a review of the literature. Insights on Learning Disabilities, 11, 129-169.

Loew S.J., Marsh, N.V. and Watson, K. (2014).The prevalence of symptoms of visual stress/Meares-Irlen syndrome in subjects diagnosed with chronic fatigue syndrome. *International Journal of Clinical and Health Psychology,14*, 87-92.

Loew, S.J., Fernández E. and Watson, K. (2013). Incidence of Meares-Irlen/visual stress syndrome in reading and learning disorders: does fluorescent lighting in classrooms affect literacy and numeracy? *Aula Abierta*, *41*, 23-32.

Loew, S.J. and Watson, K. (2013). The prevalence of scotopic sensitivity/Meares-Irlen syndrome in subjects diagnosed with ADHD: does misdiagnosis play a role? *Croatian Review of Rehabilitation Research*, *49*, 50-58.

Loew, S.J. and Watson, K. (2012).*Spectral filtering of fluorescent lighting: effects upon reading and visual discomfort in slow readers*. In: J.A. Gonzalez-Pienda, C. Rodriguez, D. Alvarez, R. Cerezo, E. Fernandez, M. Cueli, T. Garcia, E. Tuero, and Suarez, N. (Eds.), Learning Disabilities: Present and Future. Oviedo: Learning Disabilities WorldWide, Pp. 267-278.

Loew, S.J. and Watson, K. (2012).A prospective genetic marker of the visual-perception disorder Meares-Irlen syndrome. *Perceptual and Motor Skills*, *114*, 870-882.

Rodríguez, C.,Areces, D., García, T., Cueli, M., Loew, S.J. and González-Castro, P. (2015). ADHD and writing learning disabilities: overlapping disorders and educational implications. *Insights on Learning Disabilities*, *12*, 121-146.

Iglesias-García, M.T., Gutiérrez-Fernández, N., Loew, S. and Rodríguez, C. (2016 in press).Hábitos y técnicas de estudio en adolescentes con Trastorno por Déficit de Atención con o sin Hiperactividad (TDAH). *European Journal of Education and Psychology*.

Dr. Loew is a biological scientist whose primary research interests are the epidemiology of Meares-Irlen/visual stress syndrome, the overlap of symptoms with ADHD and other disorders, and the effects of fluorescent lighting upon literacy and learning in general. His research in these areas has been published in a number of peer-reviewed journals and has also been presented at several international conferences. He has recently completed a wide-ranging PhD research project investigating biophysical and genetic factors in visual stress, its role in declining rates of student literacy and numeracy, and whether increasingly brighter fluorescent lighting has enhanced that role. Dr. Loew is also one of the few (if any) researchers of visual stress who actually has the condition himself, and this has undoubtedly contributed to his reputation for novel research ideas and insights relating to reading and attention disorders.

Marisol Cueli, PhD

Affiliation: Department of Psychology, University of Oviedo
Date of Birth: 10-August-1986
Education: PhD in Psychology
Address: Department of Psychology, University of Oviedo. Plaza Feijoo s/n, 33003, Oviedo, Spain.

Research and Professional Experience: Lecture in the University of Oviedo

Publications Last 3 Years:

Marisol Cueli, Paloma González-Castro, Luis Álvarez, Trinidad García, and Julio Antonio González-Pienda. (2014). Variables afectivo-motivacionales y rendimiento en matemáticas: un análisis bidireccional. *Revista Mexicana de Psicología*, *31*(2), 153-163

Marisol Cueli, Paloma González-Castro, Jennifer Krawec, José Carlos Núñez y Julio Antonio González-Pienda. (2016). Hipatia: a hypermedia learning environment in mathematic. *Anales de Psicología*, *32*(1), 98-105.

Marisol Cueli, Paloma González-Castro, Celestino Rodríguez, José Carlos Núñez y Julio Antonio González-Pienda. (In press).Título: Intervención sobre las variables afectivo-motivacionales relacionadas con el aprendizaje en matemáticas. *Educación XXI*

Marisol Cueli, Celestino Rodríguez, Trinidad García, Débora Areces and Paloma González-Castro. (2015). Título: Experimental study on neurobiofeedback: improved ADHD concentration through nirHEG and blood fluidity. *Revista de Psicología clínica con niños y adolescentes*, 2(2), 9-21.

Paloma González-Castro, PhD

Affiliation: Department of Psychology, University of Oviedo
Date of Birth: 07-January-1968
Education: PhD in Psychology
Address: Department of Psychology, University of Oviedo. Plaza Feijoo s/n, 33003, Oviedo, Spain.

Research and Professional Experience: Lecture in the University of Oviedo

Publications Last 3 Years:

Paloma González-Castro, Celestino Rodríguez, Ángel López, Marisol Cueli, and Luis Álvarez. (2013). Attention Deficit Hyperactivity Disorder, differential diagnosis with blood oxygenation, beta/theta ratio, and attention measures. *International Journal of Clinical and Health Psychology, 13*(2), 101-109

Paloma González-Castro, Celestino Rodríguez, Marisol Cueli, Lourdes Cabeza, and Luis Álvarez. (2014). Math Competence and Executive Control Skills in Students with Attention Deficit/Hyperactivity Disorder and Mathematics Learning Disabilities. *Revista de Psicodidáctia, 19*(1), 125-143.

Paloma González-Castro, Marisol Cueli, Lourdes Cabeza, David Álvarez-García and Luis Álvarez. (2014). Improving basic math skills through integrated dynamic representation strategies. Psicothema, 26(3), 378-38.

Paloma González-Castro, Celestino Rodríguez, Marisol Cueli, Trinidad García, and David Álvarez-García. (2015). State, trait anxiety and selective attention differences in Attention Deficit Hyperactivity Disorder (ADHD) subtypes. International Journal of Clinical and Health Psychology, 15(2), 105-112.

Paloma González-Castro, Marisol Cueli, Celestino Rodríguez, Trinidad García, and Luis Álvarez. (In press, 2016).Efficacy of neurofeedback versus pharmacological support in subjects with ADHD. *Applied Psychophysiology and Biofeedback.*

Celestino Rodríguez Pérez

Affiliation: Department of Psychology, University of Oviedo

Date of Birth: 25-January-1980

Education: PhD in Psychology

Address: Department of Psychology, University of Oviedo. Plaza Feijoo s/n, 33003, Oviedo, Spain.

Research and Professional Experience: Assistant Professor at the University of Oviedo

Publications Last 3 Years:

Trinidad García, Celestino Rodríguez, Paloma González-Castro, David Álvarez, Marisol Cueli, and Julio Antonio González-Pienda. (2013). Funciones ejecutivas en niños y adolescentes con trastornos por déficit de atención con hiperactividad y dificultades lectoras. *International Journal of Psychology and Psychological Therapy, 13*(2), 179-194

Paloma González-Castro, Celestino Rodríguez, Ángel López, Marisol Cueli, and Luis Álvarez. (2013). Attention Deficit Hyperactivity Disorder, differential diagnosis with blood oxygenation, beta/theta ratio, and attention measures. *International Journal of Clinical and HealthPsychology, 13*(2), 101-109

Paloma González-Castro, Celestino Rodríguez, Marisol Cueli, Lourdes Cabeza, and Luis Álvarez. (2014). Math Competence and Executive Control Skills in Students with Attention Deficit/Hyperactivity Disorder and Mathematics Learning Disabilities. *Revista de Psicodidáctia, 19*(1), 125-143.

Trinidad García, Celestino Rodríguez, Paloma González-Castro, Luis Álvarez, and Marisol Cueli. (2014). La atención y el sacádico: Efectos clínicos en el Trastorno por Déficit de Atención con Hiperactividad (TDAH). Revista *Iberoamericana de Psicología y Salud, 5*(1), 1-21

Paloma González-Castro, Celestino Rodríguez, Marisol Cueli, Trinidad García, and David Álvarez-García. (2015). State, trait anxiety and selective attention differences in Attention Deficit Hyperactivity Disorder (ADHD) subtypes. *International Journal of Clinical and Health Psychology, 15*(2), 105-112.

Marisol Cueli, Celestino Rodríguez, Trinidad García, Débora Areces and Paloma González-Castro. (2015). Título: Experimental study on neurobiofeedback: improved ADHD concentration through nirHEG and blood fluidity. *Revista de Psicologíaclínica con niños y adolescentes, 2*(2), 9-21.

In: Dyslexia: Perspectives, Challenges and Treatment Options ISBN: 978-1-63485-328-6
Editor: Marilyn Frazier

Chapter 9

SELECTING PARTICIPANTS FOR DYSLEXIA STUDIES: COMPLEXITIES AND CHALLENGES

João Lopes[1,*], Cristina Gomes[1], Célia Oliveira[2] and Julian Elliott[3]
[1]University of Minho, Portugal
[2]Lusófona University, Porto, Portugal
[3]Durham University, Durham, County Durham, UK

ABSTRACT

The definition of, the nature of, the diagnosis of, and intervention in dyslexia are controversial. There is no consensual definition of dyslexia and although most of the specialized literature states that dyslexia has a neurodevelopmental basis, the debate seems far from exhausted. Also there is no single diagnostic procedure for dyslexia and it is not clear in what aspects interventions for dyslexia differ from those for other reading related (decoding) problems. Such disceprancies raise concerns about the constitution of samples in studies about dyslexia mainly in those studies where groups of participants with different but related reading conditions are included and compared. Reserchers apparently use different methodologies to constitute theirs samples. This makes any comparisions across studies problematic and eventually threatens the generalisability of the findings.

Keywords: dyslexia, sample constitution, poor readers, diagnosis, intervention

* School of Psychology - University of Minho: Campus de Gualtar 4710-057 Braga - Portugal
Email:joaols@psi.uminho.pt.

INTRODUCTION

Dyslexia: Definition and Nature

The word dyslexia is so familiar to most of us that it is hardly believable that there can be any doubts about the concept, about the definition, or about its diagnostic criteria. However, there seems to be many ways to define and to conceptualize dyslexia. Simply put, dyslexia is usually used to describe a word-level reading disability that has also received different labels such as "congenital word blindness" (Hinshelwood, 1907, 1911), "strephosymbolia" (Orton, 1925, 1937) or "specific reading disability," among others (Fletcher, Lyon, Fuchs, and Barnes, 2007). Although this conceptualization seems straightforward, when we try to operationalize it (e.g., for selecting research samples), a number of concerns arise: (a) is there a unique set of characteristics, a "distinct phenotypic pattern of word recognition subskills" (Stanovich, 1994, p. 588), that can reliably distinguish dyslexia from other reading related problems? (b) What processes must exactly be measured (e.g., reading, working memory, letter reversal, reading speed, reading comprehension, phonemic awareness) to reliably diagnose dyslexia?; (c) How can a researcher and/or a practitioner determine cut-off points when there are so many measures and so many definitions of dyslexia?

Is There a Unique Set of Characteristics of Dyslexia?

A clear and definite answer to this critical question is not yet available, mainly because researchers have failed to show in what way dyslexics differ from other poor readers (Rice and Brooks, 2004; Elliott and Grigorenko, 2014). In fact, the most important question to be asked about the diagnosis of dyslexia is not whether dyslexics differ from normal readers but whether they constitute a diagnosable subgroup of poor readers (Elliott and Grigorenko, 2014). Because it is hard to establish the specific phenotypic profile of dyslexics, researchers (e.g., Nelson, 2015; Leinonen et al., 2001; Partanen et al., 2012; Torppa, Eklund, van Bergen, and Lyytinen, 2015), as well as the popular media and the general public (these latter most likely because of lack of knowledge), often use the label dyslexia simply as a synonym for poor reading. However researchers typically state that, unlike other reading deficits, dyslexia appears to have a neurological and genetic basis even if its etiology is still unknown (Fisher and DeFries, 2002; Habib, 2000, Partanen et. al, 2012). In theory, the etiology of dyslexia would then be different from the etiology of other poor reading conditions. The problem is that the neurological origin of dyslexia is usually inferred (not really demonstrated) from behaviors even in samples used in research studies, and it is not clear why this origin is neurological in dyslexics but not in poor readers (Lopes, 2012). Moreover there might be an inversion of the alleged causal chain in some etiological models of dyslexia. Goswami (2015), for example, carefully scrutinized evidence for and against sensory based models of dyslexia and concluded that the sensory deficits found in dyslexics may well be caused by reduced reading experiences, not the contrary.

In part, because of these drawbacks, the DSM-V (American Psychiatric Association, 2013) board recently dismissed dyslexia as a taxonomic entity, subsuming it under the category of specific learning disability (SLD) with impairment in reading. This decision was challenged by a significant number of researchers and scientific societies (e.g., the IDA – International Dyslexia Association) that play an important role in the advocacy of dyslexia.

Such researchers and scientific societies basically contend that dismissing dyslexia as a category will leave poor readers under-recognized and therefore underserved (Wolf, 2014). Moreover, the critics argued that APA decision was not supported by evidence. Ultimately, the DSM board accepted that dyslexia could be used as a specifier once the reading problem has been identified.

The DSM-V board also ruled out any need for an IQ-performance discrepancy for the diagnosis of SLD, following strong criticism of the IQ-performance discrepancy model (e.g., Siegel and Smythe, 2008; Stanovich, 1994; Stuebing et al., 2002). Although discrepancy criterion have not been an exclusive criterion for a dyslexia diagnosis (e.g., Tassé, and Havercamp, 2006) it has long been considered by many that those with dyslexia are bright people with phonemic awareness difficulties and poor word identification skills (Siegel, 2003). Along with the alleged neurological origin of dyslexia, the notion of dyslexia as the "affliction of geniuses" (Coles, 1987) has also been considered (e.g., Martelli et. al., 2014) as a distinguishable feature of dyslexics (compared with other reading disabled students).

Since the concept of dyslexia was built upon the "intuition" (Stanovich, 1994) that reading-IQ discrepancy represented not only a distinct group of poor readers (the dyslexic group) but also a distinct etiology, the elimination of the reading-IQ discrepancy criterion in DSM-V makes the differential diagnosis of dyslexia less tenable and ultimately unnecessary. Notwithstanding such an understanding continues to be frequently used by psychologists and researchers (O'Donnell and Miller, 2011; Warnke, Schulte-Körne, and Ise, 2012). Rice and Brooks (2004) suggest that the widespread use of the reading-IQ discrepancy criterion for the selection of dyslexics samples for empirical studies (e.g., Costanzo, Menghini, Caltagirone, Oliveri, and Vicari, 2013; Dahle and Knivsberg, 2014; Dole, Hoen, and Meunier, 2012), contributes to the perpetuation of the procedure, even if IQ does not help to identify a specific reading profile (Stanovich, 1994) and does not predict children's response to reading interventions (Stuebing, Barth, Molfese, Weiss and Fletcher, 2009).

What Must Really Be Measured to Reliably Diagnose Dyslexia?

The long and varied list of symptoms and cognitive correlates of dyslexia found in the specialized literature makes the measurement and diagnosis of dyslexia particularly difficult. In the absence of a clear and operational definition of dyslexia, researchers and practitioners are confronted with multiple protocols of measurement (e.g., Bell, McCallum and Cox, 2003; Chan, Ho, Chung, Tsang and Lee, 2012). Choosing a set of measures that adequately combine validity, reliability, parsimony, cost-effectiveness, usability, etc., is a complex and highly problematic task.

Researchers tend to use an array of varied measures to select dyslexic participants for their samples on the basis of the long list of symptoms said to characterize dyslexia (Le Jan et al., 2011). These include variables such as working memory, attention, visual processing (e.g., eye tracking), auditory processing, executive functions, reading (e.g., decoding accuracy, reading speed, comprehension), and phonological awareness. Le Jan et. al. (2011) state that "...the review of the literature on dyslexia... shows that (1) on the one hand, reading and spelling tasks are good predictors of dyslexia, (2) on the other hand, some garden-variety children may have poor reading/spelling as dyslexic children but cannot be "labelled" as dyslexics" (p. 2). This statement is interesting because (a) it suggests that reading tasks are the best predictors of dyslexia, perhaps, therefore, dismissing the need for any further tests; and because (b) it asserts, with no further explanation, that some garden-variety poor readers may exhibit the very same reading problems as dyslexics even though they cannot be labeled in this way. Both findings are important because they appear to contradict many of the diagnostic practices of dyslexia. These rely on the assumption that it is imperative to measure a number of cognitive functions to diagnose dyslexia, and that it is clear in what ways garden-variety poor readers differ from dyslexics.

With regard to the use of measures that go beyond reading to diagnose dyslexia, it is imperative that researchers and practitioners substantiate their use. Indeed, although it can be argued that several cognitive variables play a role in reading problems, evidence supporting the utility of identifying and intervening in these cognitive processes is scarce to non-existent (Elliott and Grigorenko, 2014). The measurement of those processes may therefore make the evaluation of dyslexia both expensive and unfruitful.

McGuiness (1997, p. 132) stresses that "As time goes by, reading predicts reading more than anything else. When two measures nearly perfectly correlate, no other test score can contribute further to the relationship." Other authors (e.g., Stanovich, 2005; Vellutino, Fletcher, Snowling and Scanlon, 2004) suggest that rather than focusing their efforts on psychometric assessments to detect the cognitive or biological causes of reading problems, practitioners should focus on the assessment of educational variables (e.g., reading) that are both relevant and amenable to intervention.

Although challenged on the grounds of its limited use for diagnosis or intervention in respect of reading (decoding) difficulty, cognitive testing (particularly IQ testing) has shown significant resilience (Gibbs and Elliott, 2015; Stanovich, 2005). A number of reasons may explain this phenomenon. One the most important is that in some countries the determination of an individual's IQ is deemed necessary for determining eligibility for additional educational resources. This is a strong, but administrative, argument that does address issues of the reliability or validity of the diagnosis, or its irrelevance for intervention.

Another argument that is often proposed is that the assessment of IQ is more "scientific" for the diagnosis of dyslexia than the assessment of aspects of reading (e.g., phonology, reading speed, reading accuracy, word recognition, and comprehension). Stanovich (2005) forcefully refutes this argument stating that IQ testing and that the IQ/discrepancy criterion in defining dyslexia and learning disabilities represent practices "in the border of pseudoscience" (p. 103). Elliott and Grigorenko (2014) revising the evidence about the nature and role of a variety of cognitive processes that might underlie dyslexia conclude that "…it is perhaps surprising that such a vast raft of studies has resulted in only limited understanding of how various cognitive processes underpin dyslexia/reading disability" (p. 86). This means that IQ testing as well as the assessment of other cognitive correlates (e.g., attention, working memory) may be of little use for the diagnosis of learning disabilities in general and dyslexia in particular. Stuebing et al. (2009) conducted a meta-analysis of 28 scientific papers comprising 39 samples to study the predictive value of child cognitive characteristics to reading interventions and concluded that the effect sizes are small. In the light of this finding, the authors questioned the practical effect of these variables for reading assessment and for reading intervention.

How Can a Researcher and/or a Practitioner Determine Cut-Off Points?

The answer to the preceding questions seems to make the answer to this question straightforward: researchers and/or practitioners can only decide on the basis of arbitrary cut-off points (Elliott, 2014). Arriving at a diagnosis is the result of a complex decision-making process. If the relation of the measures with the construct under consideration is unclear, and if the metrics of the tests are hard to match, hesitations, delays in decision-making, and diagnostic errors are more likely (Hill and Ridley, 2001; Ketterlin-Geller and Yovanoff, 2009). In fact, the complex combination of measures that may be quite different in nature, and the problems with the metrics, increase the likelihood of diagnosing false positives and false negatives and the use of subjective cues in a specific diagnosis, even when objective cues suggested otherwise (e.g., Aspel, Willis and Faust, 1998).

Clearly reading performance operates along a continuum and the diagnosis of a category such as dyslexia relies upon determining arbitrary and questionable cut-off points (Lopes, 2012; Shaywitz, Escobar, Shaywitz, Fletcher, and Makuch, 1992). The same can be said about other alleged reading categories like garden-variety poor reading. For such reasons, some authors (e.g., Shaywitz et. al., 1992) contend that reading is more akin to obesity than to pregnancy.

The review of the literature about the definition and nature of dyslexia shows that researchers are confronted with significant challenges when they try to decide whether a specific individual (1) is a 'true dyslexic' (as opposed to a 'true poor reader').

The Constitution of Samples in Studies about Dyslexia

There appears to be little systematic pattern or procedure for inclusion and exclusion of participants in dyslexia studies. Significant differences are found in the diagnostic tools (e.g., reading tests, IQ tests, past school performance, cognitive measures), in the contexts where participants are recruited (e.g., schools, clinics, hospitals, special education), and in the professional groups that make the diagnostic (psychologist, neuropsychologist, speech therapist, phono-audiologist). It is possible to find multiple procedures, multiple criteria and multiple measures in the constitution of samples in studies about dyslexia. These include: (a) measures previously selected by the investigator, including reading tests and IQ testing (e.g., Silani et al., 2005); (b) a formal diagnosis of dyslexia previously conducted by special education services (e.g Jeffries and Everatt, 2004); (c) a documented history of dyslexia and reading tests (e.g., Milne, Hamm, Kirk, and Corballis, 2003); (d) selection on the basis of RTI models (e.g., Cestnick and Coltheart, 1999); (e) a diagnosis of dyslexia alongside a personal and family history of reading problems (e.g.Gilger, Pennington and DeFries, 1991) and (f) having attended speech therapy in the past (e.g., Robichon and Habib, 1998).

Studies also differ in the contexts sampled: (a) dyslexia centers (e.g., Rey, De Martino, Espesser, and Habib, 2002); (b) speech therapy (e.g., Crisp and Ralph, 2006); (c) resource centers for reading disabled students (e.g., Pasquini, Corriveau, and Goswami, 2007); (d) school settings (e.g., Siok, Niu, Jin, Perfetti, and Tan, 2008); (e) universities (e.g., Oganian and Ahissar, 2012), among others. Research also shows that there is a significant number of professionals who have diagnosed participants for dyslexia studies: (a) psychologists (e.g., Gallagher, Laxon, Armstrong, and Frith, 1996); (b) neuropsychologists (e.g., Dalmás and Dansilio, 2000); (c) special education teachers (e.g., Pammer and Wheatley, 2001); (d) neurologists (e.g., Nopola-Hemmi et al. 2001); (e) speech therapists (e.g., Virsu, Lathi-Nuuttila, and Laasonen, 2003); (f) fonoaudiologists (e.g., Callens, Tops, Stevens, and Brysbaert, 2014), among others.

These differences may account for the heterogeneity of the samples thus making it difficult to compare the results across samples and across studies. These drawbacks challenge researchers to be more systematic in addressing their selection procedures.

Samples in Studies about Dyslexia: The University of Minho Project

In order to more deeply understand how researchers deal with the problems of sample selection in dyslexia studies, a group of researchers based at the University of Minho (the authors of this chapter), have been conducting a series of studies on this topic. In the first phase of this project, the researchers analyzed a total of six hundred and eighty nine articles published between 1996 and 2014 (Gomes, 2015). Six hundred and seventy one of these articles concerned studies whose samples include individuals either with dyslexia only, or studies whose samples contrasted participants with dyslexia with those without reading problems. The remaining eighteen studies compared those participants deemed to have dyslexia with those considered to have reading problems other than dyslexia. All studies were collected from the Scopus database.

The authors developed an analytic framework taking into account the: a) title of the article; b) article publication year; c) journal in which the article was published; d) number of dyslexic participants in the sample; e) contexts where samples were collected; f) researchers' criteria to constitute the samples; g) measures used to select participants for the samples; and h) professional affiliation of those that conducted the participants´ selection process. A mixed qualitative and quantitative strategy was developed for data analysis. For the purpose of this chapter, only a number of findings from this study will be reported here.

Samples in Studies about Dyslexia: General Findings

Overall, the study showed that there were significant variations in the way researchers sought to constitute samples of dyslexics and of controls in their studies. There are certainly some similarities between studies but even when variables are in common use, the measures employed to operationalize these may be quite different. It is therefore difficult to compare the results of the studies and to generalize the findings.

One interesting finding was that in the majority of the studies reviewed (67%) the samples of dyslexic participants were small (<30), and in only 6% of the studies samples were large (>150). This means that studies with dyslexic participants typically had low *n´*s which may carry some generalization problems.

Another finding was that samples were collected in clinical contexts, in community settings, or constituted reused samples. About 28% of the studies did not report the contexts from where dyslexic samples were collected. This number raises to 50% for samples of participants with reading problems other than dyslexia.

It was found that researchers typically used four main methods to select participants for dyslexic samples: a formal diagnosis of dyslexia, tests selected by the researchers (e.g., reading tests) (by far the most common method), the academic history of the participants, and family history of dyslexia. In many studies these methods were used in combination. Four percent of the studies held no information about how participants were selected. For controls with reading problems other than dyslexia the only method reported involved tests selected by the researchers. Eleven percent of the studies reported no information about how participants were selected.

In around three quarters of the studies, the researchers themselves conducted the process of selecting participants. In around 15% of the studies, there was no information available about who conducted the selection process.

Samples in Studies about Dyslexia: Inclusion and Exclusion Criteria

The University of Minho study´s (Gomes, 2015) has pointed out that researchers widely vary in the inclusion criteria in samples of dyslexics and controls. This is most likely a consequence of the lack of consensus about the definition, the causes and the methods of assessment of dyslexia (Elliott, 2010; Snowling, 2013). However in a significant number of studies it is difficult to identify the conceptualization and/or the definition of dyslexia that is being employed. Elliott and Grigorenko (2014) stress that although researchers do not share a single conceptualization of dyslexia, differences of understanding are rarely made explicit in their description of their samples of dyslexic participants. Elliott and Grigorenko contend that the selection of dyslexic participants is based on poor results in one or more tests of reading only, with arbitrary cut-off points. Therefore these participants do not represent a true sub-group of poor readers selected on the basis of a specific cognitive profile.

The research group of the University of Minho also found that researchers tended to be more judicious in their selection of dyslexic participants than in the selection of controls with other reading problems. Certainly, the varied and often nonoperational definitions of dyslexia require researchers to be particularly careful in their selection of dyslexic samples in order that such groups can be distinguishable from controls.

A feature worth mentioning in studies about dyslexia is that the widely cited exclusion criterion "lack of educational opportunities" is seldom made sufficiently clear to enable a judgement to be made. Elliott and Grigorenko (2014) and Lopes (2012) argue that this criterion is based on a complex and unreliable judgment and that almost certainly, educational opportunities of this kind are rarely considered. This issue is most relevant because dyslexia is widely considered to be a neurological disorder (Boets, 2014; Dole, Meunier, and Hoen, 2014; Norton, Beach, and Gabrieli, 2015; Olulade, Flowers, Napoliello, and Eden, 2015), which means that researchers must ensure that their samples of dyslexics do not include students that simply received poor teaching (which, in itself, would be very difficult to determine). As Elliott and Grigorenko (2014), have pointed out, separating biological from environmental factors prior to undertaking a lengthy period of systematic instruction is virtually impossible.

The University of Minho study's failed to find evidence concerning the extent to which educational opportunities were controlled in research studies. Most likely researchers assumed that any student who attended school received appropriate educational opportunities. This may explain why educational opportunities are not truly an issue in research studies about dyslexia, even if this factor may threaten the validity of the sampling procedures employed.

Our analysis also demonstrated that the IQ is still routinely measured as a way to differentiate samples of dyslexics from samples of other poor readers. This is problematic as there is now powerful evidence that IQ does not predict decoding differences between supposed poor readers and dyslexic readers (Fletcher et al., 2007; Stuebing et al., 2009), that IQ does not predict reading performance (Vellutino, Scanlon, and Lyon, 2000), and that IQ scores do not predict which poor readers will be more or less resistant to intervention (Gresham and Vellutino, 2010). This continued practice is thus a threat to the integrity of the samples and to the reliability of the results.

Another important finding is that the samples of controls who are deemed to other reading problems than dyslexia are often selected on the basis of a reading test and of a cognitive test. This clearly differs from the broader array of tests typically used for the diagnosis of dyslexia. Apparently, many researchers believe that the diagnosis of dyslexia is more complicated than the diagnosis of other reading problems. The European Dyslexia Association (EDA), for instance, states that "The term 'dyslexia' indicates a more complex syndrome than just a problem with reading" (http://www.eda-info.eu/causes-of-dyslexia). However it is hard to understand why other poor readers wouldn't suffer from the emotional, motivational, and self-image problems that the EDA says are characteristic of dyslexics. Actually, since these characteristics are usually consequences, not causes, of perceived reading failure, it is highly likely that most, if not all, poor readers experience these self-defeating feelings (McGuinness, 2005).

In reporting their results of the studies conducted in the Isle of White and in inner London, Rutter and Yule (1975) concluded that "...neither in a study of children with specific reading retardation ..., nor in an investigation of a group regarded as dyslexic... has it been possible to demonstrate any clustering of the developmental anomalies said to characterize dyslexia" (p. 194). The authors also found that inner London poor readers scoring in the lower range of a battery of tests (e.g., reading, IQ) outnumber poor readers on the Isle of White by a factor of four. This calls into question the heritability of dyslexia and other reading problems and suggests a strong environmental effect in reading failure (McGuinness, 1997). Rutter and Yule (1975) conclude that "In short, there has been a complete failure to show that the signs of dyslexia constitute any meaningful pattern. It may be concluded that the question of whether specific reading retardation is or is not dyslexia can be abandoned as meaningless" (p. 194).

The Connecticut Longitudinal Study also showed that children with reading problems, independently of their IQ, performed poorly in measures of phonemic awareness and that reading scores spread along a continuum from good to bad. In the context of this same study, Shaywitz et. al. (1992), using an IQ-discrepancy model, tested children from first to sixth grade and found the diagnosis of dyslexia to be rather unstable. Of the 25 children diagnosed as dyslexics in grade 1, only 7 were considered dyslexic in grade 3, and of the 24 students diagnosed as dyslexics in grade 5, only 14 were considered to be dyslexic in grade 3. The authors therefore conclude that "Dyslexia is not an all-or-none phenomenon, but like hypertension, occurs in degrees" (p. 145). This suggests that dyslexia can hardly be conceived as a real category and that the differential diagnosis of dyslexia is quite problematic.

Contexts of Sample Collection

The University of Minho study's (Gomes, 2015) showed that most samples for dyslexia studies are collected in community and clinical settings, often without a clear conceptualization of dyslexia and with unique sets of measures. This is likely to lead to more heterogeneous samples and consequently is a threat to any generalization of results. Furthermore, a significant number of studies reuse samples from past studies which can lead to a self-reproduction of heterogeneous samples. Even more problematically, in most cases there is no information about the inclusion and exclusion criteria for the original samples.

It is worth noting that the University of Minho study's failed to find any study with samples of controls with reading problems collected in clinical settings. This suggests that researchers hold a clinical/medical perspective about dyslexia but not about poor reading in general. It may also assist in the perpetuation of the medical models of dyslexia and insufficient consideration of how this plays out in education settings.

CONCLUSION

Three main conclusions can be drawn from the literature about the samples used for studies of dyslexia:

1. The nature of the samples employed shows that there is much to clarify in this area. The procedures of researchers vary significantly from study to study and in a noteworthy number of cases it is not possible to determine how participants were selected.
2. In some studies, dyslexia seems to be conceptualized simply as a synonym for poor reading. In others it is far from clear in what specific ways so-called dyslexics differ from other poor readers for the purposes of sample allocation.
3. A very significant number of samples are still built upon the now discredited IQ-discrepancy model.

The collection of samples in dyslexia studies seems to reflect the problems of conceptualization of both dyslexia and general reading problems. Until these problems are properly addressed, current uncertainties about the homogeneity of samples and about the generalization of results will likely persist. It is therefore vital that researchers place greater emphasis both in issues of definition and conceptualization of dyslexia and in the inclusion and exclusion criteria in samples constitution.

REFERENCES

American Psychiatric Association (2013). *Diagnostic and Statistical Manual of Mental Disorders,* Fifth Edition. Arlington, VA, American Psychiatric Association.

Aspel, A. D., Willis, W. G. and Faust, D. (1998). School psychologists' diagnostic decision-making processes: Objective-subjective discrepancies. *Journal of School Psychology, 36*(2), 137-149.

Bell, S. M., McCallum, R. S. and Cox, E. A. (2003). Toward a research-based assessment of dyslexia: Using cognitive measures to identify reading disabilities. *Journal of Learning Disabilities, 36*(6), 505-516.

Boets, B. (2014). Dyslexia: Reconciling controversies within an integrative developmental perspective. *Trends in Cognitive Sciences, 18*(10), 501-503. doi: 10.1016/j.tics.2014.06.003.

Büttner, G. and Hasselhorn, M. (2011). Learning Disabilities: Debates on definitions, causes, subtypes, and responses. *International Journal of Disability, Development and Education, 58*(1), 75–87. doi:10.1080/ 1034912X.2011.548476.

Callens, M., Tops, W., Stevens, M. and Brysbaert, M. (2014). An exploratory factor analysis of the cognitive functioning of first-year bachelor students with dyslexia. *Annals of Dyslexia, 64*, 91-119.

Cestnick, L. and Coltheart, M. (1999). The relationship between language-processing and visual-processing deficits in developmental dyslexia. *Cognition, 71*, 231-255.

Chan, D. W., Ho, C. S. H., Chung, K. K. H., Tsang, S. M. and Lee, S. H. (2012). The Hong Kong Behaviour Checklist for Primary Students: Developing a brief dyslexia screening measure. *International Journal of Disability, Development and Education, 59*(2), 173-196. doi: 10.1080/ 1034912x.2012.676437.

Coles, G. (1987). *The learning mystique: A critical look at "learning disabilities."* New York: Columbine.

Costanzo, F., Menghini, D., Caltagirone, C., Oliveri, M. and Vicari, S. (2013). How to improve reading skills in dyslexics: The effect of high frequency rTMS. *Neuropsychologia, 51*, 2953-2959. doi: 10.1016/j. neuropsychologia.2013.10.018.

Crisp, J. and Ralph, M. A. L. (2006). Unlocking the nature of the phonological-deep dyslexia continuum: the keys to reading aloud are in phonology and semantics. *Journal of Cognitive Neuroscience, 18*(3), 348-362.

Dahle, A. E. and Knivsberg, A. (2014). Internalizing, externalizing and attention problems in dyslexia. *Scandinavian Journal of Disability Research, 16*(2), 179-193. doi: 10.1080/15017419.2013.781953.

Dalmás, J. F. and Dansilio, S. (2000). Visuographemic alexia: a new form of a peripheral acquired dyslexia. *Brain and Language, 75*, 1-16.

Desforges, M. and Lindsay, G. (2010). Procedures used to diagnose a disability and to assess Special Educational Needs: An International Review. In *The National Council for Special Education*, University of Warwick, Oct. 2010 (1-1999).

Dole, M., Hoen, M. and Meunier, F. (2012). Speech-in-noise perception deficit in adults with dyslexia: Effects of background type and listening configuration. *Neuropsychologia, 50*, 1543-15552.

Dole, M., Meunier, F. and Hoen, M. (2014). Functional correlates of the speech-in-noise perception impairment in dyslexia: An MRI study. *Neuropsychologia, 60*(1), 103-114. doi: 10.1016/j.neuropsychologia. 2014.05.016.

Elliott, J. (2014). Dyslexia - A problematic diagnosis. *Psychologist, 27*(6), 385.

Elliott, J. G. (2010). Dyslexia: diagnoses, debates and diatribes. *Education Canada, 46*(2), 14-17.

Elliott, J. G. and Grigorenko, E. L. (2014). *The Dyslexia debate*. New York: Cambridge University Press.

Fisher, S. E. and DeFries, J. C. (2002). Developmental dyslexia: Genetic dissection of a complex cognitive trait. *Nature Reviews Neuroscience, 3*, 767–780. http://dx.doi.org/ 10.1038/nrn936.

Fletcher, J. M., Lyon, G. R., Fuchs, L. S. and Barnes, M. A. (2007). *Learning Disabilities: From identification to intervention*. New York: Guilford Press.

Gallagher, A. M., Laxon, V., Armstrong, E. and Frith, U. (1996). Phonological difficulties in high-functioning dyslexics. *Reading and Writing, 8*, 499-509.

Gibbs, S. and Elliott, J. (2015). The differential effects of labelling: how do 'dyslexia' and 'reading difficulties' affect teachers' beliefs. *European Journal of Special Needs Education, 30*(3), 323-337. doi: 10.1080/ 08856257.2015.1022999.

Gilger, J. W., Pennington, B. and DeFries, J. C. (1991). Risk for reading disability as a function of parental history in three family studies. *Reading and Writing, 3*, 205-217.

Gomes, C. M. S. (2015). *Constituição de amostras em estudos sobre dislexia [Sample constitution in dyslexia studies]*. Master thesis, University of Minho, Braga. URL:https://repositorium.sdum.uminho.pt/bitstream/ 1822/37567/1/Cristina%20Maria%20da%20Silva%20Gomes.pdf.

Goswami, U. (2015). Sensory theories of developmental dyslexia: three challenges for research. *Nature Reviews Neuroscience, 16*(1), 43-54. doi: 10.1038/nrn3836.

Gresham, F. M. and Vellutino, F. R. (2010). What is the role of intelligence in the identification of specific learning disabilities? Issues and clarifications. *Learning Disabilities Research and Practice, 25*(4), 194-206.

Habib, M. (2000). The neurological basis of developmental dyslexia: An overview and working hypothesis. *Brain, 123,* 2373–2399. http://dx.doi. org/10.1093/brain/123. 12.2373.

Hill, C. L. and Ridley, C. R. (2001). Diagnostic decision making: Do counselors delay final judgments? *Journal of Counseling and Development, 79*(1), 98-104.

Hinshelwood, J. (1907). Four cases of congenital word blindness. *British Medical Journal, 2*, 1229-1232.

Hinshelwood, J. (1911). Two cases of congenital word blindness. *British Medical Journal, 1*, 608-609.

Jeffries, S. and Everatt, J. (2004). Working memory: its role in dyslexia and other specific learning difficulties. *Dyslexia, 10*, 196-214.

Ketterlin-Geller, L. R. and Yovanoff, P. (2009). Diagnostic assessments in mathematics to support instructional decision making. *Practical Assessment, Research and Evaluation, 14*(16).

Le Jan, G., Le Bouquin-Jeannès, R., Costet, N., Trolès, N., Scalart, P., Pichancourt, D., . . . Gombert, J. E. (2011). Multivariate predictive model for dyslexia diagnosis. *Annals of Dyslexia, 61*(1), 1-20. doi: 10.1007/s11881-010-0038-5.

Leinonen, S., Müller, K., Eeppänen, P. H. T., Mikko, A. R. O., Ahonen, T. and Eyytinen, H. (2001). Heterogeneity in adult dyslexic readers: Relating processing skills to the speed and accuracy of oral text reading. *Reading and Writing, 14*(3-4), 265-296.

Lopes, J. (2012). Biologising reading problems: the specific case of dyslexia. *Contemporary Social Science: Journal of the Academy of Social Sciences, 7*(2), 215-229. doi: 10.1080/21582041.2012.692098.

Martelli, M., De Luca, M., Lami, L., Pizzoli, C., Pontillo, M., Spinelli, D. and Zoccolotti, P. (2014). Bridging the gap between different measures of the reading speed deficit in developmental dyslexia. *Experimental Brain Research, 232*(1), 237-252. doi: 10.1007/s00221-013-3735-6.

McGuinness, D. (1997). *Why our children can't read and what we can do about it: A scientific revolution in reading*. New York: Touchstone.

McGuinness, D. (2005). *Language development and learning to read*. Cambridge: MIT Press.

Milne, R. D., Hamm, J. P., Kirk, I. J. and Corballis, M. C. (2003). Anterior-posterior beta asymmetries in dyslexia during lexical decisions. *Brain and Language, 84*, 309-317.

Nelson, J. M. (2015). Examination of the double-deficit hypothesis with adolescents and young adults with dyslexia. *Annals of Dyslexia, 65*(3), 159-177. doi: 10.1007/s11881-015-0105-z.

Nopola-Hemmi, J., Myllyluoma, B., Haltia, T., Taipale, M., Ollikainen, V., Ahonen, T., ... and Widén, E. (2001). A dominant gene for developmental dyslexia on chromosome 3. *Journal of Medical Genetics, 38,* 658-664.

Norton, E. S., Beach, S. D. and Gabrieli, J. D. E. (2015). Neurobiology of dyslexia. *Current Opinion in Neurobiology, 30*, 73-78. doi: 10.1016 /j.conb.2014.09.007.

O'Donnell, P. S. and Miller, D. N. (2011). Identifying students with specific learning disabilities: School psychologists' acceptability of the discrepancy model versus response to intervention. *Journal of Disability Policy Studies, 22,* 83-94. doi: 10.1177/1044207310395724.

Oganian, Y. and Ahissar, M. (2012). Poor anchoring limits dyslexics' perceptual, memory, and reading skills. *Neuropsychologia, 50*, 1895-1905.

Olulade, O. A., Flowers, D. L., Napoliello, E. M. and Eden, G. F. (2015). Dyslexic children lack word selectivity gradients in occipito-temporal and inferior frontal cortex. *NeuroImage: Clinical, 7*, 742-754. doi: 10.1016/j.nicl.2015.02.013.

Orton, S. T. (1925). "Word-blindness" in school children. *Archives of Neurology and Psychiatry, 14*, 285–516. doi:10.1001/archneurpsyc.1925. 02200170002001.

Orton, S. T. (1937). *Reading, writing and speech problems in children.* New York: W. W. Norton and Co.

Pammer, K. and Wheatley, C. (2001). Isolating the m(y)-cell response in dyslexia using the spatial frequency doubling illusion. *Vision Research, 41*, 2139-2147.

Partanen, M., Fitzpatrick, K., Mädler, B., Edgell, D., Bjornson, B. and Giaschi, D. E. (2012). Cortical basis for dichotic pitch perception in developmental dyslexia. *Brain and Language, 123*, 104–112.

Pasquini, E. S., Corriveau, K. H. and Goswami, U. (2007). Auditory processing of amplitude envelope rise time in adults diagnosed with developmental dyslexia. *Scientific Studies of Reading, 11*(3), 259-286.

Rey, V., De Martino, S., Espesser, R. and Habib, M. (2002). Temporal processing and phonological impairment in dyslexia: effect of phoneme lengthening on order judgment of two consonants. *Brain and Language, 80*, 576-591.

Rice, M. and Brooks, G. (2004). *Developmental dyslexia in adults: A research review.* London: NRDC.

Robichon, F. and Habib, M. (1998). Abnormal callosal morphology in male adult dyslexics: relationships to handedness and phonological abilities. *Brain and Language, 62*, 127-146.

Rutter, M. and Yule, W. (1975). The concept of specific reading retardation. *Journal of Child Psychology and Psychiatry and Allied Disciplines, 16*(3), 181-197.

Share, D. L. and Silva, P. A. (2003). Gender bias in IQ-discrepancy and post-discrepancy definitions of reading disability. *Journal of Learning Disabilities, 36*(1), 4-14.

Shaywitz, S. E., Escobar, M. D., Shaywitz, B. A., Fletcher, J. M. and Makuch, R. (1992). Evidence that dyslexia may represent the lower tail of a normal distribution of reading ability. *New England Journal of Medicine, 326*(3), 145-150. doi: 10.1056/NEJM199201163260301.

Siegel, L. S. (2003). IQ-discrepancy definitions and the diagnosis of LD: Introduction to the special issue. *Journal of Learning Disabilities, 36*(1), 2-3.

Siegel, L. S. and Smythe, I. S. (2008). The importance of phonological processing rather than IQ discrepancy in understanding adults with reading disorders. In L. E. Wolf, H. S. Schreiber, and J. Wasserstein (Eds.), *Adult Learning Disorders: Contemporary Issues* (pp. 275-300). New York: Psychology Press.

Silani, G., Frith, U., Demonet, J. F., Fazio, F., Perani, D., Price, C., ... and Paulesu, E. (2005). Brain abnormalities underlying altered activation in dyslexia: a voxel based morphometry study. *Brain, 128*, 2453-2461.

Siok, W. T., Niu, Z., Jin, Z., Perfetti, C. A. and Tan, L. H. (2008). A structural-functional basis for dyslexia in the cortex of Chinese readers. *Proceedings of the National Academy of Sciences, 15*(14), 5561-5566.

Snowling, M. J. (2013). Early identification and interventions for dyslexia: a contemporary view. *Journal of Research in Special Educational Needs, 13*(1), 7–14. doi:10.1111/j.1471-3802.2012.01262.x.

Stanovich, K. E. (1994). Annotation: Does Dyslexia Exist? *Journal of Child Psychology and Psychiatry and Allied Disciplines, 35*(4), 579–595.

Stanovich, K. E. (2005). The future of a mistake: Will discrepancy measurement continue to make the learning disabilities field a pseudoscience? *Learning Disability Quarterly, 28*, 103-106.

Stuebing, K. K., Barth, A. E., Molfese, P. J., Weiss, B. and Fletcher, J. M. (2009). IQ is not strongly related to response to reading instruction: A meta-analytic interpretation. *Exceptional Children, 76*(1), 31-51.

Stuebing, K. K., Fletcher, J. M., LeDoux, J. M., Lyon, G. R., Shaywitz, S. E. and Shaywitz, B. A. (2002). Validity of IQ-discrepancy classifications of reading disabilities: A meta-analysis. *American Educational Research Journal, 39*(2), 469-518.

Tassé, M. J. and Havercamp, S. M. (2006). The role of motivation and psychopathology in understanding the IQ-Adaptive Behavior discrepancy. *International Review of Research in Mental Retardation, Vol. 31* (pp. 231-259).

Torppa, M., Eklund, K., van Bergen, E. and Lyytinen, H. (2015). Late-emerging and resolving dyslexia: A follow-up study from age 3 to 14. *Journal of Abnormal Child Psychology, 43*(7), 1389-1401. doi: 10.1007/s10802-015-0003-1.

Vellutino, F. R., Fletcher, J. M., Snowling, M. J., and Scanlon, D. M. (2004). Specific reading disability (dyslexia): What have we learned in the past four decades? *Journal of Child Psychology and Psychiatry, 45*, 2-40.

Vellutino, F. R., Scanlon, D. M. and Lyon, R. (2000). Differentiating between difficult-to-remediated poor readers. More evidence against the IQ-Achievement discrepancy definition of reading disability. *Journal of Learning Disabilities, 33*(3), 223-238.

Virsu, V., Lahti-Nuuttila, P. and Laasonen, M. (2003). Crossmodal temporal processing acuity impairment aggravates with age in developmental dyslexia. *Neuroscience Letters, 336*, 151-154.

Warnke, A., Shulte-Korne, G. and Ise, E. (2012). Developmental dyslexia. In M. E. Garralda and J. Raynaud (Eds.), *Brain, mind, and developmental psychopathology in childhood* (pp. 173-198). Lanham, MD: Jason Aronson Publishing.

Wolf, M. (2014). *Marcus Aurelius and the continuing dyslexia debate.* https://eida.org/marcus-aurelius-and-the-continuing-dyslexia-debate/

About the Authors

João Lopes holds a PhD in Psychology, and he is a hired Professor in the School of Psychology of the University of Minho. His research interests focuses in the areas of learning disabilities, reading instruction, classroom behavior problems and classroom management. He wrote more than a dozen books on these subjects. He authored "Conceptualization, assessment and intervention in reading problems: The sophisticated arquitecture of a misconception, 2010 (Psiquilíbrios), and co-authored "Reading teaching in primary grades: Teachers' beliefs, teachers' knowledge and teachers' background", 2014 (Francisco Manuel dos Santos Foundation), with Louise Spear-Swerling, Célia Oliveira, Gabriela Velasquez, Leandro Almeida, Luísa Araújo, Jamie Zibulsky and Elaine Cheesman.

Cristina Gomes is an Educational Psychologist. She holds a Master degree in Psychology from the Universtity of Minho. She currently is a member of the "Learning and Behavior Problems Research Group" at the University of Minho and she conducts research in the area of reading problems. She has been actively involved in the project of samples constitution in dyslexia studies.

Célia Oliveira holds a PhD in Experimental Psychology at the University of Minho. As a school psychologist she focused on the developmental problems of handicapped children and on the learning problems of school-aged children. She currently teaches Psychology at the O'Porto Lusófona University. She co-authored "Reading teaching in primary grades: Teachers' beliefs, teachers' knowledge and teachers' background", 2014 (Fundação Francisco Manuel dos Santos), with João Lopes, Louise Spear-Swerling, Gabriela Velasquez, Leandro Almeida, Luísa Araújo, Jamie Zibulsky and Elaine Cheesman.

Julian Elliott is Principal of Collingwood College, and Professor of Educational Psychology, at Durham University. He is a Fellow of the Academy of Social Sciences, a Chartered Psychologist, and an Associate Fellow of the British Psychological Society. His research primarily operates at the interface of educational psychology as both a discipline and a profession. His most recent book (co-authored with Rod Nicolson), Dyslexia: Developing the Debate. London: Bloomsbury Press, 2016, follows on from his earlier The Dyslexia Debate, co-authored with Elena Grigorenko (Cambridge University Press, 2014).

In: Dyslexia: Perspectives, Challenges and Treatment Options ISBN: 978-1-63485-328-6
Editor: Marilyn Frazier

Chapter 10

CHILDREN'S LITERATURE AS A RESOURCE TOOL TO MEET THE PSYCHOSOCIAL-EMOTIONAL NEEDS OF CHILDREN WITH DYSLEXIA

Chiew Hong Ng[1,*], Noel Kok Hwee Chia[1] and Patricia Mui Hoon Ng[3]
[1]National Institute of Education,
Nanyang Technological University, Singapore
[2]Research Associate, Katong School, Singapore

ABSTRACT

Educators and counselors have always been concerned about meeting the needs of children with dyslexia especially in addressing reading problems as well as coping with psychosocial-emotional issues. Although a lot of research has been done on difficulties with accurate and/or fluent word recognition, poor spelling and decoding abilities of children with dyslexia and how these affect the development of language and literacy skills, very little is written or studies being done on how to help children with dyslexia cope with their socio-emotional struggles and, hence, their psychological well-being. In this chapter, the authors have chosen to discuss the use of children's literature as a resource tool to help such children address their psychosocial-emotional needs.

Keywords: children's literature, psychosocial-emotional needs, children with dyslexia

INTRODUCTION

Many may have heard about dyslexia as a reading disability, but those who have not come across a learner with dyslexia may not understand how it can affect one's life and socio-emotional well-being, much less know what the symptoms are. In its simplest sense, Chia

* Corresponding author: chiewhong,ng@nie.edu.sg.

(2015) has explained that dyslexia means difficulty with words as the term is derived from *dys* which means "bad or difficult" and *lexis* which refers to "words."

Dyslexia was first described in a seminal work – *A case of congenital word-blindness (inability to learn to read* – by Morgan (1896) in the British Medical Journal (cited in Pennington, Peterson, and McGrath, 2009). However, there was little development in the knowledge of the cognitive phenotype until almost a quarter of a century ago when progression was made towards neuropsychological deficits in phonological representation. Earlier theories had focused on the reversals of symbols that was termed *strephosymbolia* or twisted symbols by Orton (1925, 1928). Orton (1928) referred to the so-called congenital word blindness as a specific disability in reading and argued that it was unrelated to subnormal intelligence. Elaborating on the condition which he believed to be a physiological variant due to the persistence of the activity of the non-dominant cerebral hemisphere, he reported that children with strephosymbolia demonstrate an ability to read from a mirror and produce mirror writing. He also offered that the prognosis was good with proper instruction that incorporates directional kinesthetic training.

According to Pennington, Peterson and McGrath (2009), children affected by dyslexia can learn to read given appropriate and adequate intervention, though they may remain as slow readers and poor spellers for the whole of their lives. Nevertheless, these researchers also reported that future educational and occupational success is likely for those who are bright. Children with dyslexia can learn to read, provided they are given adequate and appropriate learning support, which includes the three basic strategies for dealing with written words (see Frith, 1986, for detail): (1) logographic strategy as an instant word recognition based on noticeable graphic features, analogous to the "Chinese" way of identifying Chinese characters known as *hanzhi*; (2) alphabetic or letter-to-sound strategy as analyzing a word strictly by putting together the sound of each letter sequentially to conjure up a word as it appears or as it is spelled; and (3) orthographic strategy as an "instant recognition of morphemic parts of a word taking into account letter order, but not letter sound; rather, if any sound at all, it is the sound of morphemes or of whole words" (Frith, 1986, p. 72). In this chapter, though we do address reading issues related to dyslexia, our main focus here is on how children's literature can be used, not so much as a teaching resource for remedial reading, but as a resource tool to address the psychosocial-emotional needs of children with dyslexia. We use the term *resource tool* to refer to the rich resource of children's literature as an assistive device.

Diagnostic Profile for Dyslexia

There is often confusion between learning disability and learning difficulty because the two terms have been used interchangeably most of the times in literature. In general, *learning disability*, according to the Foundation for People with Learning Disabilities (2001), means "significantly reduced ability to understand new or complex information, to learn new skills" (para. 8) or acquire new knowledge, and also includes "reduced ability to cope independently which starts before adulthood with lasting effects on development" (para. 9). In other words, "learning disability is a condition that affects learning and intelligence across all areas of life" (Dagan, Burke, Davies, and Chinn, 2015, p. 11). The terms "*learning difficulty* and/or *specific learning difficulty* describe difficulties such as dyslexia and dyspraxia" (Foundation for People with Learning Disabilities, 2001, para. 3) and it "is a condition that makes specific areas of learning difficult, but does not affect the overall intelligence of an individual" (Dagan, Burke, Davies, and Chinn, 2015, p. 11). Tannock (2014) explained that *disorder* is a medical term while *disability* is an educational term used by educators and also by psychologists and therapists.

In the Educator's Diagnostic Manual of Disabilities and Disorders (EDM), Pierangelo and Giuliani (2007) described dyslexia as one of the many Specific Learning Disabilities (SLD) under the Individuals with Disabilities Education Act of 2004 (IDEA 2004). Since the advent of IDEA 2004, schools in the U.S. have been required to provide an Individualized Education Program (IEP) for affected students. The description of a disability to be stated in the IEP can be found in the EDM. Using the EDM, dyslexia is first described as a learning disability (LD) at Level 1 and then as a specific LD known by the term *Dyslexia* (LD 4.0) at Level 2. Further subtyping of each category is described at sequential levels, hence the EDM allows for the discovery of specific traits to be more easily categorized or identified from the existing categories.

The EDM refers to LD as a neurobiological disorder in the structure of an individual's brain and the way it works. This disorder would often affect one's ability to read, write, listen, speak, reason, and do mathematics. To identify an LD, learning problems that are primarily the result of visual, hearing, or motor disabilities are to be precluded. On top of that, learning problems attributed primarily to mental retardation, emotional disturbance, or environmental, cultural, or economic disadvantage must also be ruled out.

For the risk factors in dyslexia, deficits in phonological representation and word recognition should be tested (Torgesen, 1999). Pennington, Peterson and McGrath (2009) recommended that school work and observations should also be used to triangulate the diagnosis of dyslexia. They also pointed out that since dyslexia is familial and inheritable, the risk profile should be checked with medical records and information given by the family.

The Effects of Dyslexia on Reading

Pennington, Peterson and McGrath (2009) pointed out that genetic breakthroughs in the research of dyslexia had found that children with dyslexia experienced problems in printed word recognition, and so those without word recognition problems in reading comprehension are differentiated as poor comprehenders from poor decoders. To illustrate this assumption, Figure 1 shows a model of reading disabilities where reading has only two components – decoding and comprehension – occurring in a continuum. Within the continuum of reading disabilities, dyslexia can be described as the polar opposite of hyperlexia (Aaron, 1989; Chia, Poh, and Ng, 2009; Gough and Tunmer, 1986; Ng, 2013; Ng and Chia, 2013). Hyperlexia is also known as direct dyslexia (Tyre and Young, 1994). Thus, dyslexia is perceived as a disorder with poor word recognition but good comprehension on the assumption that conceptual understanding can still be achieved by other means such as listening comprehension. The types of conceptual and social deficits in hyperlexia (Healy, 1982) are in stark contrast to dyslexia. Occupying the section in the continuum between dyslexia and hyperlexia is the non-specific reading disabilities (NSRDs) which include those who are both poor decoders and comprehenders (see Figure 1).

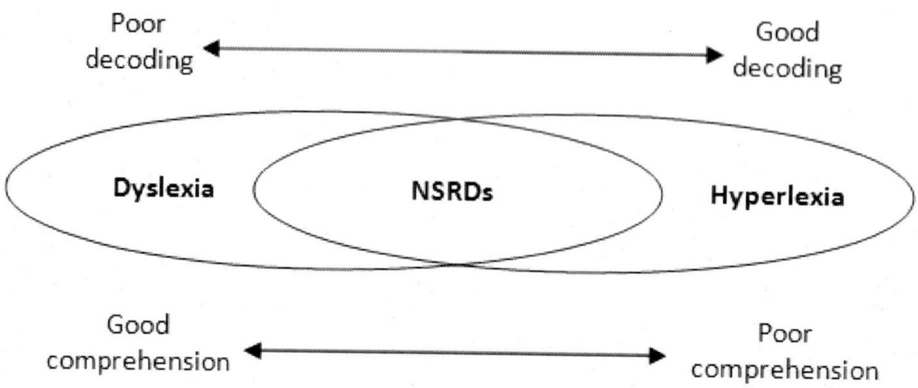

Figure 1. Bipolarity of reading disabilities (Chia, Poh, and Ng, 2009).

Nonetheless, there are details in the cognitive analysis of reading comprehension that have made dyslexia seem far more complex than the simplified assumption of poor decoding ability. This can be seen in the model of reading comprehension by Pennington, Peterson and McGrath (2009) as shown in Figure 2 that highlights how deficits in phonological memory could affect reading comprehension.

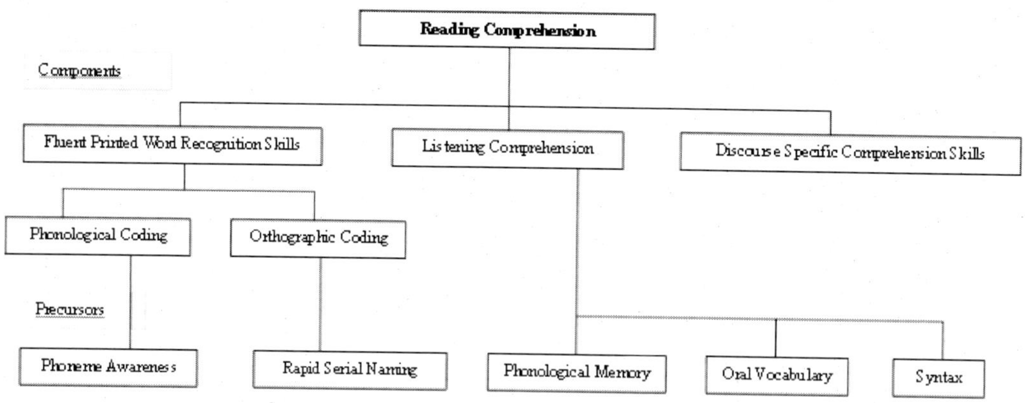

Figure 2. Reading comprehension: Cognitive components and their precursors (adapted from Pennington, Peterson, and McGrath, 2009).

Pennington, Peterson and McGrath (2009) have also noted that dyslexia is one of the three types of abnormal language development sharing the common risk factors etiologically, and hence, co-morbidities occur. The other two types are speech sound disorder that impairs the development of speech production, and language impairment that affects the expression and/or comprehension of spoken language.

According to Figure 2, there are two levels of components that make up reading comprehension. To begin, there are three cognitive components needed for reading comprehension: (1) fluent printed word recognition skills, (2) listening comprehension, and (3) discourse specific comprehension skills. Printed word recognition skills can be divided into two sub-components: (1) phonological coding and (2) orthographic coding. The former refers to the use of letter-sound correspondences to decipher the pronunciation of words that are new to the reader, while the latter refers to the use of word-specific patterns to recognize new words and their pronunciation. As dyslexia is found to be characterized by both phonological and orthographic types of deficits, it can be diagnosed by identifying deficits in accuracy and speed of printed word recognition and decoding.

Currently, the best approach to treat dyslexia is the systematic phonics instruction, which the National Reading Panel (2000) has found to produce significant benefits for students with learning difficulties, disabled readers, as well as low-achieving students without disabilities, and concluded that "systematic phonics instruction provides beginning readers, at-risk readers, disabled readers, and low-achieving readers with a substantial edge in learning to read over alternative forms of instruction not focusing at all or only incidentally on the alphabetic system" (p. 137).

Since spoken language precedes reading in development, a deeper probe can be made in terms of phonemic awareness and rapid serial naming of letters and/or numbers or a mix of both letters and numbers (e.g., the Letter-Number Sequencing subtest in the Wechsler Intelligence Scale for Children-Fourth Edition). On the one hand, phonemic awareness refers to the ability of the child to operationalize the structure of a word according to its sound. For example, "mat" without the "m" would give the sound "at." Rapid serial naming, on the other hand, is a processing speed measure. Broader spoken language skills such as phonological memory, oral vocabulary, and syntax are precursors of listening comprehension skills. We can thus draw the implication that the three cognitive components, i.e., fluent printed word recognition skills, listening comprehension, and discourse specific comprehension skills, are needed for reading comprehension and all their precursors are the key areas that should be targeted for early intervention.

According to Rief and Stern (2010), among the LDs, reading disorders are the most common and dyslexia largely accounts for reading disorders. The U.S. Department of Education (2004) has provided the different disability categories and it has been found that students with LD topped the percentage of total number of students receiving special education services at 47.2% (Pierangelo and Giuliani, 2007). The speech and language impairments, which can co-exist with dyslexia, ranked the next highest at 18.8%. Locally, the Dyslexia Association of Singapore (2009) estimates that about 3-10% of the population in Singapore has dyslexia, and about 20,000 of them are in the primary and secondary schools, making an average of 1 to 2 students with dyslexia in a class of 40.

EFFECTS OF DYSLEXIA ON PSYCHOSOCIAL-EMOTIONAL FUNCTIONING

Peck's (1982) report on the U.S. findings from a suicide prevention center have shown that half of the age 10 to 14 years old victims of suicide and attempted suicide had the diagnosis of being hyperactive, perceptually impaired, or dyslexic. Compiling from sources such as the Washington Literacy Council and National Institute for Literacy, Vinson (2012) provided a profile of the functionally illiterate, i.e., those who are unable to read well enough to complete a job application or understand directions and news reports. They make up 85% of juvenile offenders, high school dropouts as well as unwed mothers; and 68% to 75% of prisoners in state and federal systems, welfare recipients and those arrested. On the impact of academic underachievement, 66% of students who are not proficient readers by fourth grade will end up on welfare or in jail; 90% of welfare recipients are high school dropouts. All in all, a total of 32 million adults in the U.S. have been found to lack basic prose literacy skills. On the basis of these reports, it is crucial for psychosocial-emotional intervention to take place early for children with dyslexia and help them adapt in society. Only then can problems be nipped in the bud, or, at least, reduced in magnitude when these children grow up.

With inclusion becoming increasingly pervasive in many countries, it is also important for educators and counselors to understand the interaction between psychosocial-emotional concerns and learning disabilities and the impact of that interaction on children's psychosocial-emotional functioning in the inclusive school context. According to Abrams (1986), "[T]he vast majority of children with learning disabilities have some emotional problem associated with the learning difficulty" (p. 190) and that "[C]onstant failure and frustration may lead to strong feelings of inferiority, which in turn, may intensify the initial learning deficiency" (p. 189). Hiebert, Wong and Hunter (1982) found that students with learning disabilities, as early as in Grade 3, displayed negative academic self-concepts. It is paramount for educators to meet the psychological and emotional needs of children with dyslexia. Sabornie (1994) has stated, in no uncertain terms, that "[E]ducators' lack of concern for social-affective problems among pupils is analogous to educational neglect" (p. 268).

Research studies (e.g., Humphrey and Mullins, 2002; Riddick, 1995, 1996) have indicated that the experience of dyslexia could have a negative impact on learners' self-concept because learners with dyslexia often manifest lower levels of self-esteem. Manzo and Manzo (1993) described "deep emotional conflicts or fears that otherwise would give rise to considerable anxiety are disowned or put aside by converting them into an external expression of some type that results in a feeling of detachment, which seems to be relaxed indifference or *la belle* indifference as it sometimes is called in psychiatric literature" (p. 409). This behavioral or attitudinal problem has been termed as Conversion Reaction Syndrome and has been found in some individuals with dyslexia as well as others with specific neurological impairment. Denckla (1972) described such individuals as sweet, sloppy and silly. Lyon and Watson (1981) as well as Satz and Morris (1981) have identified such individuals as having related motivational and emotional challenges.

Perhaps the Whole Language Approach (Pearson, 2000; Westwood, 1999, 2004), which has been a predominant approach for early literacy teaching and learning in English-speaking countries, can offer educators a plausible solution to help unmotivated children with dyslexia develop a positive attitude towards reading. The Whole Language Approach advocates a literacy-rich environment to combine speaking, listening, reading, and writing, and emphasizes the meaning of texts over the sounds of letters. Readers have to interpret the meaning of a text and construct a personal meaning using their prior knowledge. Moreover, the approach encourages a love for reading and children's literature through guided reading and reading aloud activities. It "reflects a constructivist philosophy of learning in which children are viewed as inherently active, self-regulating learners who construct knowledge for themselves, with little or no explicit decoding instruction" (National Inquiry into the Teaching of Literacy, 2005, p. 12).

In addition to the motivational and emotional challenges displayed by students with dyslexia, research studies (e.g., Edwards, 1994; Humphrey, 2001, 2002, 2003; Riddick, 1995; 1996) have found that many of these students also experience teasing and bullying and feelings of exclusion by their peers. According to Humphrey (2001), peer bullying has a negative impact on self-esteem. In a study done on middle school students with and without learning disabilities, Sabornie (1994) found that students with learning disabilities felt more lonely, integrated less well in school, were stigmatized by the LD label, and were victimized (e.g., physically assaulted, had their possessions removed) compared to those without disabilities. The participants in Glazzard's (2010) study, too, talked about the need for schools to address all forms of bullying seriously.

However, the findings in Glazzard's (2010) and Riddick's (1995) studies suggested that the diagnosis of dyslexia and the ownership of the LD label might have a positive impact on these students' self-esteem. The participating students in Glazzard's (2010) study identified the official diagnosis of dyslexia as the turning point when they realized they had a genuine specific difficulty rather than a general learning difficulty and, as a result, their self-esteem was boosted. Still many educators, counselors and parents are skeptical of these findings and more studies are required to validate Glazzard's (2010) and Riddick's (1995) findings.

Another study done by Riddick (1996) found that a lot of research into self-esteem has focused on children with reading disabilities (including dyslexia) or learning difficulties in general. Prater (2003), in researching the portrayal of characters with learning disabilities in storybooks, found that 72.2% of the characters had a reading disability too. Humphrey (2002) expressed the view that children with dyslexia in mainstream schools had lower levels of self-esteem related to reading ability than their peers without dyslexia or those with dyslexia in special units. Humphrey and Mullins (2002) argued that children with dyslexia associate strongly reading ability and intelligence as they perceive themselves as lacking in intelligence because they struggle with reading.

Value of Children's Literature in Meeting Psychosocial-Emotional Needs

LD can lead to children experiencing greater anxiety. For example, Margalit and Zak (1984) found that children with LD tended to feel more often that events beyond their control were happening to them while Margalit and Raviv (1984) found that they had more frequent somatic complaints. Chandler (1994) suggested that for some children, "school achievement has become equated with self-competency, and the loss of competence has led to feelings of inadequacy, depression, withdrawal and an uncaring attitude [while]… poor school performance [leads] to dependency and learned helplessness as a maladaptive style of coping" (p. 163). High levels of anxiety and stress have been identified as the most indicative behavioral correlates of dyslexia and a 'panic' reaction is experienced by some people with dyslexia when placed in situations where they cannot cope (Lucid Research Limited, 2006).

One way to address the anxiety and stress experienced by children with dyslexia is through using children's literature, which can help them cope with a wide range of emotions such as trauma in life, loss, inadequacy, teach and encourage resilience and give them the opportunity to see that though others struggle with similar issues, still they can attain academic success eventually. Children can "learn from literature how other people handle their problems, characters [protagonists] in books can help children deal with similar problems, as well as understand other people's feelings" (Norton and Norton, 2011, p. 3).

Children's literature enables readers to better understand the human experience of self and others vicariously by engaging its readers in the lives, values, and struggles of protagonists who are very different or very similar to themselves (Rosenblatt, 1983). The vicarious experiences of children's literature lead to personal development as well as pleasure (Norton and Norton, 2011).

Children's literature can help to develop emotional intelligence and Golman (1995) has identified five basic elements of emotional intelligence that children need: (1) self-awareness, (2) managing emotions, (3) handling anxiety in appropriate ways, (4) motivating oneself, and (5) sensitivity toward others. Researchers (e.g., Andrews, 1998; Biaska and Lynch, 1998; Dobo, 1982; Favazza and Odom, 1997) have suggested using fictional books that include characters with disabilities to teach children about disabilities, encourage a healthy attitude toward people with disabilities, and create an awareness or understanding of a given disability for students without disabilities. According to Altieri (2008), "literature can help all children understand how much they have in common with students with disabilities and can help with uneasiness caused by ignorance" (p. 48). In fact, the study done by Altieri (2008) specifically looked at contemporary, realistic fiction books or children's literature (published in the United States between 1993 and 2003), which could take place in today's world, portraying school-age protagonists with dyslexia so that the educational field can better understand how the storybooks describe dyslexia and the school experience through looking at how the dyslexia was depicted and understood, instructional methodology implemented, characteristics related to the self-concept of the character with dyslexia, and the portrayal of the protagonist's teachers.

Many of the characters with dyslexia described in storybooks displayed low self-esteem in 70 per cent out of 72 storybooks reviewed by Altieri (2008) that have included demeaning comments about the abilities of students with dyslexia.

Here are some examples of storybooks written about protagonists with dyslexia. For example, the protagonist in *The Wrong Side of the Pattern* (Litchman, 1997) expresses feelings of poor self-esteem when she calls herself "baby" and "stupid."

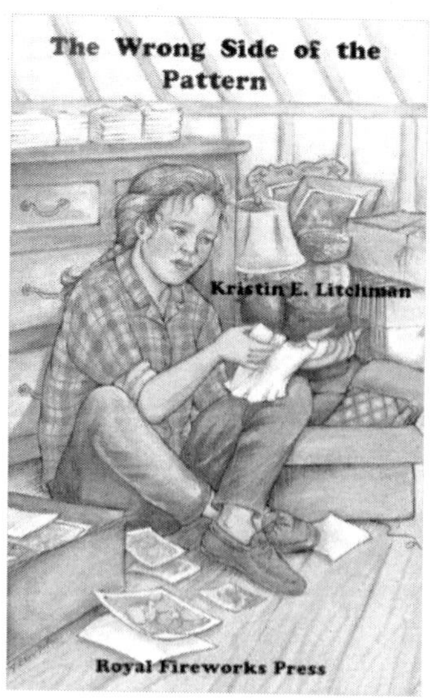

In another example, in *Sarey by Lantern Light* (Beckhorn, 2003), the protagonist Sarey constantly worries about whether people at school would ever pick her as a partner because she has dyslexia. In a third example, the protagonist Buddy in *Dolphin Sky* (Rorby, 1996) talks about how the children pick on her because she cannot read properly and gets directions reversed. In another interesting storybook, *How Dyslexic Benny Became a Star: A Story of Hope for Dyslexic Children and Their Parents* (Griffith, 1998), the author describes how the protagonist as a loner copes with dyslexia.

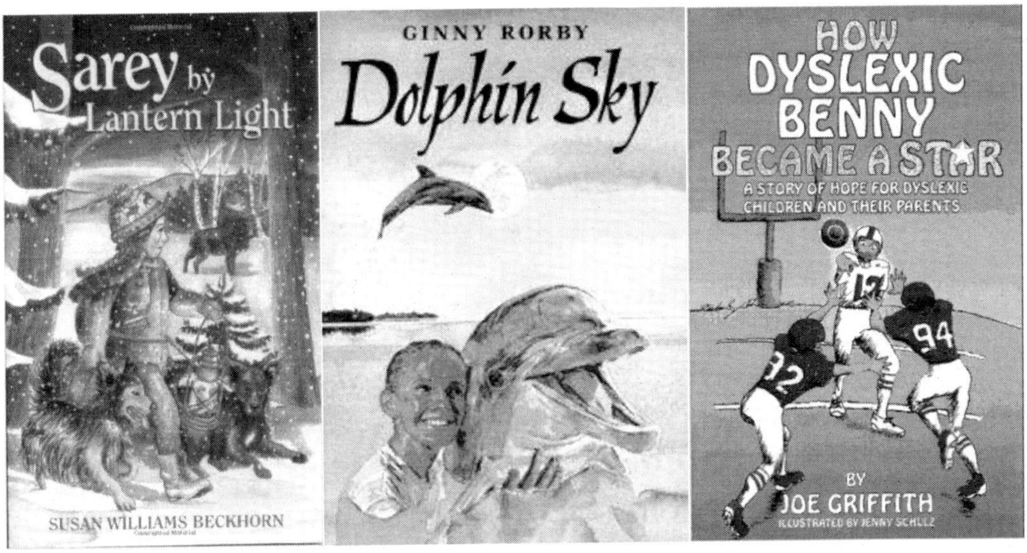

VALUE OF CHILDREN'S LITERATURE IN READING DEVELOPMENT

Children's literature may be defined as those storybooks specifically written for children to be read as literature and to give children spontaneous pleasure, and not merely to instruct them (Darton, 1982; Egoff, 1981). Morrow (1992) found that children, who are exposed to literature at a younger age, tend to develop sophisticated language structures, vocabulary and syntax. Through children's literature, children gain knowledge and discover how language works in terms of how written language differs from spoken language.

According to Olen (1990), storybooks used in reading aloud to children help to stimulate "children's interest, emotional development, imagination, develops the children's vocabulary and makes them more sensitive to language" (p. 382). Storybooks with repetitive language are excellent for enticing listeners to join in during oral reading. If the authors of these storybooks use well-formed, relatively short sentences rich in varied vocabulary, such books can offer children the opportunity to hear new vocabulary items embedded in varied grammatical sentences and children will learn how words are used in various ways (Dickinson, Griffith, Golinkoff, and Hirsh-Pasek, 2012).

Reading storybooks helps children learn language because it requires the participants to be active and engage in responsive interactions about word meanings. This is especially so through dialogic reading which encourages interactions about stories read. Dialogic reading occurs when adults and children engage in conversations about the books read (Arnold, Lonigan, Whitehurst, and Epstein, 1994; Valdez-Menchaca and Whitehurst, 1992) with the adults taking on the role of providing feedback, prompting children to voice their thoughts, feelings and opinions through questions and engaging in discussions about the book read (Whitehurst et. al, 1994). When educators and children engage in dialogic reading around a book, they are engaging in a language-based activity involving varied vocabulary and diverse sentences structures (Dickinson, Griffith, Golinkoff, and Hirsh-Pasek, 2012).

In schools, adequate academic as well as psychosocial-emotional support for children with dyslexia can create a brighter and better future for them. However, there are many different facets to this disability such that both educators and parents cannot assume that the needs of one child with dyslexia are the same as another. To address these differing needs, suggestions are offered in terms of looking at selection criteria for non-fiction books that can get these children excited and capture their interest to start reading something first. Similarly, there are also suggestions on how to select appropriate fiction books that portray protagonists with special needs (including dyslexia) to meet the psychosocial-emotional needs of readers with dyslexia.

Meeting Psychosocial-Emotional Needs of Children with Dyslexia Through Children's Literature

To meet the psychosocial-emotional needs, educators should consider several key factors when selecting contemporary realistic fiction books that portray characters (preferably protagonists) with dyslexia. When educators and parents review storybooks, they need to assess if these books positively and accurately portray individuals with dyslexia. Next, they must determine if the positive qualities of these books outweigh the negative characteristics. Here is the list of guidelines specifically prepared for selecting storybooks for readers with dyslexia, modified from the list provided by Altieri (2008):

- What is the portrayal of other characters (including the protagonists) in the storybook? According to Altieri (2008), other characters should show respect and support for the character with dyslexia. This is because when "the protagonist experiencing the reading difficulty is a child or adolescent, the portrayal of the family may also play a pivotal role in the story" (p. 53) since family support is essential for adolescents or children experiencing dyslexia McNulty (2003).
- How do other characters go about helping the protagonist with the reading difficulty? Because children do not learn the same way, educators need to use more than one particular method of teaching as well as offer high-quality teaching (Altieri, 2008). Educators need to keep in mind affective factors and ensure an environment that builds self-esteem and encourages the learner (Jordan, 1996) as well as promotes talents and interest in learning (Pierson, 1999).
- Is the problem with reading solved with a simple, quick solution or does the storybook present the problem as a challenge that the protagonist must continue to address? There is no quick-fix approach to solve issues resulting from the dyslexic

condition. However, appropriate methods can reduce the psychosocial-emotional problems. Still, a student with dyslexia must learn to cope with the chronic condition for lifetime (Clark and Uhry, 1995; Jordan, 1996).

- What terms does the author use in talking about dyslexia? According to McNulty (2003), people in the stories should encourage characters with dyslexia and should not label them as lazy, mentally retarded, or stupid. Altieri (2008) emphasizes that "blame and labels do not have a place when discussing children with dyslexia or any learning disability" (p. 53) and that educators should highly encourage "people first" language (Andrews, 1998), which requires a focus on the person first and the label second. Therefore, "instead of using the phrase *dyslexic child,* the author should say the *child with dyslexia*" (Altieri, 2008, p. 53).

In engaging children with dyslexia in the reading process, educators should not underestimate the power of discussion and reflection in reading. With discussion and reflection, even books that educators might have reservations selecting can find a place in the curriculum or at home because they provide teachable moments while adults help the students navigate the books and think about what they are reading. When Salende and Moe (1983) studied fourth, fifth, and sixth graders, they concluded that literature can be highly successful in enabling a positive attitude change toward disabled individuals provided that in using books that feature characters with disabilities, there are follow-up discussions or activities to create the positive attitude. Hiebert, Wong and Hunter (1982) have also suggested that teachers should systematically build "'positive affect and hopeful expectation, utilizing self-instruction or some other procedure for promoting positive affect" (p. 342) through asking children to visualize a pleasant experience or situation before they begin reading.

In terms of types of children's literature to be selected, educators, parents and caregivers can use books that explain dyslexia to help the children understand their specific disability and how to overcome challenges in learning or social integration. For instance, in the illustrated picture storybook *It's Called Dyslexia* (Moore-Mallinos, 2007) told from a child's point of view, the protagonist in the story knows the alphabet, but she often mixes up the letters or writes them backwards. The teacher explains that she has dyslexia, and that she can be helped to read and write correctly so she should never give up. There is also a parent's section at the back of the book. In *My Name is Brain Brian* (Betancourt, 1992), children at Brian's school make fun of him because of his numerous mistakes when reading aloud and while writing on the board. However, a caring teacher recognizes the symptoms of dyslexia and sets out to get Brian the help he needs. Brian is initially embarrassed but after listening to the teacher's explanation, he understands that he needs the extra help simply because his brain learns differently and he is actually smart. *So You Think You've Got Problems* (Birkett, 1993) is an easy-to-read book for children with dyslexia of all ages. It explains, simply and sympathetically, what is dyslexia and how children with dyslexia can overcome their problems through help as well as how they are not alone and that there are others experiencing the same difficulties.

According to Norton and Norton (2011), children with dyslexia should be offered vicarious experiences through children's literature so that they can learn how to handle their problems from characters in storybooks dealing with similar problems. At the same time, children without dyslexia can also read and learn about the feelings of these characters with dyslexia and how they struggle to cope with their daily challenges. In this way, both children with and without dyslexia can share and appreciate the various life challenges faced by the characters with dyslexia in these storybooks and understand how they go about coping with their daily struggles while still deriving pleasure from reading (Norton and Norton, 2011).

For example, in *Whispers in the Graveyard* by (Breslin, 1994), Solomon is a boy with dyslexia who likes to hide from his home and school problems in the local graveyard. He finds the inner strength to face his problems and overcome an ancient and evil power released when workmen start to disturb the graves. In another example, the protagonist Sam in the comic-book *Moving the Goalposts* (Childs, 1998) is the star goalkeeper who has dyslexia. The book portrays Sam's literacy difficulties in an authentic manner in narrating how Sam overcomes his learning problem when he has to write and read out a match report during the school assembly. In a third example, the main character with dyslexia in *How to Write Really Badly* (Fine, 1996) has an extraordinary talent for model making and is an unexpected source of support for the know-it-all narrator of the story, Chester, who at first is scornful of Joe. Finally, in the fourth example, Frankie Ruggles DBNS (Dyslexic but not Stupid), who is the protagonist in *Ghost Writer* (Jarman, 2008), becomes involved in trying to help a boy from 100 years before who may have been dyslexic too.

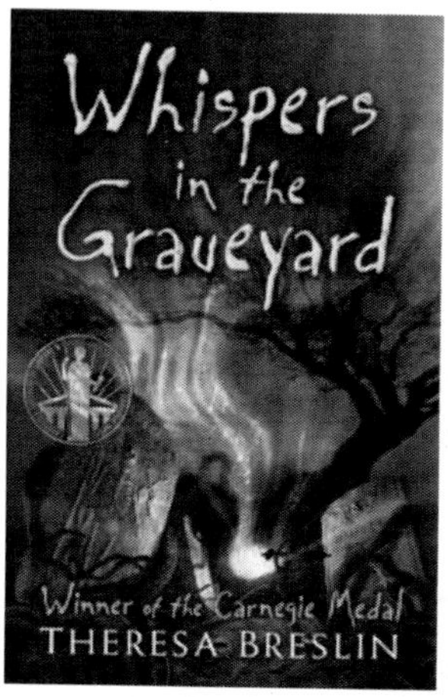

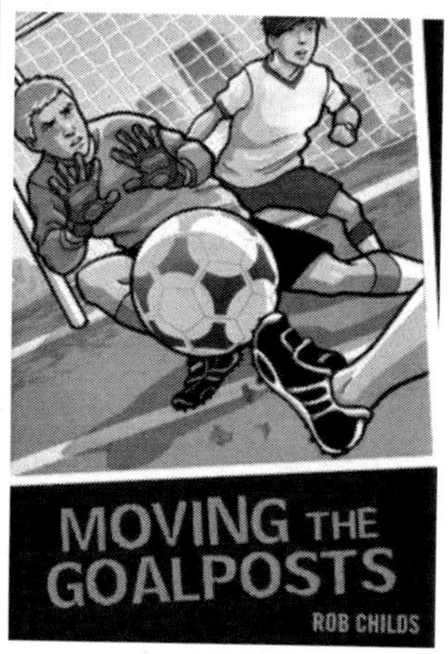

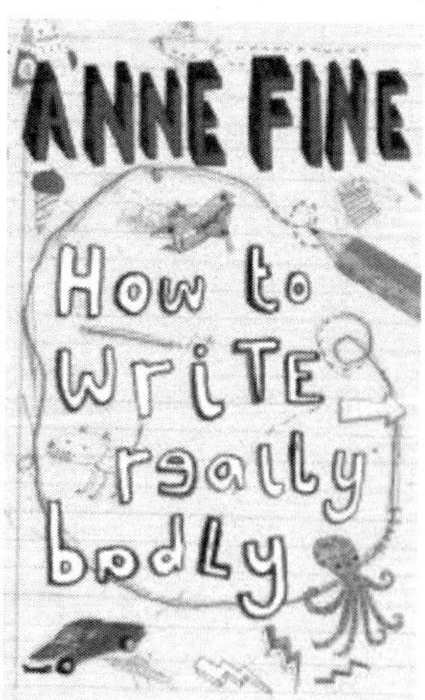

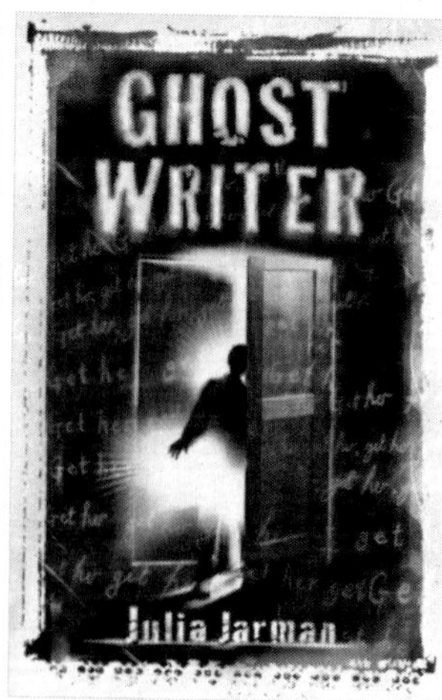

CONCLUSION

In the regular classroom lesson, children's literature offers a good teaching resource for educators, especially when it is used in reading classes. In this chapter we have traced the reading and social-emotional difficulties faced by children with dyslexia, and highlighted the value of children's literature in teaching language skills to children with dyslexia. We have also shown how children's literature can be employed as an effective tool to address affective needs where selected reading materials are used as therapeutic adjutants to help students with dyslexia to understand their psychosocial-emotional problems by learning how the characters (preferably protagonists) with dyslexia in storybooks are coping with their daily life struggles.

We have also looked at selection criteria in terms of how in selecting appropriate storybooks from a wide range offered by children's literature to be used with readers with dyslexia, three considerations must be noted: (1) the storybooks must be specifically dyslexia-friendly; (2) they must feature characters with dyslexia or those who struggle with reading; and (3) they must have a high interest level and low reading age.

REFERENCES

Aaron, P. G. (1989). *Dyslexia and hyperlexia: Diagnosis and management of developmental reading disabilities*. NY: Kluwer Academic/Plenum Publishers.

Abrams, J. C. (1986). On learning disabilities: Affective considerations. *Journal of Reading, Writing, and Learning Disabilities*, 2, 189-196.

Altieri, J. L. (2008). Fictional characters with dyslexia: What are we seeing in books? *Teaching Exceptional Children*, 41(1), 48-54.

Andrews, S. E. (1998). Using inclusive literature to promote positive attitudes toward disabilities. *Journal of Adolescent and Multi-Literacy*, 41, 420-426.

Arnold, D. H., Lonigan, C. J., Whitehurst, G. J., and Epstein, J. N. (1994). Accelerating language development through picture book reading: replication and extension to a videotape training format. *Journal of Educational Psychology*, 86(2), 235-243.

Beckhorn. S. W. (2003). *Sarey by lantern light*. Camden, ME: Down East Books.

Betancourl. J. (1993). *My name is Brain Brian*. NY: Scholastic.

Biaska, J. K., and Lynch, E. C. (1998). Is everyone included: Using children's literature to facilitate the understanding of disabilities. *Young Children*, 53(2), 36-39.

Birkett, R. (1993). *So, you think you've got problems?* UK: Egon Publishers.

Breslin, T. (1994). *Whispers in the graveyard*. London, UK: Methuen Young Books.

Chandler, L. A. (1994). Emotional aspects of learning problems: Implications for assessment. *Special Services in the Schools*, 8(2), 161-165.

Chia, N. K. H. (2015). *Difficulties in word recognition and reading: Dyslexia/specific learning disability*. In Ng, C. H. (Co-Ed.), Series on learning difficulties in school-aged children (Paper No. 1) (pp. 1-49). Singapore: Pearson Education/Prentice-Hall.

Chia, N. K. H., Poh, P. T. C., and Ng, A. G. T. (2009). Identifying and differentiating children with hyperlexia and its subtypes: A meta-analysis of results from WISC-III subtests and standardized reading tests. *Journal of the American Academy of Special Education Professionals*, 1, 71-99.

Childs, R. (2010). *Moving the goalpost*. London, UK: A and C Black Publishers Ltd.

Clark, D., and Uhry, J. (1995). *Dyslexia: Theory and practice of remedial instruction.* Baltimore: York.

Dagan, D., Burke, C. K., Davies, J., and Chinn, D. (2015). *Learning disabilities: Positive practice guide*. London, UK: Foundation for People with Learning Disabilities.

Darton, F. J. H. (1982). *Children's books in England: Five centuries of social life*. 3rd ed. London: Cambridge University Press.

Denckla, M. B. (1972). Clinical syndromes in learning disabilities: the case for "splitting' versus 'lumping." *Journal of Learning Disabilities*, 5, 400-406.

Dickinson, D. K., Griffith, J. A., Golinkoff, R. M., and Hirsh-Pasek, K. (2012). How reading books fosters language development around the world. *Child Development Research.* Retrieved on 1 December 2015 from http://www.hindawi.com/journals/cdr/2012/602807/.

Dobo, P. J. (1982).Using literature to change attitudes toward the handicapped. *The Reading Teacher*, 36, 290-292.

Dyslexia Association of Singapore. (2009). *About dyslexia.* Retrieved from http://www.das.org.sg/dyslexia-myths.html

Edwards, J. (1994). *The scars of dyslexia: Eight case studies in emotional reactions.* London, UK: Cassell.

Egoff, S. A. (1981). *Trends and patterns in contemporary children's literature*. Chicago, IL: American Library Association.

Favazza. P. C., and Odom, S. I. (1997). Promoting positive attitudes of kindergarten age children toward people with disabilities. *Exceptional Children*, 63, 405-418.

Fine, A. (1996). *How to write really badly*. USA: Mammoth

Foundation for People with Learning Disabilities (2001). *What does the term 'learning disability' mean?* Retrieved from http://www. learningdisabilities.org.uk/help-information/about-learning-disabilities/ definition-learning-disability/.

Frith, U. (1986). A developmental framework for developmental dyslexia. *Annals of Dyslexia*, 36, 69-81.

Glazzard, J. (2010). The impact of dyslexia on pupils' self-esteem. *British Journal of Learning Support*, 25(2), 63-69.

Golman, D. (1995). *Emotional intelligence*. NY: Bantam Books.

Gough, P. B., and Tunmer, W. E. (1986). Decoding, reading, and reading disability. *Remedial and Special Education*, 7, 6-10.

Griffith, J. (1998). *How dyslexic Benny became a star: A story of hope for dyslexic children and their parents*. Dallas, TX: Yorktown Press.

Healy, J. M. (1982). The enigma of hyperlexia. *Reading Research Quarterly*, 17, 319-338.

Hiebert, B., Wong, B., and Hunter, M. (1982). Affective influences on learning disabled adolescents. *Learning Disabilities Quarterly*, 5(4), 334-343.

Humphrey, N. (2001). *Self-Concept and self-Esteem in developmental dyslexia: Implications for teaching and learning*. Unpublished PhD thesis, Liverpool John Moores University.

Humphrey, N. (2002). Teacher and pupil ratings of self-esteem in developmental dyslexia. *British Journal of Special Education*, 29(1), 29-36.

Humphrey, N. (2003). Facilitating a positive sense of self in pupils with dyslexia: the role of teachers and peers. *Support for Learning*, 18(3), 130-136.

Humphrey, N., and Mullins, P. (2002) Personal constructs and attribution for academic success and failure in dyslexia. *British Journal of Special Education,* 29(4), 196-203.

Jarman, J. (2008). *Ghost writer*. London, UK: Andersen Press.

Jordan, D. (1996). *Overcoming dyslexia in children, adolescents, and adults*. Austin, TX: Pro-Ed.

Litchman. K, (1997). *The wrong side of the pattern*. Unionville, NY: Royal Fireworks Press.

Lucid Research Ltd (2006). *Undesrstanding dyslexia: Introductory notes. Fact Sheet 13.* Lucid Research Ltd. Retrieved from: www.Lucid-Research.com.

Lyon, R., and Watson, B. (1981). Empirical derived subgroups of learning disabled readers: Diagnostic characteristics. *Journal of Learning Disabilities,* 14, 256-261.

Manzo, A. V., and Manzo, U. C. (1993). *Literacy disorders: Holistic diagnosis and remediation*. Orlando, FL: Holt, Rinehart and Winston.

Margalit, M., and Raviv, A. (1984). LDs' expressions of anxiety in terms of minor somatic complaints. *Journal of Learning Disabilities*, 17, 226-228.

Margalit, M., and Zak, 1. (1984). Anxiety and self-concept of learning disabled children. *Journal of Learning Disabilities*, 17, 537-539.

McNulty, M. A. (2003). Dyslexia and the life course. *Journal of Learning Disabilities,* 36, 363-381.

Moore-Mallinos, J. (2007). *It's called dyslexia* (Live and Learn Series). Dublin, Ireland: O-Brien Press.

Morrow, M. (1992). The impact of a literature-based program on literacy achievement, use of literature and attitudes of children from minority backgrounds. *Reading Research Quarterly*, 27(3), 255-274.

National Inquiry into the Teaching of Literacy (2005). *Teaching reading*. Canberra, Australia: Commonwealth of Australia.

National Reading Panel (2000). *Teaching children to read: An evidence-based assessment of the scientific research literature on reading and its implications for reading instruction: Reports of the subgroups.* Washington, DC: National Institute of Child Health and Development.

Ng, P. M. H. (2013). A brief updated examination on the enigma of hyperlexia. *The Journal of Reading and Literacy*, 5, 39-50.

Ng, P. M. H., and Chia, N. K. H. (2013). *Teaching reading comprehension to children with hyperlexia* (With 40 passages ready for use). Singapore: Pearson.

Norton, D. E., and Norton, S. E. (2011). *Through the eyes of a child: An introduction to children's literature.* (8th edition). Boston: Pearson.

Olen, S. I. I. (1990). Promoting reading aloud to the parents and other child-minders of pre-school children. *South African journal of library and information science*, 58(4), 382-387.

Orton, S. T. (1925). 'Word-blindness' in school children. *Archives of Neurology and Psychiatry*, 14, 581-615.

Orton, S. T. (1928). Specific reading disability – strephosymbolia. *Journal of the American Medical Association*, 90, 1095-1099.

Pearson, P. D. (2000). Reading in the 20th century. In T. Good (Ed.), *American education: Yesterday, today and tomorrow*. Yearbook of the National Society for the Study of Education (pp. 152-208). Chicago, IL: University of Chicago Press.

Peck, M. (1982). Youth suicide. *Death Education*, 6(1), 29-47.

Pennington, B. F., Peterson, R. L., and Mcgrath, L. M. (2009). Dyslexia. In B. F. Pennington (Ed.), *Diagnosing learning disorders: A neuropsychological framework* (2nd ed., pp. 45-82). NY: The Guilford Press.

Pierangelo, R., and Giuliani, G. (2007). *The educator's diagnostic manual of disabilities and disorders*. San Francisco, CA: Jossey-Bass.

Pierson, J. M. (1999). Transforming engagement in literacy instruction: The role of student genuine interest. *Annals of Dyslexia*, 49, 307-329.

Prater. M. A. (2003). Learning disabilities in children's and adolescent literature: How are characters portrayed? *Learning Disability Quarterly*, 26, 47-62.

Morgan, W. P. (1896). A case of congenital word-blindness (inability to learn to read). *British Medical Journal*, ii, 1543-1544.

Riddick, B. (1995). Dyslexia: dispelling the myths. *Disability and Society*, 10(4), 457-473.

Riddick, B. (1996). *Living with dyslexia*. London, UK: Routledge.

Rief, S. F., and Stern, J. M. (2010). *The dyslexia checklist: A practical reference for parents and teachers* (1st Ed.). San Francisco, CA: Jossey-Bass.

Rorby. G. (1996). *Dolphin sky*. NY: G. P. Putnam's Sons.

Rosenblatt, L. M. (1983). The reading transaction: What for? In R. Parker and F. Davis (Eds.), *Developing literacy: Children's use of language* (pp. 118-135). Newark, DE: International Reading Association.

Sabornie, E. J. (1994). Social-affective characteristics in early adolescents identified as learning disabled and nondisabled. *Learning Disability Quarterly*, 17(4), 268-279.

Salende, S. J., and Moe, L. (1983). Modifying non handicapped students' attitudes toward their handicapped peers through children's literature. *Journal for Special Education*, 19, 22-27.

Satz, P., and Morris, R. (1981). Learning disability subtypes: A review. In E. Pirozzolo and M. Wittrock (Eds.), *Neuropsychological and cognitive processes in reading* (pp. 109-141). NY: Academic Press.

Tannock, R. (2014). *DSM-5 changes in diagnostic criteria for specific learning disabilities: What are the implications?* Retrieved from: http:// dyslexiahelp.umich.edu/sites/default/ files/IDA_DSM-5%20Changes.pdf/.

Torgesen, J. K. (1999). Assessment and instruction for phonemic awareness and word recognition skills. In H. Catts and A. G. Kamhi (Eds.), *Language and reading disabilities* (pp. 133-135). Boston, MA: Allyn and Bacon.

Tyre, C., and Young, P. (1994). *Specific learning difficulties*. Staffordshire, UK: QED.

U.S. Department of Education, (2004). *Individuals with Disabilities Education Act (IDEA) data*. Washington, DC: Author. Retrieved February 1, 2015, from http://wwwIDE Adata.org/PartBdata.asp.

Valdez-Menchaca, M. C., and Whitehurst, G. J. (1992). Accelerating language development through picture book reading: a systematic extension to Mexican day care. *Developmental Psychology*, 28(6), 1106-1114.

Vinson, B. P. (2012). *Preschool and school-age language disorders*. Clifton Park, NY: Cengage Learning.

Westwood, P. (1999). Constructivist approaches to mathematical learning: A note of caution. In D. Barwood, D. Greaves, and P. Jeffrey. *Teaching numeracy and literacy: Interventions and strategies for 'at risk' students*. Victoria, Australia: Australian Resource Educators' Association.

Westwood, P. S. (2004). *Learning and learning difficulties: A handbook for teachers.* Victoria, Australia: Australian Council for Educational Research.

Whitehurst, G. J., Arnold, D. S., Epstein, J. N., Angell, A. L., Smith, M., and Fischel, J. E. (1994). A picture book reading intervention in day care and home for children from low-income families. *Developmental Psychology*, 30(5), 679-689.

In: Dyslexia: Perspectives, Challenges and Treatment Options ISBN: 978-1-63485-328-6
Editor: Marilyn Frazier

Chapter 11

DIAGNOSTIC INTERVENTIONS BY OPERATIONALIZING THE DEFINITION OF DYSLEXIA

Noel Kok Hwee Chia
National Institute of Education,
Nanyang Technological University, Singapore

ABSTRACT

Throughout the historical development in dyslexia research since 1676, many terms have been used to describe this specific learning disability and research has always been rather unclear and inconsistent. In its broadest sense, dyslexia can refer to the reading problems that theoretically include from straining the eyes to read under inadequate light to specific cerebral defects or minimal brain damage associated with the inability to interpret visual symbols. The definition of dyslexia continues to be a controversial subject for academic discourse with so many contradictory empirical findings in the literature due to many factors that interfere with the development of language and literacy skills. There obviously are many possible causes of dyslexia and its various subtypes. Without an agreed-on definition of dyslexia, it is challenging to come up with best interventions for this specific reading disability. Since there is no one best intervention strategy, professionals working in the field of dyslexia have to be trained in many different approaches just to treat different aspects of the disability. Often whatever little success achieved in the intervention may be more of a Pyrrhic victory, resulting in many other socio-emotional challenges such as stress, resistance to reading, lack of interest and low motivation. One possible way to circumvent this problem is to operationalize the current acceptable definition of dyslexia in order to better understand the disability and plan appropriate interventions targeting at its various symptoms.

Keywords: diagnosis, dyslexia, intervention, operating definition, symptoms

INTRODUCTION

The first form of specific learning difficulty to be described in medical research literature was probably reading difficulty, which grew out of several clinical cases done by physicians and psychologists interested in brain functions and in the effects of brain injury on cognitive abilities, in both children and adults, in the late 19th century.

Long before the formal establishment of dyslexia as a field of educational practice in the 1960s, the medical paradigm took an intrinsic theoretical perspective of learning difficulties, disabilities and/or disorders (Spear-Swerling and Sternberg, 1998). Although all the three terms – difficulties, disabilities and disorders in learning – seem to be similar, they actually are not and, strictly speaking, should not be used interchangeably. Difficulty, when it is used, concerns a specific learning problem (e.g., sounding a voiced *th* and a voiceless *th*, spelling words that end with *–ch* or *–tch*, and counting 1 to 20 in ascending or descending order); disability refers to an inability to perform certain tasks that end up affecting a part of or the rest of the learning process (e.g., word recognition and decoding in the reading process, or spelling and transcription in the writing process) as a result of developmental delay or immaturity; and disorder refers to some form of "a neurological impairment or of an acquired causation" (Chia, 2012, p. 80).

However, in Australia, the National Health and Medical Research Council (NHMRC, 1990) defined and differentiated between the two terms: learning difficulties and learning disabilities. The former is used as a generic term referring to the substantial 10 to 16 per cent of the Australian population of children and adolescents with problems in developmental and academic skills that may be resulted from "intellectual disability, physical and sensory defects, emotional difficulties, inadequate environmental experiences, lack of appropriate educational opportunities" (NHMRC, 1990, p. 2). The latter refers to the much smaller proportion of two to four per cent of the Australian population of children and adolescents with developmental and academic skills that are significantly below expectation for their age and general ability. They included "severe and prolonged directional confusion, sequencing and short-term retention difficulties … but are not considered to be the direct result of intellectual disability, physical and sensory defects or emotional difficulties (NHMRC, 1990, p. 2). The Foundation for People with Learning Disabilities (FPLD), UK, has also differentiated between learning difficulty (LD) and learning disability (LD): the former "is a condition that makes specific areas of learning difficult, but does not affect the overall intelligence of an individual" (Dagan, Burke, Davies, and Chinn, 2015, p. 11), while the latter "is a condition that affects learning and intelligence across all areas of life" (Dagan, Burke, Davies, and Chinn, 2015, p. 11).

Unlike NHMRC and FPLD, the National Joint Committee on Learning Disabilities (NJCLD, 1994), founded in 1975 and is based in the United States, did not differentiate among the three terms (i.e., difficulties, disabilities and disorders) but used all the three terms interchangeably as follows:

> "a heterogeneous group of *disorders* manifested by significant *difficulties* in the acquisition and use of listening, speaking, reading, writing, reasoning, or mathematical abilities. These *disorders* are intrinsic to the individual and presumed to be due to central nervous system dysfunction. Problems in self-regulatory behaviors, social perception, and social interaction may exist with learning *disabilities* but do not by themselves constitute

a learning *disability*. Even though a learning *disability* may occur concomitantly with other handicapping conditions or environmental influences, it is not the result of those conditions or influences" (NJCLD, 1994, p. 65-66).

DYSLEXIA RESEARCH: A BRIEF HISTORICAL BACKGROUND

According to Guardiola (2001), the history of dyslexia research has undergone four major stages of development, although they are not clearly differentiated. The first stage, known as the *Origins of Dyslexia*, began around 1676 and lasted until the end of the 19th century, identified the first subjects with reading and language deficits. The second stage, known as the *Study of Developmental Dyslexia*, took place between 1895 and 1950, and it was during this period that the causes and symptoms of dyslexia were carefully studied and analyzed. The third stage, known as the *Evolution of the Concept of Dyslexia*, which occurred between 1950 and 1970, opened the field of dyslexia studies to cover clinical, research, and educational approaches. It was during this third stage that more studies (e.g., Boder, 1976; Mattis, French, and Rapin, 1975; Myklebust and Johnson, 1962) were done to identify the various subtypes of dyslexia. Finally, the fourth stage, known as the *Modern Theories of Dyslexia*, began somewhere around 1970 and continues till today, has led to the establishment of our current knowledge and understanding of dyslexia (see Guardiola, 2001, for detail).

Table 1. Six Phases of Historical Development in Dyslexia Research

Duration (Years)	Four stages of research studies (Guardiola, 2001)	Six phases of dyslexia research
1676-1895	Stage 1: The Origins of Dyslexia	Phase 1: The Enigma of Dyslexia
1895-1899	Stage 2: The Study of Developmental Dyslexia	
1900-1910		Phase 2: Deciphering the Dyslexia Code
1911-1920		
1921-1930		
1931-1940		Phase 3: The Search for an Answer
1941-1950		
1951-1960	Stage 3: The Evolution of the Concept of Dyslexia	
1961-1970		Phase 4: Armada of Terms, Definitions and Theories of Dyslexia
1971-1980	Stage 4: The Modern Theories of Dyslexia	
1981-1990		Phase 5: From Divided Opinions to Consensus
1991-2000		Phase 6: The Operating Definition of Dyslexia
2001-2010		
2011-beyond		

However, in this chapter, unlike Guardiola's (2001) four stages of historical development of dyslexia studies, I have proposed six developmental phases of dyslexia research (see Table

1), beginning from 1676, when the physician John Schmidt described the first account of word blindness, and until the second decade of the 21st century when research in the cognitive neuroscience has shed lights on subtypes of dyslexia in children (see Katzir, Kim, Wolf, Morris, and Lovett, 2008, for detail) as well as linkage analysis and genetic association studies (e.g., Bishop, 2009; Paracchini, Steer, and Buckingham, 2008; Shastry, 2007) have identified genetic markers for dyslexia such as DCDC2 and KIAA0319 on chromosome 6 and DYX1C1 on chromosome 15.

Phase 1 - From 1676-1899: The Enigma of Dyslexia

The genesis of the dyslexia studies began with the first recorded case of the loss of reading ability described as word blindness (or aphasia) in 1676 by the physician, John Schmidt (cited in Elliott and Grigorenko, 2014). In 1825, Professor Lordat of Montpelier, France, described about the temporal loss of his ability to comprehend or make sense of print (cited in Guardiola, 2001). Thirty six years later, Broca (1861) concluded in his study that the left anterior area of the brain was critical for language production. Thirteen years later, a study done by Wernicke (1874) described lesions in the posterior portion of the left temporal lobe of the brain resulting in great difficulty in comprehending speech. The brain research studies by Broca (1861) and Wernicke (1874) have often been regarded as the foundation for dyslexia studies (Lerner, 1993; Smith, 1991; Torgesen, 1991). Their early research interest, using clinical and autopsy studies of adults suffering from strokes and other brain injuries, took an intrinsic perspective focusing on a variety of human abilities (e.g., language or spatial abilities) in relation to specific cortical areas of the brain, and had contributed to a long established line of research in psychology and medicine. During that period, such serious science constituted a substantial improvement over the popularized pseudo-medicine of phrenology that had erroneously believed brain functions could be deduced from the measuring of bumps on a person's head and the shape of a person's skull (Gail, 1835).

In Germany, Kussmaul (1877), a physician, described a man of normal intelligence with adequate education but was unable to learn to read, and he called this problem *reading blindness*. Ten years later, Berlin (1884), another German physician, coined the term *dyslexia* from Greek, which means "difficulty with words," to describe this isolated reading difficulty. Unfortunately, by the 1930s, the word *dyslexia* was widely used in an inconsistent way to refer to many things. For instance, some still refer it to specific reading difficulty alone, while others would combine reading and writing difficulties to mean dyslexia. There are still others who use the term for all types of specific learning difficulty. Today, when dyslexia is used, it is often accompanied by the preceding adjective "developmental" to mean that it is of constitutional origin rather than due to external insults or injuries (Aaron, 1989).

Dejerine (1891, 1892), a French neurologist, provided the most complete accounts of sudden but circumscribed loss of reading ability due to neurological impairment in literate adults, along with his post-mortem findings. His first report (Dejerine, 1891) indicated that the ability to read was located in an area of the left cerebral cortex known as angular gyrus, which together with the adjacent visual cortex, played an important role in the reading and writing processes. Dejerine's (1892) second report extended his definition of reading disability to include the loss of ability to read musical notations.

Hinshelwood (1895), a Scottish eye surgeon, published the first British report describing about a specific reading difficulty in a child and called the condition *word blindness*. Twelve years later, Hinshelwood (1907) wrote that dyslexia "is not due to cerebral disease, nor is there any history of difficulties at birth" (p. 1231) and concluded that the reading deficit was the result of some faulty neurological development.

Another British doctor, Morgan (1896), published his paper on "Congenital Word Blindness" in the British Medical Journal describing a 14-year-old boy called Percy F. with reading disability which he considered its etiology to be congenital and attributed it to defective development of the left angular gyrus. During this phase of dyslexia research, studies (e.g., Abell, 1894; Cattell, 1885; Quantz, 1887) on word blindness were more concerned with eye movements and reading speed. Although it was recognized that some children were slow readers, an extrinsic perspective was adopted to attribute these children's tardiness to external factors including materials and methods used in teaching reading and the amount of classroom time devoted to it.

Phase 2 - From 1900s-1930s: Deciphering the Dyslexia Code

Morgan's paper is often taken as an important turning point that marked the beginning of serious attempts by several British ophthalmologists, like Thomas (1905), Fisher (1905, 1910), and Stephenson (1907), in their respective published papers to identify word blindness. There were also reports on patients with reading problems published in other countries such as the Netherlands (e.g., Lechner, 1903), Argentina (e.g., Wernicke, 1903), and Germany (e.g., Foerster, 1905; Peters, 1908; Warburg, 1911); and the United States of America (e.g., Orton, 1925, 1928; Schapringer, 1906, cited in Anderson and Meier-Hedde, 2001).

Uhl (1916) published the first report in the United States of an attempt to diagnose and treat individual reading problems. This was followed by Bronner (1917) who described several cases of reading disabilities resembling two categories of reading disorders, namely developmental dyslexia and hyperlexia. Other terms such as developmental alexia and congenital word blindness began to appear in research studies (e.g., Dearborn, 1925; Fildes, 1921; Lord, 1925; Schmitt, 1918; Wallin, 1920) describing reading disability in children. Orton (1928), an American neurologist, coined the term *strephosymbolia*, which means "twisted symbols," to describe the disorder.

Orton (1925) also proposed the first theory of how specific reading difficulty arose from the intrinsic perspective, putting a great emphasis on the development of dominance of one side of the brain. According to Orton (1925, 1928), the brain is divided into two hemispheres, where the Left Hemisphere (LH) regulates language functions and the Right Hemisphere (RH) dominates a few other language functions, but in individuals with dyslexia neither of the hemispheres dominates language functions. However, this has not been proved.

It was also during this phase of development in dyslexia research, especially in the 1920s, that saw a dramatic turn of events within a quarter of a century, when educationists began to take a serious interest on reading disability. Gates (1922), C.T. Gray (1922) and W.S. Gray (1922) published their three respective monographs addressing the issue of reading disability from an educational perspective. In the 1930s, Strauss and Werner (1939), for example, emphasized the importance of treating each child with learning disability individually in order to assess his/her specific educational needs within a learning context such as classroom or school. It was their work that eventually gave the impetus to the establishment of clinical and educational services for children with dyslexia, first in North America, and later in Europe, Oceania and the rest of the world.

Phase 3 - From 1940s-1950s: The Search for an Answer

Around the turn of the 20th century and right into the 1950s saw clinical research that was more directly relevant to dyslexia studies. Early researchers such as W.P. Morgan, James Hinshelwood, Samuel Orton, Grace Fernald, Alfred Strauss and Heinz Werner were frequently cited as being among the early pioneers of the dyslexia research by others in the 1980s (e.g., Aaron, 1989; Gearheart and Gearheart, 1989) and 1990s (e.g., Chia, 1992, 1996; Lerner, 1993; Smith, 1991; Spear-Swerling and Sternberg, 1998). Nearly all of these pioneering figures in the dyslexia studies were physicians or psychologists. During that period, educationists played very minor or no role in the dyslexia field (Spear-Swerling and Sternberg, 1998). Indeed *learning disabilities* – a term preferred by the educationists – was not coined until 1960s (see Hammill, 1993, for detail) – although "reading disability" or "dyslexia" was used long before then.

During the 1940s, the world witnessed the horrors of the Second World War as well as the rise of nationalism among the former British colonies with the decline of the once "invincible" British Empire. Very little, if any, significant research studies (e.g., Gesell and Amatruda, 1947; Strauss and Lehtinen, 1947) on dyslexia were carried out during that decade. However, one noteworthy classic book *Psychopathology and Education of the Brain Injured Child* by Strauss and Lehtinen (1947) was published in the United States and regarded by many as the foundation of the field of learning disabilities (including dyslexia). Alfred Strauss, a psychiatrist, had previously worked with brain-injured adults in Germany before he migrated to the United States in 1937. He collaborated with Laura Lehtinen to study institutionalized children with brain injury which caused behavioral, perceptual and thinking disorders with characteristics such as abnormal responses to environmental stimuli, disorganization, distractibility, hyperactivity, higher levels of motor activity, motor problems, perseveration, and perceptual disturbances (Strauss and Lehtinen, 1947). These characteristics became known as the Strauss Syndrome.

In the 1950s, interest on dyslexia research turned to genetics for an intrinsic explanation of its cause, which has been assumed to be due to hereditary transmission. In one study done by Hallgren (1950) on family histories of approximately 300 children with substantial learning deficits, he found that 88 per cent of them had an immediate family member with dyslexia. Hence, Hallgren (1950) suggested dyslexia was hereditary. In three other studies on dyslexia in identical and fraternal twins conducted by Hermann (1959), his findings showed a 100 per cent correlation in identical twins, and only a 33 percent correlation among fraternal twins. As a result, Hermann (1959) redefined dyslexia as a defective capacity for acquiring, at the normal time, a proficiency in reading and writing, corresponding to the average performance. Like Hallgren (1950), Hermann (1959) took an intrinsic perspective to conclude that dyslexia is indeed hereditary, often accompanied by difficulties with other symbols, and the condition exists in absence of intellectual defect of the sensory organs.

From the 1870s through several decades until the 1950s, the early guiding pioneers of the dyslexia field were mainly physicians and psychologists, who tended to be oriented toward intrinsic explanations of poor reading (and of other learning problems) rather than toward extrinsic explanations. Moreover, physicians had a natural tendency to frame their intrinsic view on dyslexia specifically akin to pathogenesis, i.e., an illness or disease. As a result, it was not surprisingly, to note that many labels (e.g., alexia, aphasia, dyslexia, dysphasia) used by the early authorities for what educationists would call "reading disability" or "learning disabilities" have a distinctly medical, if not downright grim, cast: "dyslexia" (Berlin, 1884); "congenital word-blindness" (Morgan, 1896; and much later, Hinshelwood, 1917); "strephosymbolia" (Orton, 1937); and "brain-injured" or "cripple-brained" (Strauss, 1943; Strauss and Lehtinen, 1947).

Phase 4 - From 1960s-1970s: Armada of Terms, Definitions and Theories on Dyslexia

Between the decades of 1960s and 1970s, the term dyslexia gained credence as a biological disorder that was certifiable as well as a physical condition that could be diagnosed and treated. As a result, there was an armada of terms, definitions and theories to explain dyslexia (Plessis, 2002). For an example, Kirk (1963) proposed the term *learning disabilities* instead of dyslexia to the group of parents who helped to found the Association for Children with Learning Disabilities. In another example, Clements (1966) promoted the use of the term *minimal brain dysfunction* to distinguish between children with serious neuropathology and the minimally affected. One of the early texts on *Learning Disabilities* of the same title by Johnson and Myklebust (1967) used the term *psycho-neurological learning disabilities* to replace dyslexia. Another term *central processing dysfunction* was used by Chalfant and Scheffelin (1969) to refer to many types of learning disorders relating to a range of skills they thought were important in the neuro-physiological use of information. Tomatis (1969) proposed *auditory system deficit* exclusively as the main problem in his theory of dyslexia.

The period of 1960s saw many theories being put forth to explain the condition of dyslexia and they include the following: visual perception deficits (e.g., Frostig and Horne, 1964; Frostig, Lefever, and Whittlesey, 1964), poor perceptuo-motor coordination (e.g., Roach and Kephart, 1966), and auditory perception and language deficits (e.g., Kirk, McCarthy, and Kirk, 1968). For example, the theories basing on the visual perception deficit (e.g., Birch, 1962; Getman, 1965; Justisen, 1960) argued that subtle vision impairment might be the cause of dyslexia. Although serious eye problems do interfere with a child's ability to read, eye problems are not the same thing as dyslexia and should not be mistaken for the cause of dyslexia. Children with 20/20 vision may be dyslexic, but there are also those children with short-sightedness, long-sightedness or astigmatism who may not have difficulty learning to read. In other words, it is always possible for a child to have dyslexia and eye problems at the same time, but eye problems do not cause dyslexia (Ott, 1997; Stanley, 1994).

While different professions refer to similar conditions with different names, the term learning disabilities or specific learning disability (or *dyslexia* which is still the preferred term used in countries such as the United Kingdom, Malaysia and Singapore) gained widespread acceptance due to federal legislation (Federal Register, 1977) in the United States, but there have been two large groups reported in the research literature: those presumed to have brain damage and those to have a genetic etiology. Whatever terms, definitions or theories proposed to explain the condition of dyslexia, the World Federation of Neurology (1968) provided the "traditional" definition of dyslexia as follows: "a disorder in children who, despite conventional classroom experience, fail to attain the language skills or reading, writing, and spelling commensurate with their intellectual abilities" (Waites, 1968, pp. 21-22). This can be summarized in the following Table 2.

Table 2. Intrinsic and Extrinsic Factors of Dyslexia

Intrinsic factors	Extrinsic factors	
	In spite of …	… the following shortcomings are noted
Constitutional origin	• Conventional instruction • Adequate intelligence • Socio-cultural opportunities	• Difficulty in learning to • Read • Write • Spell

One significant event that took place in the 1960s was The Invalid Children's Aid Association on Word Blindness or Specific Developmental Dyslexia Conference 1962 held in New York. At the conference, paper presentations used terms such as *alexia*, *dyslexia* and *word blindness* interchangeably and synonymously to describe the loss of reading ability caused by lesions in different parts of the brain. These papers reflected the commonalities found in dyslexia cases. In summary, two key points were noted in the conference papers: (1) the lower continuum of reading level was represented by retarded readers; and (2) reading retardation (extrinsic perspective) was the result of poor teaching, non-stimulating environment, emotional disturbance, and lack of motivation. The broad area of agreement made by the panel of experts at the conference was that dyslexia is a constitutional or genetically determined disorder.

In 1971, Bateman suggested that the extrinsic term *teaching disabilities* or "dysteachia" – coined by Armstrong (1987) to refer to children suffering from "pedagogical illness" or inappropriate teaching strategies – should be used to replace the intrinsic term LDs. His reason was that LDs are caused by the inadequate skills of the adults, who are supposed to teach the children, instead of putting the blame on children with mysterious brain dysfunctions. It was Bateman's (1971) attempt to argue that poor or inadequate teaching could result in LDs among students and it is a bold move towards adopting an interactive perspective to explain the condition of dyslexia.

With the beginning of the 1970s, research studies (e.g., Hier et al., 1978; Holmes, 1973, 1978; Witelson, 1977) took a neurological approach to define and identify dyslexia and its subtypes. Marshall and Newcombe (1973), for example, took a cognitive neuropsychological perspective in identifying two types of reading failure: (1) deep dyslexia, i.e., individuals with this reading failure perform poorly in decoding which involves grapheme-phoneme conversion skills but can understand written words better than pronounce them; and (2) surface dyslexia, i.e., individuals with this reading failure can convert print into sound but cannot understand the written word correctly (see Figure 1).

According to Jorm (1979), developmental dyslexia resembled deep dyslexia because the underlying cause of the problem in both cases is a disability in the phonological conversion of print. However, Ellis (1979) disagreed and argued that an individual with developmental dyslexia hardly ever commits semantic errors (e.g., father → dad, mother → mum or mom) in

dyslexia as "a learning difficulty that primarily affects the skills involved in accurate and fluent word reading and spelling" (Rose, 2009, p. 30), including the following points:

- Characteristic features of dyslexia are difficulties in phonological awareness, verbal memory and verbal processing speed.
- Dyslexia occurs across the range of intellectual abilities.
- Dyslexia is best thought of as a continuum, not a distinct category, and there are no clear cut-off points.
- Co-occurring difficulties may be seen in aspects of language, motor co-ordination, mental calculation, concentration and personal organization, but these are not, by themselves, markers of dyslexia.

(Rose, 2009, p. 30)

The BDA Management Board adopted the definition but included an additional paragraph as follows: "A good indication of the severity and persistence of dyslexic difficulties can be gained by examining how the individual responds or has responded to well-founded intervention" (BDA, 2016, para. 5). The BDA definition of dyslexia is also adopted by the Dyslexia Association of Singapore.

This latest BDA definition of dyslexia shows some similarities to the one adopted by the International Dyslexia Association (IDA) Board of Directors on November 12, 2002. The IDA operating definition of dyslexia is as follows:

> "Dyslexia is a specific learning disability that is neurological in origin. It is characterized by difficulties with accurate and/or fluent word recognition and by poor spelling and decoding abilities. These difficulties typically result from a deficit in the phonological component of language that is often unexpected in relation to other cognitive abilities and the provision of effective classroom instruction. Secondary consequences may include problems in reading comprehension and reduced reading experience that can impede the growth of vocabulary and background knowledge." (Lyon, Shaywitz, and Shaywitz, 2003, p. 2)

On the one hand, there are some similar or common key features found in both BDA and IDA definitions of dyslexia, which are widely used and cited throughout the world, as shown in Table 3 below:

Table 3. BDA and IDA Definitions of Dyslexia

BDA definition	IDA definition
• a learning difficulty	• a specific learning disability
• affects the skills involved in accurate and fluent word reading and spelling	• difficulties with accurate and/or fluent word recognition and by poor spelling and decoding abilities
• are difficulties in phonological awareness,	• difficulties typically result from a deficit in the phonological component of language
• occurs across the range of intellectual abilities	• unexpected in relation to other cognitive

On the other hand, some of the features are stated in one of the two definitions but not in the other (see Table 4 below).

Table 4. Omitted Features in BDA and IDA Definitions of Dyslexia

BDA definition	IDA definition
• verbal memory and verbal processing speed	• is neurological in origin
• best thought of as a continuum, not a distinct category, and there are no clear cut-off points	• abilities and the provision of effective classroom instruction
• Co-occurring difficulties may be seen in aspects of language, motor co-ordination, mental calculation, concentration and personal organization, but these are not, by themselves, markers of dyslexia	• Secondary consequences may include problems in reading comprehension and reduced reading experience that can impede the growth of vocabulary and background knowledge
• Severity and persistence of dyslexic difficulties can be gained by examining how the individual responds or has responded to well-founded intervention	

In the recently published fifth edition of the Diagnostic and Statistical Manual of Mental Disorders (DSM-5; American Psychological Association, 2013), the various names of learning disorder including dyslexia were no longer used. The diagnosis of Learning Disorder has been changed to Specific Learning Disorders (or Specific Learning Disabilities). The word *disorder* is a medical term used in DSM-5 while the term *Learning Disabilities* is an educational term used in the Educator's Diagnostic Manual of Disabilities and Disorders (EDM; Pierangelo and Giuliani, 2007) and also by many psychologists (Tannock, 2014).

THE OPERATING DEFINITION OF DYSLEXIA

There are several definitions, descriptions and models of dyslexia. For example, Hynd and Hynd (1984) proposed their neurolinguistic model of dyslexic subtypes composing of surface, phonological and deep dyslexia. The model put forth by Gough and Tunmer (1986) consists of three types of reading disability: those with the inability to decode; those with the inability to comprehend; and those who exhibit both problems. Aaron (1989) proposed his model basing on the types of reader revolving around two major components of reading ability: decoding and comprehension: (1) normal readers who have no problems with decoding and comprehension; (2) dyslexic readers who have poor decoding but no problem with comprehension; (3) non-specific reading disabled, who have a mix of problems with decoding and comprehension of varying degrees of severity; and (4) hyperlexic readers who have good decoding but impaired comprehension. Chia (1996) proposed his tri-continua model of dyslexia where the first continuum of reading deficits – congenital, developmental and acquired – concerns the nature of occurrence or onset of dyslexia and each may be appropriate for certain contexts or purposes; the second continuum concerns the way a reader processes a given text: directly via grapheme-phoneme correspondence or indirectly via reliance on context-driven process (i.e., prior knowledge) for reading; and the third continuum of reading deficits falls between one end of deficits located in the phonologicsal core and the other opposite end of deficits located in the logographic/visual core. Table 5 shows the different terms used for dyslexia over the past decades.

Table 5. Different Terms used to describe Dyslexia

Examples of Researcher/s (Year)	Examples of Different Terms used to describe Dyslexia
Kussmaul (1877)	Reading blindness
Berlin (1887)	Dyslexia
Dejerine (1892)	Reading disability
Hinshelwood (1895)	Word blindness
Morgan (1896)	Congenital word blindness
Schmitt (1918)	Developmental alexia
Orton (1928)	Strephosymbolia
Strauss (1943)	Brain injury
Johnson and Myklebust (1967)	Psycho-neurological learning disability
Chalfant and Scheffelin (1969)	Central processing dysfunction
Marshall and Newcombe (1973)	Surface dyslexia, deep dyslexia
Hynd and Hynd (1984)	Deep dyslexia, surface dyslexia, phonological dyslexia
Wilsher and Taylor (1986)	Perceptual dysfunction
Tyre and Young (1994)	Specific learning difficulties, direct dyslexia
Chia (1996)	Dyslexic syndrome
IDEA (2004)	Specific learning disability
Moats and Tolman (2009)	Reading disabilities
DSM-5 (APA, 2013)	Specific learning disorder

Among these definitions of dyslexia, I have chosen to use the comprehensive IDA definition in my illustration to show how to operationalize this definition in order to formulate an operational intervention. The BDA definition of dyslexia is more elaborated and is just as good, too.

To test out an operating definition of dyslexia in order to establish its nosology (see Pennington, 1991, for more detail), we need both Validation and Verification which are complementary aspects of testing the fitness of the definition for the purpose. I refer to this overall checking process as the V and V procedure. However, it is not within the scope of this chapter to delve further on this issue but to provide a brief explanation why the V and V procedure is needed. The first V is Validation and it asks the question: "Are we trying to define the right thing?" In other words, the question to be asked about dyslexia will be: “Is the operating definition of dyslexia specified to the actual traits of that condition?” The second V is Verification and it asks the question: "Have we defined what we were trying to describe about dyslexia?" In other words, the question to be asked about dyslexia will be: “Does the operating definition of dyslexia conform to a set of specifications used to identify it?”

There are three basic components to establish the operating definition of dyslexia and they are: (1) Identification of the phenomenon (or condition of dyslexia) through establishing a theoretical concept; (2) Validation of the condition (of dyslexia) with appropriate tests to determine the existence of dyslexia, its duration and quantity; and (3) Procedure of the above two components should be repeatable by others in the dyslexia research.

Therefore, it is important for teachers as well as interventionists to know the agreed-on operating definition of dyslexia essential for their professional practice in order to provide the best intervention programs for these individuals with this specific learning disability (Brown-Waesche, Schatschneider, Maner, Ahmed, and Wagner, 2011, p. 296). In order to come up with a good intervention program for dyslexia, the following points should be taken into consideration: (1) If we know sufficiently enough about dyslexia and recognize its traits/symptoms, we can plan a targeted intervention to address this disability. (2) If we recognize some tell-tale signs of something not right but do not know sufficiently enough about dyslexia and its subtypes (if any), we can only administer symptomatic intervention. (3) If we know next to nothing about dyslexia or any of its subtypes at all and have no ideas what the tell-tale signs are that something is not right about the development of a child with dyslexia, i.e., not progressing normally, we can expect to have a sure chaotic intervention.

Returning to the IDA operating definition of dyslexia, it is defined as "a specific learning disability that is neurological in origin. It is characterized by difficulties with accurate and/or fluent word recognition and by poor spelling and decoding abilities. These difficulties typically result from a deficit in the phonological component of language that is often unexpected in relation to other cognitive abilities and the provision of effective classroom instruction. Secondary consequences may include problems in reading comprehension and reduced reading experience that can impede the growth of vocabulary and background knowledge" (Lyon, Shaywitz, and Shaywitz, 2003, p. 4). When this operating definition is being analyzed by asking the two V questions described earlier, we begin to notice several symptoms popping out of the definition before us. These symptoms described in the definition can be classified under four categories. We need to know them and what each category of symptoms means in order to understand dyslexia and, more importantly, how we can deal with the disability. The four categories of symptoms for dyslexia are: (1) core symptoms: These are the definite non-variant traits found to be present and are observable in individuals with dyslexia; (2) causal symptoms: These are the underlying neurological/genetic traits of dyslexia; (3) consequential symptoms: These are the traits that result from the core and/or causal traits of dyslexia; (4) co-existing symptoms: These are also other possible traits found to be co-existent with the current core and/or causal traits of dyslexia.

Table 6 shows the four categories of symptoms that define dyslexia according to the IDA operating definition. The three core symptoms – difficulties in accurate or fluent word recognition, poor spelling and poor decoding abilities – become the classical triad of impairments for dyslexia. The underlying cause of this triad of impairment is the phonological processing deficit that constitutes the main causal symptom for dyslexia. As a result, problems in reading comprehension and reduced reading experience become the consequential symptoms. The co-existent symptoms of poor reading comprehension and reduced reading experience are impeded vocabulary development as well as background knowledge.

Table 6. Four Categories of Symptoms according the IDA Definition of Dyslexia

Core symptoms	Causal symptoms	Consequential symptoms	Co-existing symptoms
• Difficulties in accurate/fluent word recognition • Poor spelling ability • Poor decoding ability	• Deficit in phonological component of language	• Problems in reading comprehension • Reduced reading experience	• Impeded growth of vocabulary • Impeded background knowledge

From Operating Definition of Dyslexia to Operational Application of Diagnostic Intervention

The first step to take in planning any appropriate diagnostic intervention or treatment for dyslexia is to operationalize the definition of dyslexia by establishing a standard operating procedure to address the symptoms of dyslexia in a systematic and organized way.

From the operating definition of dyslexia, various traits of this specific learning disability are identified and classified under the four categories of symptoms. From the categorisation of the symptoms, teachers and interventionists can see clearly the three core symptoms of dyslexia or the triad of impairments in dyslexia (i.e., difficulties in accurate/fluent word recognition, poor spelling and decoding abilities) which their teaching or intervention should be focusing on. Underlying this triad of impairments is the deficit in phonological processing (or letter-to-sound correspondence). One standardized test which is a practical measure for identifying individuals with significant phonological processing difficulties is the Phonological Assessment Battery (PhAB) (Frederickson, Drith, and Reason, 1997), which consists of six subtests that are designed to assess different aspects of phonological processing: (1) alliteration test which assesses the ability to isolate the initial sounds in single syllable words; (2) naming speed tests (include picture naming test and digit naming test) which assess the speed of phonological production; (3) rhyme test which assesses the ability to identify the rhyme in single syllable words; (4) spoonerisms test which assesses if an examinee can segment single syllable words and then blend the segments to provide new words or word combinations; (5) fluency test which assesses the retrieval of phonological information from long-term memory; and (6) non-word reading test which assesses the ability to decode letter strings.

On the top priority in the proposed operating procedure to devise a good intervention program for dyslexia is to determine the causal (underlying) symptoms that are causing the disability. As already mentioned earlier, a deficit in phonological processing is thought to be the main underlying cause of dyslexia (Wright and Conlon, 2009). Phonological processing is the cognitive ability to sense a word by sight or hearing, decipher by segmenting the word into its discrete sounds, and then corresponding each sound with its appropriate letter that constitutes the word. The phonological processing deficit "is thought to have an adverse effect on the word recognition system by interfering with the ability to establish links between spoken sounds and written letters" (Chia and Houghton, 2011, p. 143). Hence, training in phonolgocial awareness coupled with systematic phonics instruction in letter-sound/grapheme-phoneme correspondences is crucial for helping students with dyslexia to develop efficient word recognition, decoding and spelling skills (Mather and Wendling, 2012).

The next step is to treat the core symptoms of dyslexia according to the degree of severity of each symptom. As already mentioned earlier, the three core symptoms identified in the IDA definition of dyslexia are difficulties in accurate/fluent word recognition, poor spelling and decoding abilities. In order to determine the severity of each of the difficulties, relevant standardized tests should be administered to determine the equivalent age for each of the three components: word recognition age (WRA), word expression/reading age (WEA/RA) and spelling age (SpA). These equivalent ages are matched against an individual's chronological age (CA) or mental age (MA), if there is one available from the individual's psychological assessment report. If the WRA, WEA/RA and SpA are three years behind CA or MA, there is a cause for concern that the individual concerned does display specific learning difficulties in word recognition, decoding and spelling abilities. In assessing word recognition, the Word Recognition and Phonic Skills Test-Second Edition (WRaPS-2) (Moseley, 2003), for example, can be used to assess a student's word recognition and phonic skills. The standardized test can also help to pinpoint problems in the initial stages of learning to read. The Burt Word Reading Test (NZCER, 1981) is another example that can be used to assess the student's word expression or decoding skill. The term *decoding* (also known as basic reading skills) refers "to the ability to use the systematic correspondences between sounds and spellings to acquire a repertoire of words that can be recognised by sight" (Mather and Wendling, 2012, p. 148). There is a difference in testing word recognition (silent decoding) and word expression (oral decoding). In assessing word recognition, a list of words is shown to the examinee. The examiner will say the target word first and then says it in a given sentence before repeating the target word again. The examinee will have to recognise and choose the correct word spoken by the examiner from the list. In assessing word expression, the examinee will be shown a list of words and has to read each word aloud, starting from the top row and then moving from left to right before going down to the next row. Reading aloud is an effective way to develop an individual's phonemic awareness and linguistic ability to read (Adams, 1990). Finally, in assessing spelling performance, the Single Word Spelling Test (Socre and Masterson, 2001), for example, can be used to identify gaps in a student's spelling skills and track the student's progress in spelling development over time. It also provides teachers and interventionists useful information for effective planning of spelling instruction.

The above discussion about first two categories of symptoms must be taken seriously by teachers and interventionists in planning an appropriate remedial reading or intervention program. It also suggests that the best intervention approach has to be structured, systematic, sequential, multisensory, synthetic phonics instruction covering the basic concepts of reading, spelling and writing (Ritchey and Goeke, 2006; Rose and Zirkel, 2007). According to Uhry and Clark (2005), although there are many different phonics intervention strategies, they incorporate three main principles: (1) letter-sound/graphem-phoneme correspondences are taught explicitly and directly; (2) a pre-planned scope and sequence of phonograms, which are unit symbols of the phonetic writing system to represent a word, syllable or phoneme; and (3) the letter-sound correspondences are practiced in isolation as well as in a given text.

However, not all the phonics intervention strategies are suitable for remedial teaching for students with dyslexia. Among them, according to Mather and Wendling (2012), there are four that best cater to the learning needs of students with dyslexia: analytic phonics, synthetic phonics, phonics-through-analogy and phonics-through-spelling. The analytic phonics strategy uses a whole-to-part sequence to teach analysis of letter-to-sound patterns once the words have been identified as whole entities (Ehri, 2006). This strategy involves segmenting a word into its constitutent phonological elements before blending them together to pronounce the word in its entirety. Unlike the analytic phonics, the synthetic phonics strategy uses a part-to-whole sequence to learn the phonological elements or sounds of the constituent letters through explicit instruction and blend them to pronounce the word in its entirety. Phonics-through-analogy strategy often uses word families and involves learning new words by analogy to words already known. For instance, if an individual knows the rime *-op* as in the word p*op*, he/she can easily relate it to new consonant-vowel-consonant (CVC) words such as h*op*, t*op* and c*op* as well as consonant blend-vowel-consonant words such as dr*op*, st*op* and pl*op*. Finally, phonics-through-spelling strategy involves three steps to spell words phonetically: (1) segment a word into its constitutent letter sounds or phonemes; (2) choose the letter symbols or graphemes that spell those phonemes; and (3) write the word out.

Following up in the next step is to address the consequential (secondary) symptoms of dyslexia in order to keep the individual's self-esteem up with the correct approach to motivate him/her to do his/her very best. In the IDA definition, the two consequential symptoms are problems in reading comprehension and reduced reading experience. These symptoms are not the causes of dyslexia but the results of it. Since a student with dyslexia is not reading too well, his/her reading comprehension suffers as a result. This, in turn, impacts the student's interest in reading as well as the motivation to read. As a result, the student's reading experience suffers, too. One good example of a standardized test for reading comprehension is the McLeod Assessment of Reading Comprehension (McLeod and McLeod, 1999), which "assesses reading comprehension by means of the cloze procedure in which an examinee reads a series of passages and supplies words that have been deleted from sentences within each passage" (p. 112). The other only standardized test on reading experience available to date is a very dated but excellent Graded Test of Reading Experience taken from the Standard Reading Tests (Daniels and Diack, 1958). It is good for teachers and interventionists to take note of these two diagnostic tests as they can provide useful information on the progress of a student with dyslexia, especially in terms of his/her response to the remedial teaching or intervention. If the results of the two assessments show a significant improvement in both reading comprehension and reading experience after a period of intensive intervention, it is certainly a good indication that the student with dyslexia is making a good progress.

Intervention strategies used in teaching reading comprehension should involve explicit instruction and may include the following steps (NSW Department of Education and Training, 2010): (1) select an appropriate text that is slightly lower the student's expected reading level and of high interest; (2) select an appriopriate strategy and explain to the student how it is used; (3) model the strategy so that the student understands how it works; (4) provide guided support such as reading aloud or have a reading buddy work with the student; (5) give the student time to do his/her own independent practice using the selected strategy; and (6) ask the student to reflect on how using the strategy helped him/her understand the text better. Examples of reading comprehension strategies include making connections between the text and their own prior knowledge/experience or brainstorming prior knowledge such as LINK (List, Inquire, Note, and Know) strategy (Vaughan and Estes, 1986), predicting using Anticipation Guide strategy (Herber, 1978) to forecast the main ideas in a given passage through the use of statements that activates the students' thoughts and opinions, questioning using K-W-L (Know/Want to Know/Learned) method (Ogle, 1986) with a further extension into what is now known as K-W-L Plus strategy (Carr and Ogle, 1987), visualizing such as You-Ought-to-Be-in-Pictures strategy, which "prepares students to read a passage using pictures to process new learning through extensive use of mental imagery" (Buehl, 2001, p. 149), and summarizing of main ideas or events.

One way to enhance positive reading experience can be done through peer tutors or reading buddies program where two or more individuals read together. For example, an older or better student partners with a student with dyslexia and read with him/her at a specific time at a cozy reading corner or resource room. This can help to develop a love of reading for students with dyslexia and also promote a greater motivation to read.

Besides those individuals with dyslexia, there is a unique group of individuals who can read very well, and their reading age is significantly higher than their chronological or mental age. However, they perform extremely poorly in their reading comprehension. Tyre and Young (1994) termed this anomaly *direct dyslexia* because such an individual is able to process print using the whole word recognition skills and convert it into speech using phonological skills. Direct dyslexia is also known as hyperlexia, which is often associated with autism spectrum disorder. It is not within the scope of the chapter to delve into this condition. One example of an intervention strategy that can help this group of students with direct dyslexia or hyperlexia is mind mapping (Barron, 1969). Another example is the scaffolding interrogatives method (SIM for short) (see Ng and Chia, 2013, for more detail). This method requires the student "to read sentence by sentence, and then to chart each sentence in several columns of what interrogatives with sentential contents" (Chia, 2002, p. 14). The chart helps to scaffold the student's textual comprehension. When the student finishes reading the passage, textual meaning is built. "The completed chart provides a new format of reorganized ideas based upon the original text, to aid comprehension" (Chia, 2002, p. 14).

Other than phonological processing deficit and reading comprehension impairment, a third group of individuals with normal language comprehension but impaired reading ability has been identified by Moats and Tolman (2009). The individuals in this group are observed to be hesitant in speaking because of difficulty naming words or difficulty in word retrieval and hence, their fluency or naming speed is very much affected. Different terms have been used to describe this anomalous condition such as anomia, dysnomia, anomic aphasia, and dysphasia. Figure 2 shows how the three groups of individuals with different reading disabilities in terms of phonological processing impairment (dyslexia), language comprension impairment (hyperlexia) and fluency/naming speed impairment (dysnomia, which is also known as anomia and anomic aphasia) are associated with each other as they share some common learning difficulties.

Lastly, it is also good to treat the co-existing symptoms that are giving problems to a student with dyslexia who is already struggling to read. These co-existent symptoms are impeded vocabulary development as well as background knowledge as a result of poor reading comprehension and reduced reading experience. Like the consequential symptoms, they are not the causes of dyslexia. One excellent standardized assessment of vocabulary development is the Comprehensive Receptive and Expressive Vocabulary Test-Third Edition (CREVT-3) (Wallace and Hammill, 2013). It is a good measure of both receptive and expressive word knowledge to identify individuals who are significantly lagging behind their peers in word knowledge as well as to note discrepancies between receptive and expressive vocabulary. The test is also useful in documenting the progress of a student with dyslexia in his/her vocabulary development after having undergone an intervention program. With improvement in word recognition and decoding skills, students with dyslexia should be able to perform well in their reading comprehension, reading experience, receptive and expressive vocabulary development and background knowledge acquisition.

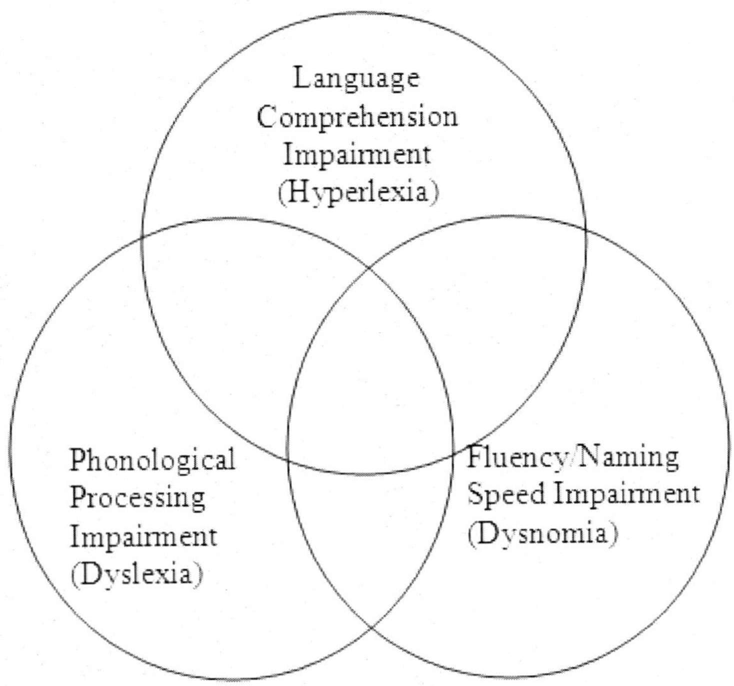

Figure 2. Three Groups of Reading Disabilities (adapted from Moats and Tolman, 2009).

There are several intervention strategies that can help students with dyslexia to build up their vocabulary. One good example is the Frayer strategy that provides a format to help deepening an understanding of a given concept (Frayer, Frederick, and Klausmeier, 1969). It uses a visual way of distinguishing between items with features that represent or define the concept and those lacking some key features of the concept. Another example is the Word Family Tree (Buehl, 1999) strategy that can be used by students with dyslexia to connect a key term or word "to its origins, to related words sharing a common root, to words that serve a similar function, and to situations in which the student might expect the word to be used" (Buehl, 2001, p. 146). Mind maps, for example, are also a popular strategy that offers a visual representation to perceive essential features inter-connected within the given context of the larger picture.

Table 7 summarizes what has been discussed above on the examples of different standardized tests that can be used to assess the three core symptoms of dyslexia, its consequential/secondary as well as co-existing symptoms and, also, the appropriate intervention strategies recommended for with each of the difficulties.

Table 7. A Summary of Standardized Tests and Intervention Strategies

Core Symptoms of Dyslexia		
Difficulties in fluent/accurate word recognition	Poor decoding (basic reading skills)	Poor spelling skills
Standardized Test, e.g.: Word Recognition and Phonic Skills Test-2nd Ed.	*Standardized Test,* e.g.: Burt Word Reading Test	*Standardized Test,* e.g.: Single Word Spelling Test
Intervention Strategy, e.g.: Analytic phonics, synthetic phonics	*Intervention Strategy,* e.g.:Phonics-through-analogy, word families	*Intervention Strategy,* e.g.:Phonics-through-spelling
Causal Symptoms of Dyslexia		
Deficit in phonological processing		
Standardized Test, e.g.: Phonological Assessment Battery		
Intervention Strategy, e.g.: Analytic phonics, synthetic phonics, phonics-through-analogy, and phonics-through-spelling		
Consequential Symptoms of Dyslexia		
Problems in reading comprehension	Reduced reading experience	
Standardized Test, e.g.: McLeod Assessment of Reading Comprehension	*Standardized Test,* e.g.: Graded Test of Reading Experience	
Intervention Strategy, e.g.: LINK method, K-W-L, K-W-L Plus	*Intervention Strategy,* e.g.: Peer tutoring, reading buddy program	
Co-existing Symptoms of Dyslexia		
Impeded growth of vocabulary	Impeded growth of background knowledge	
Standardized Test, e.g.: Comprehensive Receptive and Expressive Vocabulary Test-3rd Ed.	*Standardized Test,* e.g.: Not applicable	
Intervention Strategy, e.g.: Frayer method, mind maps, Word Family Trees	*Intervention Strategy,* e.g.: Participation in group discussion and group activities that involve sharing of ideas	

CONCLUSION

All students with dyslexia regardless of its degree of severity require proper interventions involving letter-to-sound (grapheme-to-phoneme) correspondence conducted in a systematic, explicit and intensive way to teach word recognition, decoding and spelling skills. The longer any student with dyslexia struggles with the triad of impairments without any effective intervention, the greater would be the negative impact on his/her self-esteem and motivation to read, spell or write. This, in turn, will also affect reading comprehension and reading experience, and impede vocabulary development and growth of background knowledge. Finally, both teachers and interventionists must take note that for any intervention to be successful, their students with dyslexia must engage in meaningful activites involving reading, spelling and writing so that they enjoy what they are learning as well as being able to express and communicate their ideas confidently.

REFERENCES

Aaron, P. G. (1989). Dyslexia and hyperlexia: Diagnosis and management of developmental reading disabilities. NY: Kluwer Academic/Plenum Publishers.

Abell, A. M. (1894). Rapid reading and slow reading. Educational Review, 8, 283-287.

Adams, M. J. (1990). Beginning to read: Thinking and learning about print. Cambridge, MA: MIT Press.

American Psychological Association (2013). Diagnostic and Statistical Manual of Mental Disorders-Fifth Edition (DSM-5). Washington, DC: The Author.

Anderson, P. L., and Meier-Hedde, R. (2001). Early case reports of dyslexia in the United States and Europe. Journal of Learning Disabilities, 34(1), 9-21.

Armstrong, T. (1987). Describing strengths of children identified as 'learning disabled' using Howard Gardner's theory of multiple intelligences as an organizing framework. Unpublished PhD dissertation. California Institute of Integral Studies.

Barron, R. (1969). The use of vocabulary as an advance organiser. In H. Herber and P. Sanders (Eds.), Research in reading in the content areas: First year report (pp. 29–30). Syracuse, NY: Syracuse University Press.

Bateman, B. (1971). The essentials of teaching. San Rafael, CA: Dimensions Publishing.

Berlin, R. (1884). Uber dyslexie [About dyslexia]. Archiv fur Psychiatrie, 15, 276-278.

Birch, H. G. (1962). Dyslexia and the maturation of visual function. In J. Money (Ed.), Reading disability (pp. 161-169). Baltimore, MD: The Johns Hopkins University Press.

Bisgaard, M. L., Eiberg, H., Moller, N., Niebuhr, E., and Morh, J. (1987). Dyslexsia and chromosome 15 heteromorphism:Negative LOD score in a Danish material. Clinical Genetics, 32, 118-119.

Bishop, D. V. M. (2009). Genes, cognition, and communication: insights from neurodevelopmental disorders. Annals of the New York Academy of Sciences, 1156, 1-18.

Boder, E. (1976). School failure: Evaluation and treatment. Pediatrics, 58(3), 394-403.

British Dyslexia Assocaition (1996). The dyslexia handbook. Reading, UK: The Author.

British Dyslexia Assocaition (2016). Dyslexia: Definitions. Retrieved from: http://www.bdadyslexia.org.uk/dyslexic/definitions.

British Dyslexia Assocaition Management Board (2007, October). Definition of dyslexia. Retrieved from: http://www.bdadyslexia.org.uk/dyslexic/ definitions.

Broca, P. (1861). Perte de la parole. Ramollisement chronique et destruction partielle du lobe anterior gauche du cerveau. Bulletin et Memoires de la Societe d'Anthropologie de Paris, 2, 219.

Bronner, A. F. (1917). The psychology of special abilities and disabilities. Boston, MA: Little, Brown and Co.

Brooks, L. (1997). Dyslexia: 100 years on brain research and understanding. Staines, Middlesex, UK: The Dyslexia Institute.

Brown-Waesche, J.S., Schatschneider, C., Maner, J.K., Ahmed, Y. and Wagner, R.K. (2011). Examining agreement and longitudinal stability of reading disability using the affected-status agreement index. Journal of Learning Disability, 44, 296-307.

Buehl, D. (1999). Word family trees: heritage sheds insight into words' meaning and use. WEAC News and Views, 35(2), 14.

Buehl, D. (2001). Classroom strategies for interactive learning (2nd ed.). Newark, DE: International Reading Association.

Carr, E. M., and Ogle, D. (1987). K-W-L plus: A strategy for comprehension and summarization. Journal of Reading, 28, 626-631.

Cattell, J. M. (1885). The inertia of the eye and brain. Brain, 8, 295-312.

Chalfant, J., and Scheffelin, M. (1969). Central processing dysfunction in children: A review of research. NINDS Monograph No. 9. Washington, DC: US Government Printing Office.

Chia, N. K. H. (1992). Defining and understanding developmental dyslexia. Education Today, 43(3), 12-17.

Chia, N. K. H. (1996). The tri-continua model of dyslexic syndrome. Education Today, 46(3), 33-40.

Chia, N.K.H. (2002). Effectiveness of scaffolding interrogatives method (SIM): A strategy to improve a hyperlexic child's reading comprehension: A case study. The Educational Therapist, 23(3), 12–19.

Chia, N. K. H. (2012, Spring-Summer). What is LD in special needs education? Journal of the American Academy of Special Education Professionals, 78-86.

Chia, N. K. H. and Houghton, S. (2011). The effectiveness of Orton-Gillingham based instruction with Singaporean children with specific reading disability (dyslexia). British Journal of Special Education, 38(3), 143-149.

Clark, L. (2009, January 15). The dyslexia 'myth': It's a wicked excuse used to cover up bad teaching, claims Labour MP. Mail Online. Retrieved from: www.dailymail.co.uk/news/article-1116644/The-dyslexia-myth-Its-wicked-excuse-used-cover-bad-teaching-claims-Labour-MP.html.

Clements, S. D. (1966). Minimal brain dysfunction in children: Terminology and identification, phase one of a 3-phase project. NINDS Monograph No. 3. Washington, DC: US Government Printing Office.

Dagan, D., Burke, C. K., Davies, J., and Chinn, D. (2015). Learning disabilities: Positive practice guide. London, UK: Foundation for People with Learning Disabilities.

Daniels, J. C., and Diack, H. (1958). Standard reading tests. St Albans, UK: Hart-Davis Educational.

Dearborn, W. F. (1925). The etiology of word blindness. In E. |Lord, L. Carmichael and W. F. Dearborn (Eds.), Special disabilities in learning to read and write. Harvard Monographs in Education, Vol.II, Series I, No. 1. Cambridge, MA: Harvard University Press.

DeFries, J. C., Fulker, D. W., and LaBuda, M. C. (1987). Reading disability in twins: Evidence for a genetic etiology. Nature, 329, 537-539.

Dejerine, J. C. (1891). Sur un Cas de Cécité Verbale avec Agraphie, Suivi d'Autopsie. Memorires de la Societe de Biologie, 3, 197-201.

Dejerine, J. (1892). Contribution a l'etude anatomoclinique et Clinique des differences varieties de cecite verbale. Memorires de la Societe de Biologie, 4, 61-90.

Department of Education and Science (1972). The Tizard report. London, UK: HMSO.

Department of Education and Science (1975). The Bullock report. London, UK: HMSO.

Department of Education and Science (1978). The Warnock report. London, UK: HMSO.

Department of Education and Science (1981). The Tansley and Panckhurst report. London, UK: HMSO.

Duara, R., Kushch, A., Cross-Glenn, K., Barker, W. W., Jallad, B., Pascal, S., Loewenstein, D. A., Sheldon, J., Rabin, M., and Levin, B. (1991). Neuroanatomic differences between dyslexia and normal readers on magnetic imaging scans. Archives of Neurology, 48, 410-416.

Dunne, D. W. (2000, May). Research shows brains of dyslexics change as reading improves. Education World, 1-3.

Ehri, L. C. (2006). Alpbetics instruction helps children learn to read. In R. M. Joshi and P. G. Aaron (Eds.), Handbook of orthography and literacy (pp. 649-677). Mahwah, NJ: Erlbaum.

Elliott, C. D. (1990). Definition and identification of specific learning difficulties. In P. D. Pumfrey and C. D. Elliott (Eds.), Children's difficulties in reading, spelling and writing (pp. 91-104). Basingstoke, UK: Falmer Press.

Elliott, J. G., and Grigorenko, E. L. (2014). The dyslexia debate: Cambridge studies in cognitive and perceptual development. New York, NY: Cambridge University Press.

Ellis, A. W. (1979). Developmental and acquired dyslexia: Some observations on Jorm (1979). Cognition, 7, 413-420.

Evans, B. J. W., and Drasdo, N. (1990). Review of ophthalmic factors in dyslexia. Ophthalmic and Physiological Optics, 10, 123-132.

Evans, B. J. W., and Drasdo, N. (1991). Tinted lenses and related therapies for learning disabilities: An overview. Ophthalmic and Physiological Optics, 2, 206-217.

Farmer, M.E. and Klein, R.M. (1995). The evidence for a temporal processing deficit linked to dyslexia: A review. Psychonomic Bulletin and Review, 2(4), 460-493.

Federal Register (1977, December 20). Volume 42, No. 163, p. 65083. Washington, DC: US Government Printing Office.

Ferrei, C. A.,and Wainwright, R. B. (1984). Breakthrough for dyslexia and learning disabilities. Pompano Beach, FL: Exposition Press.

Fildes, L. G. (1921). A psychological inquiry into the nature of the condition known as congential word blindness. Brain, 44, 286-304.

Finucci, J. M. (1986). Follow-up studies of developmental dyslexia and other learning disabilities. In S. Smith (Ed.), Genetics and learning disabilities (pp. 97-121). San Diego, CA: College-Hill Press.

Fisher, J. H. (1905). Case of congenital word blindness: Inability to learn to read. Ophthalmological Review, 24, 315-318.

Fisher, J. H. (1910). Congenital word blindness: Inability to learn to read. Transactions of the Ophthalmological Society of the United Kingdom, 30, 216.

Foerster, R. (1905). Beitrage zur pathologie des lesens und schreibens (congenital wort-blindheit bein einen schwachsinnigen). Neurol Centralbl, 24, 235-236.

Frayer, D., Frederick, W., and Klausmeier, H. (1969). A schema for testing the level of cognitive mastery. Working Paper No. 16. Madison, WI: Wisconsin Research and Development Center.

Frederickson, N., Frith, U., and Reason, R. (1997). Phonological assessment battery: Manual and test materials (PhAB). Windsor, UK: NFER-Nelson.

Frostig, M., and Horne, D. (1964). The Frostig program for the development of visual perception. Chicago, IL: Follett.

Frostig, M., Lefever, D. W., and Whittlesey, J. R. B. (1964). The Marianne Frostig developmental test of visual perception. Palo Alto, CA: Consulting Psychologists Press.

Gail, F. J. (1835). On the functions of the brain and of each of its parts: With observations on the possibility of determining the instincts, propensities, and talents, or the moral and intellectual dispositions of men and animals, by the configuration of the brain and head. Volume 1. Boston, MA: Marsh, Capen and Lyon.

Galaburda, A. M. (1985). Developmental dyslexia: A review of biological interactions. Annals of Dyslexia, 35, 21-34.

Galaburda, A. M. (1993). Dyselxia and development: Neurological aspects of extraordinary brains. Cambridge, MA: Harvard Univesity Press.

Galaburda, A. M. (1994). Developmental dyslexia and animal studies: At the interface between cognition and neurology. Cognition, 50, 133-149.

Galaburda, A. M., Rosen, G. D., and Sherman, G. F. (1989). The neural origin of developmental dyslexia: Implications for medicine, neurology, and cognition. In A. M. Galaburda (Ed.), From reading to neurons (pp. 377-388). Cambridge, MA: MIT Press.

Gates, A. I. (1922). The psychology of reading and spelling with special reference to disability. Teachers College Contribution to Education (No. 129). New York, NY: Columbia University.

Gearheart, B. R., and Gearheart, C. J. (1989). Learning disabilities: Educational strategies. Columbus, OH: Merrill.

Geschwind, N., and Galaburda, A. M. (1985a). Cerebral lateralization: Biological mechanisms, associations, and pathology. (2). A hypothesis and a program of research. Archives of Neurology, 42, 428-459.

Geschwind, N., and Galburda, A. M. (1985b). Cerebral lateralization: Biological mechanisms, associations, and pathology. (2). A hypothesis and a program of research. Archives of Neurology, 42, 521-552.

Geschwind, N., and Galaburda, A. M. (1985c). Cerebral lateralization: Biological mechanisms, associations, and pathology. (2). A hypothesis and a program of research. Archives of Neurology, 42, 634-654.

Gesell, A., and Amatruda, C. S. (1947). Developmental diagnosis (2nd ed.). New York, NY: Hoeber Publishing.

Getman, G. N. (1965). The visuo-motor complex in the acquisition of learning skills. In J. Hellmuth (Ed.), Learning disorder, Vol. 1 (pp. 49-76). Seattle, WA: Special Child Publishers.

Gillingham, A., and Stillman, B. (1970). Remedial training for children with specific difficulty in reading, spelling and penmanship. Cambridge, MA: Eductors Publishing Service.

Goldberg, E., and Costa, L. D. (1981). Hemispheric differences in the acquisition and use of descriptive systems. Brain and Language, 14, 144-173.

Gough, P. B., and Tunmer, W. (1986). Decoding, reading, and reading disability. Remedial and Special Educaiton, 7(1), 6-10.

Gray, C. T. (1922). Deficiencies in reading ability: Their diagnosis and remedies. Boston, MA: D. C. Heath.

Gray, W. S. (1922). Remedial cases in reading: Their diagnosis and treatment. Educational Monographs Supplementary No. 221. Chicago, IL: University of Chicago Press.

Guardiola, J. G. (2001). The evolution of research on dyslexia. Annuario de Psicologia, 32(1), 3-30.

Hallgren, B. (1950). Specific dyslexia (congenital word-blindness): A clinical and genetic study. Acta Psychiatrica et Neurologica, Supplement 65, 1-287.

Hammill, D. (1993). A brief look at the learning disabilities movement in the United States. Journal of Learning Disabilities, 26, 295-310.

Herber, H. (1978). Teaching reading in content areas (2nd ed.). Englewood Cliffs, NJ: Prentice-Hall.

Hermann, K. (1959). Reading disability: A medical study of word blindness and related handicaps. Springfield, IL: Charles C. Thomas.

Heward, W. L., and Orlansky, M. D. (1992). Exceptional children: An introductory survey of special education (4th ed.). New York, NY: Merrill.

Hickey, C. (1997). Dyslexia: Language training course for teachers and learners. Staines, Middlesex, UK: The Dyslexia Institute.

Hier, D. B., LeMay, M., Rosenberg, P. B., and Perlo, V. P. (1978). Developmental dyslexia: Evidence for a subgroup with a reversal of cerebral asymmetry. Archives of Neurology, 35(2), 90-92.

Hinshelwood, J. (1895). Word-blindness and visual memory. The Lancet, 2, 1564-1570.

Hinshelwood, J. (1907). Four cases of congenital word-blindness occurring in the same family. The British Medical Journal, 2, 1229-1232.

Hinshelwood, J. (1917). Congenital word-blindness. London, UK: Lewis.

Hoeft, F., Meyler, A., Hernandez, A., Juel, C., Taylor-Hill, H., Martindale, J.L., McMillon, G., Kolchugina, G., Black, J.M., Faizi, A., Deutsch, G.K., Siok, W.T., Reiss, A.L., Whitfield-Gabrieli, S. and Gabrieli, J.D.E. (2007). Functional and morphometric brain dissociation between dyslexia and reading ability. Proceedings of the National Academy of Sciences of the United States of America, 104(10), 4234-4239.

Holmes, J. M. (1973). A neurolinguistic study of traumatic and developmental disorders of reading. Unpublished PhD thesis, University of Edinburgh, UK.

Holmes, J. M. (1978). Regression and reading breakdown. Baltimore, MD: John Hopkins University Press.

Hoirnsby, B. (1996). Overcoming dyslexia: A straightforward guide for families and teachers. London, UK: Vermilion.

Hynd, G. W., and Hynd, C. R. (1984). Dyslexia: Neuroanatomical/ Neurolingusitic perspectives. Reading Research Quarterly, 19, 482-489.

Hynd, G. S., Marshall, R., and Gonzalez, J. (1991). Learning disabilities and presumed central nervous system dysfunction. Learning Disabilities Quarterly, 14, 283-296.

International Dyslexia Association (2002). The International Dyslexia Association: Finding the answers. Baltimore, MD: The Author.

Irlen, H. (1983). Successful treatment of learning disabilities. Paper presented at the 91st Annual Convention of American Psychological Association at Anaheim, Califiornia, USA.

Johnson, D. J., and Myklebust, H. R. (1967). Learning disabilities: Educational principles and practices. New York, NY: Grune and Stratton.

Jorm, A. F. (1979). The cognitive and neurological basis of developmental dyslexia: A theoretical framework and review. Cognition, 7, 19-32.

Justisen, C. G. (1960). Visual perception of form and school achievement. Ed.D thesis. University of Maryland, USA.

Katzir, T., Kim, Y. S., Wolf, M., Morris, R., and Lovett, M. W. (2008). The varieties of pathways to dysfluent reading: Comparing subtypes of children with dyslexia at letter, word, and connected text levels of reading. Journal of Learning Disabilities, 41(1), 47-66.

Kavale, K. A., and Forness, S. R. (1992). History, definition and diagnosis. In N. N. Singh and I. L. Beale (Eds.), Learning disabilities: Nature, theory and treatment (pp. 121-130). New York, NY: Springer-Verlag.

Kirk, S. A. (1963). Behavioral diagnosis and remediation of learning disabilities. In S. A. Kirk (Ed.), Proceedings of the conference on explanation into problems of the perceptually handicapped child: First annual meeting. Vol. 1. Chicago, IL: Council for Exceptional Children.

Kirk, S. A., McCarthy, J. J., and Kirk, W. D. (1968). Illinois test of psycholinguistic abilities (Re. ed.). Urbana, IL: University of Illinois Press.

Kushch, A., Gross-Glenn, K., Jalklaad, B., Lubs, H., Rabin, M., Feldman, E., and Duara, R. (1993). Temporal lobe surface area measurements on MRI in normal and dyslexic readers. Neuropsychologia, 31, 811-821.

Kussmaul, A. (1877). Disturbance of speech. Cyclopedia of Practical Medicine, 14, 581-875.

Lechner, C. S. (1903). Aangeboren woordblindheid. Ned Tijdschr. Geneeskunde, 39, 235-244.

Lerner, J. W. (1993). Learning disabilities: Theories, diagnosis and teaching strategies. Boston, MA: Houghton Mifflin.

Lipton, D. J. (1999). Indivbiduals with disabilities education act amendments of 1997 and IDEA regulations of 1999: Summary of changes. Berkeley, CA: DREDF.

Lord, E. E. (1925). The study and training of a child who was word blind. In E. Lord, L. Carmichael and W. Dearborn (Eds.), Special disabilities in learning to read and write. Harvard Monographs in Education, Vol. II, Series I, No. 1. Cambridge, MA: Harvard University Press.

Lyon, G. R. (1995). Toward a definition of dyslexia. Annals of Dyslexia, 45, 3-27.

Lyon, G. R., Shaywitz, S. E., and Shaywitz, B. A. (2003). A definition of dyslexia. Annals of Dyslexia, 53, 1-14.

Manzo, A. V., and Manzo, U. C. (1994). Literacy disorders: Holistic diagnosis and remediation. Orlando, PL: Holt, Rinehart and Winston.

Marshall, J. C., and Newcombe, F. (1973). Patterns of paralexia. Journal of Psycholinguistic Research, 2, 179-199.

Mather, N., and Wendling, B. J. (2012). Essentials of dyslexia assessment and intervention. Hoboken, NJ: John Wiley and Sons.

Mattis, S., French, J. H., and Rapin, I. (1975). Dyslexia in children and young adults: Three independent neuropsychological syndromes. Developmental Medicine and Child Neurology, 17(2), 150-163.

McLeod, J., and McLeod, R. (1999). McLeod assessment of reading comprehension. Retrieved fromhttp://www.arizonansforchildren.org/User Files/File/Diagnostics/mcleod_diag.pdf.

Miles, E. (1989). The Bangor dyslexia teaching system. London, UK: Whurr Publishers.

Miles, E. (1995). Can there be a single definition of dyslexia? Dyslexia, 1(1), 37-45.

Moats, L., and Tolman, C. (2009). Excerpted from language essentials for teachers of reading and spelling: The challenges of learning to read. Module 1. Boston, MA: Sopris West.

Morgan, W. P. (1896). A case of congenital word-blindness. British Medical Journal, ii, 1543-1544.

Moseley, D. (2003). Word recognition and phonic skills: Manual (2nd ed.). London, UK: Hodder Murray.

Myklebust, H. R., and Johnson, D. (1962). Dyslexia in children. Exceptional Children, 29(1), 14-25.

National Health and Medical Research Council (NHMRC) (1990). Learning difficulties in children and adolescents. Canberra: Australian Government Publishing Service.

National Joint Committee on Learning Disabilities (NJCLD) (1994). Learning disabilities: Issues on definition. Collective perspectives on issues affecting learning disabilities: Position papers and statements (pp. 61-66). Austin, TX: Pro-Ed.

New Zealand Council for Educational Research (1981). Burt word reading test. Wellington, NZ: The Author.

Newman, S. (1989). Ocular dominance, saccadic eye movements and reading. Dyslexia Contact, 8(1), 12-13.

Ng, A. G. T. (1996). Dyslexia: What is it really? Education Today, 46(2), 54-56.

Ng, P.M.H. and Chia, N.K.H. (2013). Teaching reading comprehension to children with hyperlexia: With 40 passages ready for use. Singapore: Pearson/Prentice-Hall.

Nicholson, R. I. (1996). Developmental dyslexia: Past, present and future. Dyslexia, 2(3), 190-207.

Njiokitjien, C., Desonneville, L., and Vaal, J. (1994). Callosal size in children with learning disabilities. Behavioral Brain Research, 64(1-2), 213-218.

NSW Department of Education and Training (2010). Teaching comprehension strategies: Curriculum K-12. NSW, Australia: The Author.

Ogle, D. (1986). K-W-L: A teaching model that develops active reading of expository text. The Reading Teacher, 39, 564-570.

Orton, S. T. (1925). Word-blindness in school children. Archives of Neurology and Psychiatry, 14, 582-615.

Orton, S. T. (1928). Specific reading disability – strephosymbolia. Journal of the American medical Assocaition, 90, 1095-1099.

Orton, S. T. (1937). Reading, writing and speech problems in children. New York, NY: Norton.

Orton, J. (1966). The Orton-Gillingham approach. In J. Money (Ed.), The disabled reader: Education of the dyslexic child (pp. 119-145). Baltimore, MD: Johns Hopkins University Press.

Ott, P. (1997). How to detect and manage dyslexia. Oxford, UK: Heinemann Educational Publisher.

Paracchini, S., Steer, C. D., Buckingham, L., Morris, A. P., Ring, S., Scerri, T., Stein, J., Pembrey, M. E., Ragoussis, J., Golding, J., and Monaco, A. P., (2008). Association of KIAA0319 dyslexia susceptibility gene with reading skills in the general population. American Journal of Psychiatry, 163, 1576-1584.

Pennington, B. F. (1991). Diagnosing learning disorders: A neuropsychological framework. New York, NY: The Guilford Press.

Peters, A. (1908). Ueber kongenitale Wortblindheit. Münchener Medizinische Wochenschroft, 55, 1116-1119.

Pierangelo, R., and Giuliani, G. (2007). The educator's diagnostic manual of disabilities and disorders. San Francisco, CA: Jossey-Bass.

Plessis, S. D. (2002). Dyslexia: Is the shoe perhaps on the wrong foot? New York, NY: Audibox.

Prasse, D. P. (1986). Litigation and special education: An introduction. Exceptional Children, 52, 311-312.

Quantz, J. O. (1887). Problems in the psychology of reading. Psychological Review Monograph Supplements, No. 2.

Richards, T.L. (2001). Functional MRI and spectroscopic imaging of the brain: Application of fMRI and fMRS to reading disabilities and education. Learning Disability Quarterly, 24(3), 189-203.

Ritchey, K. D., and Goeke, J. L. (2006). Orton-Gillingham and Orton-Gillingham-based reading instruction: A review of literature. The Journal of Special Education, 40(3), 171-183.

Roach, E. G., and Kephart, N. C. (1966). The Purdye perceptual-motor survey. Columbus, OH: Merrill.

Rose, J. (2009). Identifying and teaching children and young people with dyslexia and literacy difficulties. An independent report from Sir Jim Rose to the Secretary of State for Children, Schools and Families. Retrieved from: http://webarchive.nationalarchives.gov.uk/20130401151715/http://www.education.gov.uk/publications/eOrdering Download/00659-2009DOM-EN.pdf.

Rose, T. E., and Zirkel, P. (2007). Orton-Gillingham methodology for students with reading disabilities: 30 years of case law. The Journal of Special Education, 41(3), 171-185.

Rosner, J., and Rosner, J. (1987). The Irlen treatment: A review of the literature. Optician, 25, 26-33.

Rumsey, J. M., Nace, K., Donohue, B., Wise, D., Maisog, J. M., and Andreason, P. (1997). A positron emission tomographic study of impaired word recognition and phonological processing in dyslexic men. Archives of Neurology, 54, 562-573.

Schapringer, A. (1906, February). Cited in Anderson, P. L., and Meier-Hedde, R. (2001). Early case reports of dyslexia in the United States and Europe. Journal of Learning Disabilities, 34(1), 9-21.

Schmitt, C. (1918). Developmental alexia: Congenital word-blindness or inability to learn to read. Elementary School Journal, 18, 680-700.

Selikowitz, M. (1995). Dyslexia and other learning difficulties: The facts. New York, NY: Oxford University Press.

Serafini S, Steury K, Richards T, Corina D, Abbott R, and Berninger V. (2001). Comparison of fMRI and fMR spectroscopic imaging during language processing in children. Magnetic Resonance in Medicine, 45(2), 217–225.

Shastry, B. S. (2007). Developmental dyslexia: An update. Journal of Human Genetics, 52, 104-109.

Shaywitz, B. (1995). Sex differences in the functional organization of the brain for language. Nature, 373, 607-609.

Shaywitz, B.A., Shaywitz, S.E., Pugh, K.R., Mencl, W.E., Fullbright, R.K., Skudlarski, P., Constable, R.T., Marchione, K.E., Fletcher, J.M., Lyon, G.R. and Gore, J.C. (2002). Disruption of posterior brain systems for reading in children with developmental dyslexia. Biological Psychiatry, 52(2), 101-110.

Shaywitz, S. (1996, November). Dyslexia. Scientific American, 98-105.

Slingerland, B. H. (1976). A multisensory approach to language arts for specific language disability children. Cambridge, MA: Educators Publishing Service.

Smith, C. R. (1991). Learning disabilities: The interaction of learner, task, and setting. Needham Heights, MA: Allyn and Bacon.

Socre, L., and Masterson, J. (2001). Single word spelling test. York, UK: NFER-Nelson.

Solan, H. A., and Ficarra, A. P. (1990). A study of perceptual and verbal skills of disabled readers in grades 4, 5 and 6. Journal of Amercian Optometrists Association, 61, 628-634.

Spear-Swerling, L., and Sternberg, R. J. (1998). Off track: When poor readers become learning disabled. Boulder, CO: Westview Press.

Stanley, G. (1994). Visual deficit models of dyslexia. In G. Hales (Ed.), Dyslexia matters (pp. 19-29). London, UK: Whurr Publishers.

Stanovich, K. E. (1986). Matthew effects in reading: Some consequences of individual differences in the acquisition of literacy. Reading Research Quarterly, 21, 360-364.

Stanovich, K. E. (1991). Discrepancy definitions of reading disability: Has intelligence led us astray? Reading Research Quarterly, 26, 7-29.

Stanovich, K. E. (1994). Annotation: Does dyslexia exist? Journal of Child Psychology and Psychiatry, 35, 579-595.

Stein, J., and Walsh, V. (1997). To see but not to read: The magnocellular theory of dyslexia. Trends in Neurosciences, 20(4), 147-152.

Stephenson, S. (1907). Six cases of congenital word-blindness affecting three generations of one family. The Ophthalmoscope, 5, 482-484.

Strauss, A. A. (1943). Diagnosis and education of the cripple-brained, deficient child. Exceptional Children, 9, 163-168.

Strauss, A. A., and Lehtinen, L. (1947). Psychopathology and education of the brain injured child. New York, NY: Grune and Stratton.

Strauss, A. A., and Werner, H. (1939). Disorders of conceptual thinking in the brain-injured child. Journal of Nervous and Mental Disease, 96, 153-172.

Sundet, K. (1986). Sex differences in cognitive impairment following unilateral brain damage. Journal of Clinical and Experimental Neurospsychology, 8(1), 51-61.

Tallal, P. (1996). Language comprehension in language-learning impaired children. Amercian Association for the Advancement of Science Newsletter, 271(5245), 8.

Tannock, R. (2014). DSM-5 changes in diagnostic criteria for specific learning disabilities: What are the implications? Retrieved from: http://dyslexia help.umich.edu/sites/default/files/IDA_DSM-5%20 Changes.pdf/.

Thomas, C. J. (1905). Congenital word-blindness and its treatment. The Ophthalmoscope, 3, 380-385.

Tomatis, A. (1969). Dyslexia. Ottawa, Ontario, Canada: University of Ottawa Press.

Tonnessen, F. E. (1997). How can we best define dyslexia? Dyslexia, 3, 78-92.

Torgesen, J. K. (1991). Learning disabilities: Historical and conceptual issues. In B. Y. L. Wong (Ed.), Learning about learning disabilities (pp. 3-37). San Diego, CA: Academic Press.

Travis, J. (1996). Let the games begin. Science News, 149(7), 104.

Tyre, C., and Young, P. (1994). Specific learning difficulties. Staffordshire, UK: QED.

Uhl, W. L. (1916). The use of the results of reading tests as bases for planning remedial work. Elementary School Journal, 17, 266-275.

Uhry, J. K., and Clark, D. B. (2005). Dyslexia: Theory and practice of instruction (3rd ed.). Austin, TX: Pro-Ed.

US Department of Education (2006). Individuals with Disabilities Education Act (IDEA) 2004, Section 300.8 Child with a Disability. Washington, DC: The Author.

Vaughan, J., and Estes, T. (1986). Reading and reasoning beyond the primary grades. Boston, MA: Allyn and Bacon.

Waites, L. (1968). Dyslexia International World Federation of Neurology: Report of research group on developmental dyslexia and world illiteracy. Bulletin of the Orton Society, 18, 21-22.

Wallace, G., and Hammill, D. D. (2013). Comprehensive receptive and expressive vocabulary test (3rd ed.). Torrance, CA: Western Psychological Services.

Wallin, J. E. (1920). Congential word-blindness: Some analysis of cases. The Training School Bulletin, 71, 37-47.

Warburg, F. (1911). Ueber die angeborene Wortblindheit und die Bedeutnung ihrer Kenntines fuer den Unterricht Zeit. Kinderforsch., 16, 97.

Wernicke, O. (1874). Der aphasiche symptomenkomplex. Breslau, Germany: Cohn and Weigert.

Wernicke, O. (1903). Ceguera verbal congénital. Revista de la Sociedad Médica Argenitna, 11, 477-485.

Wilkins, A. (1996). Helping reading with color. Dyslexia Review, 7, 3.

Williams, J. (1977). The impact and implication of litigation. In G. Markel (Ed.), Proceedings of the University of Michigan Instgitute on the Impact and implications of State and Federal Legislation affecting Handicapped Individuals (pp. 147-159). Ann Arbor, MI: University of Michigan School of Education.

Wilsher, C. R., and Taylor (1986). Remedies for dyslexia: Proven and unproven. Early Child Development and Care, 27, 287-299.

Witelson, S. (1977). Developmental dyslexia: Two right hemisphere and none left? Science, 195, 309-311.

World Federation of Neurology (1968). Report of research group on developmental dyslexia and world illiteracy. Bulletin of the Orton Society, 18, 21-22.

In: Dyslexia: Perspectives, Challenges and Treatment Options ISBN: 978-1-63485-328-6
Editor: Marilyn Frazier

Chapter 12

NEUROPSYCHOLOGICAL REHABILITATION AS PART OF TREATMENT FOR DEVELOPMENTAL DYSLEXIA

Ricardo Franco de Lima* and Sylvia Maria Ciasca
Department of Neurology, State University of Campinas (UNICAMP), Campinas, Brazil

ABSTRACT

Individuals with developmental dyslexia have multiple neurocognitive deficits. Among them, there can be highlighted the difficulties in executive functions (EF) that impair the study competences and academic skills. Therefore, the aim of this chapter was to describe the development of the neuropsychological rehabilitation program in executive functions for students with dyslexia. The elaboration of neuropsychological rehabilitation program involves of the following stages: (1) Theoretical basis (cognitive neuropsychology, cognitive behavior therapy, self-regulated learning models); (2) Definition of session structures (planning, execution and evaluation); (3) Development of support materials (informative materials, record-keeping forms, games, strategy support material, and cards containing a summary of each strategy learned); evaluation by three expert judges; revision; and elaboration of the final version of the application guide. The final program consists of at least thirty sessions divided into four modules: (1) Psychoeducation; (2) Orientation for parents and teachers; (3) Executive functions applied to study competences; and (4) executive functions applied to reading comprehension. The central goal of the program is to stimulate executive functioning in students with developmental dyslexia. In addition, the program should promote self-regulated learning, especially for study competencies (use of time, organization of the study environment and materials, homework, note-taking, and preparing for exams) and reading comprehension. The chapter discusses aspects of intervention with young students with dyslexia and implications of the proposed program for the practice of clinical neuropsychology.

Keywords: developmental dyslexia, executive functions, neuropsychological rehabilitation

* Corresponding author: Ricardo Franco de Lima. Email: ricardolima01@yahoo.com.br.

DEVELOPMENTAL DYSLEXIA

Developmental dyslexia (DD) is a specific learning disorder of neurobiological origin that affects reading development, in a manner that cannot be explained by intellectual performance, sensory alterations, or inadequate schooling (World Health Organization - WHO, 2008; American Psychiatric Association - APA, 2014). When defining DD, the International Dyslexia Association (IDA) emphasizes impairments to word decoding, fluent recognition of words, and, therefore, reading comprehension (Lyon et al., 2003). Figure 1 displays the diagnostic guidelines proposed in the International Classification of Diseases (ICD-10; WHO, 2008) and in the Statistical Manual of Mental Disorders (DSM-5; APA, 2014).

Proper DD diagnosis requires multidisciplinary input that takes into account the guidelines indicated above as well as the individual's clinical profile. The evaluation must be conducted by professionals in the areas of neuropsychology, speech therapy, psychopedagogy, neurology, and child/teenager psychiatry. Moreover, clinical observation and careful consideration of quantitative and qualitative test results constitute crucial steps of the diagnosis process (Ciasca et al., 2015).

Different theoretical models explain the cognitive phenotype of DD (Badian, 1997; Wolf and Bowers, 1999; Stein, 2001; Fawcett, 2001; Facoetti et al., 2003; Soriano-Ferrer, 2004; Heim et al., 2008; Menguini et al., 2010). However, the prevailing hypothesis presupposes the existence of a phonological deficit, characterized by difficulties in the grapheme-phoneme conversion, phonological conscience, verbal memory, lexical access and, consequently, comprehension (Soriano-Ferrer, 2004). Beyond language-related aspects, other models focus on automation deficits (Wolf and Bowers, 1999), orthographic abilities (Badian, 1997), magnocellular (Stein, 2001; Heim et al., 2008) and motor systems (Fawcett et al., 2001) as well as visual-spatial attention (Facoetti et al., 2003; Menguini et al., 2010). Among altered cognitive domains in DD, the executive functions (EF) have been the focus of study for many researchers in Brazil (Lima et al., 2013a; Lima et al., 2013b) and abroad (Varvara et al., 2014; Moura et al., 2015), because of their involvement in higher reading processes such as comprehension (Sesma et al., 2009).

The EF represent a multifactorial construct comprising cognitive abilities that help in the autonomous involvement with goal-oriented tasks (Diamond, 2013). From an operational perspective, the EF participate in every step of such tasks, including goal setting; planning; prioritizing; organizing; selecting strategies; self-monitoring and recognizing mistakes; having cognitive flexibility to change strategy; having inhibitory, attentional and interference control; and self-evaluating (Sánchez-Carpintero and Narbona, 2004).

A number of cognitive models have been developed with the objective of differentiating principal and secondary EF components (Tirapu-Ustárroz et al., 2008; Kluwe-Schiavon et al., 2012). Miyake et al. (2000) described a psychometric model that divides the EF into three components: cognitive flexibility (alternation of the mental state), operational memory (information updating and monitoring), and inhibitory control (inhibition of overbearing answers). Recently, Diamond (2013) proposed a model based on a review of different studies. According to the author, inhibitory control, mental flexibility and operational memory provide an adequate initial description of the EF. Subsequently, more complex processes are derived such as planning, reasoning and problem solving.

ICD-10 (OMS, 2008) F81.0 – Specific reading disability	DSM-5 (APA, 2014) 315.00 – Specific learning disability with negative effects on reading
(A) The individual's reading performance lies below the expected given the age, overall intelligence, and school year. Performance must be evaluated with the use of standardized tests of reading comprehension taken separately by each individual; (B) In the initial stages of learning, individual may have difficulties in reciting the alphabet, naming letters, rhyming, analyzing and categorizing sounds; (C) The individual has difficulties in oral reading: omissions, substitutions, additions, inversions, phonetic or syllabic inversions, slow reading, and clear difficulties in the graphem-phonem conversion; (D) The individual has limited reading comprehension: difficulty remembering texts, or making inferences based on texts; difficulty using common knowledge to develop answers to questions about texts.	(A) The individual has difficulty in learning and applying academic abilities, as indicated by at least one symptom persisting for over six months, in spite of interventions (lack of precision when reading words, lack of fluency or slow reading, poor reading comprehension); (B) The individual's affected abilities fall substantially and qualitatively below the expected for her or his chronological age, affecting academic or professional performance, as assessed by standardized tests and broad evaluations. (C) The individual might have difficulties starting in her or his school years, but these difficulties will only become apparent when the level of demand exceeds the individual's limited capacity. (D) The individual's difficulties cannot be explained by intellectual deficits, poor eye sight, untreated hearing impairment, other mental or neurologic conditions, psychosocial adversities, lack of proficiency in the language of instruction, or inadequate schooling.

Figure 1. Guidelines for the diagnosis of developmental dyslexia (DD).

Figure 2 summarizes deficits to the EF in individuals with DD that were described in comparative studies. These findings lend support to the hypothesis that DD involves multiple neurocognitive alterations, and not only a dysfunction to phonological processing. The deficits described in Figure 2 have a deeper negative impact on academic performance, especially in situations involving reading, comprehension, and writing.

Based on the current evidence, researchers could aim at developing DD interventions that would take EF alterations into account. Available intervention programs usually emphasize the language aspect using phonological remediation (Galuschka et al., 2014). Thus, intervention in other areas, such as neuropsychology, represents a fertile field for investigation and development.

NEUROPSYCHOLOGICAL REHABILITATION AND DYSLEXIA

Different terms are used to define interventions in patients with congenital or acquired lesions, or in those with functional alterations. In neuropsychology, the most common include cognitive rehabilitation, cognitive training, and neuropsychological rehabilitation (Wilson, 2008; Ciccerone et al., 2011; Gindri et al., 2012; Wilson, 2013).

Studies	Participants	Tests	Results
Helland and Asbjørnsen (2000)	Dyslexia group (DG) = 43 Control group (CG) = 20	Dichotic listening test; Wisconsin Card Sorting Test (WCST)	Deficits in all tests.
Brosnan et al. (2002)	Study 1. DG = 9 (mean age – MA = 34 yrs) CG=9 (MA = 30 yrs) Study 2. DG = 30 (MA = 14 yrs); CG = 30 (MA = 13.8 yrs) Study 3. DG = 15 (MA = 23 yrs); CG = 15 (MA = 24 yrs) Study 4. DG = 16 (MA = 9.9 yrs); CG = 16 (MA = 9.9 yrs)	Digit Span (WAIS-R); Group-embedded figures test (GEFT); Verbal fluency test (FAS); Tower of Hanoi; Figure arrangement (WAIS-R). To-be-recalled (TBR) list GEFT. Digit Span (WAIS-R); Battery subtests CANTAB FAS; Digits (WISC-III); Long-term memory evaluation.	Deficits to the verbal operational memory, inhibitory control, and verbal fluency. Similar to study 1. Deficits to the verbal operational memory. Deficits to the verbal operational memory, verbal fluency, and to the recovery of temporally-organized information.
Reiter et al. (2005)	DG = 42 CG = 42 (MA = 10.8 yrs)	Visual working memory task; Digit span (reverse order); Digit span (direct order); Flexibility task; Go/No Go test; Stroop Color Word Test (SCWT); Tower of London (ToL); Modified card sorting test (MCST); Trail Making Test (TMT); S-word test; Animal test; Five-point test	Deficits to the verbal and figurative operational memory, inhibition of inappropriate reactions, figurative and verbal fluency, and flexibility.
Lima et al. (2013a)	DG = 20 (MA = 9.70 yrs) CG = 20 (MA = 9.05 yrs)	Code, search for arithmetic symbols, and digits subtests (WISC-III); Distraction resistance index and processing speed index (WISC-III); Canceling Tests (CT), TMT A/B, SCWT, ToL, WCST, FAS	Deficits to visual-spatial attention and EF components: flexibility, inhibition control, use of strategies, verbal operational memory, and verbal fluency.
Lima et al. (2013b)	DG = 31 (MA = 9.70) CG = 30 (MA = 9.05)	Code, search for arithmetic symbols, and digits – indirect order subtests (WISC-III); processing speed index (WISC-III); TC; TMT-A/B; SCWT; ToL, WCST; FAS	Deficits to attention and flexibility, inhibition control, use of strategies, verbal operational memory, verbal and phonological fluency, and planning
Varvara et al. (2014)	DG = 65 (MA = 11.4) CG = 65 (MA = 11.9)	Colored Progressive Matrices; reading battery subtest for DD diagnosis; Category fluency test; Phonological fluency test; Spoonerism task; "map mission" and "code transmission task" subtests of the "Test of everyday attention for children"; subtests of the PROMEA (Prove di Memoria e Apprendimento per l'Eta Evolutiva); WCST	Deficits to different EF components: verbal category and phonological fluency, visual-spatial and hearing attention, phonological conscience, verbal and visual short-term memories, and verbal operational memory.
Moura et al. (2015)	DG = 50 (MA = 9.80) CG = 50 (MA = 9.82)	Code and Search for Symbols subtests (WISC-III), TMT-A and B subtests, Tower test, semantic and phonemic verbal fluency of the Coimbra Neuropsychological Assessment Battery (BANC)	Deficits to speed processing, flexibility, and verbal fluency after adjusting for intelligence level.

Figure 2. Summary of EF deficits found in individuals with DD in different comparative studies.

The term "neuropsychological rehabilitation" (NR) has been applied to the broad clinical process that aims at improving cognitive and behavioral deficits stemming from brain damage or functional alterations (Lopez-Luengo, 2001; Ginarte-Aria, 2002; Wilson, 2013). It is expected that NR might promote change to important areas that affect the patient's daily life, i.e., that it might have ecological value (Abrisqueta-Gomez, 2012), and not only an effect on the restitution of impaired cognitive functions.

The activities developed in NR programs are systematic and might involve cognitive training, learning the use of compensatory strategies, organization and routine planning, as well as the practice of functional activities. The NR can be conducted individually or in groups, with the use of modules complemented with psychoeducational and psychotherapeutic activities and orientation. Furthermore, an adequate program requires the participation of a multidisciplinary team (Abrisqueta-Gomez, 2012).

Setting goals among patient, family members and team represents a crucial step in the NR, which allows for the identification of priorities, progress evaluation, and the sub-division of the program in phases. The acronym SMART(ER) summarizes these principles: specific, measurable, achievable, realistic, timely, evaluation and review (Wilson, 2008; 2009; Miotto, 2015). In addition to cognitive aspects, emotional and psychosocial difficulties can also be included among the NR goals (Wilson, 2008).

Important methodological aspects must be taken into account during an NR program (López-Luengo, 2000; Ginarte-Arias, 2002): the evaluation must identify altered and preserved areas; goals should be individual and adapted to patient needs; the family must be involved; the program must take into account intervening variables; training starts with nuclear aspects and gradually includes activities from daily life; in the beginning activities should demand less attention; the program must make use of materials that are part of the patient's life; materials as well as visual, hearing and tactile stimuli should be diversified and could include technological resources; the level of difficulty should be adjusted to allow the patient to finish each session with more positive than negative results; instructive and educational components should be included; metacognitive training should be conducted, after the patient understands what is the cognitive function and the available strategies to work on it; sessions should take place sequentially and hierarchically; materials should motivate the patient; the therapist should give feedback on the performance and patient progress, rewarding success; the program should be generalizable to daily life and not only target test improvements; intervention efficacy should be monitored with systematic registers, and instruments to evaluate the perception of improvement.

Among theoretical principles that lend subsidies to NR programs, transference is indicated as one of the main objectives (Barnett and Ceci, 2002; Gindri et al., 2012; Nikaedo, 2015). In general, transference represents an improvement to a specific cognitive domain, task or ability (Barnett and Ceci, 2002; Gindri et al., 2012; Nikaedo, 2015). The NR may be complemented with the principles set forth in the International Classification of Functioning, Disability and Health (ICF; WHO 2003). Such principles target the reduction of functional consequences of neurological deficits and disadvantages that individuals might have when performing, for example, academic activities (Loschiavo-Alvares et al., 2011).

Among children and teenagers, NR or cognitive training studies more commonly focus on Attention Deficit and Hiperactivity Disorder (ADHD) or traumatic brain injury (TBI) (Yelin, 1996; Tucha et al., 2011). In contrast, few researchers have investigated NR as a tool for the treatment of DD.

An integrating review of the literature searched for NR studies conducted with children and/or teenagers affected by DD, to identify the most commonly used programs, their theoretical basis and efficacy. The databases available from Pubmed, PsycNET, Scopus and Proquest Central were surveyed with the following key-words: *Neuropsychological* OR *cognitive* AND *Intervention* OR *Treatment* AND *Dyslexia* OR *Reading Disorder* OR *Reading Problems* OR *Reading Difficulties* AND *Children* OR *Child*. Results included 506 registered studies. Subsequently, abstracts were read and analyzed according to the following criteria: (a) study objective should be to investigate an NR intervention method targeting individuals with DD; (b) study participants should have a DD diagnosis; (c) the study should focus on NR and not on the remediation of a specific function; (d) the abstract should be available; (e) studies should be in English or Spanish; (f) studies should have been performed with a randomized, controlled clinical method; or should constitute a case study; (g) studies should have been conducted in the last 30 years (i.e., starting in 1987) (Lima et al., 2013c).

After initial abstract analysis, 494 studies were eliminated, and 12 studies were included in the study sample. This body of work was published between 1987 and 2011, five were Italian (42%), three were from the United States (25%), two were from the Netherlands (17%), one from Australia and one from the United Kingdom (8% each). Sample sizes varied from six to 135 participants. Among the studies, three included a combination of intellectual evaluation and reading (25%), three included attention evaluation and reading (25%), in two 8%an evaluation of different types of memory and reading was conducted (17%), another two only evaluated reading (17%), one included a complete neuropsychological evaluation with instruments for the different cognitive functions (8%), and one had instruments for intellectual, reading, and behavioral scale evaluations (Lima et al., 2013c).

Ten of the studies (83%) applied or were based on the model developed by Bakker and colleagues (Bakker, 1990; Bakker et al., 1995). Among the 12 studies, three (25%) used the two versions (Hemisphere Specific Stimulation - HSS e Hemisphere Alluding Stimulation - HAS); three (25%) only used the HSS; one (8%) used a combination of the Bakker model with educational principles; one (8%) used the same model coupled to cognitive and information processing psychology; one (8%) compared visual HSS (VHSS) with traditional speech therapy; one (8%) compared HSS to Reading-focused training (RT); one (8%) used Computerized Perceptual Therapy Program; and one (8%) used intervention with a neuropsychological approach (Lima et al., 2013b).

Currently, Bakker model programs are often used by Italian researchers aiming at the stimulation of in hemispheres with the tachitoscopic presentation of words to the visual fields (visual training), with stimuli to the left or right hand (tactile training), or, still, with verbal stimuli and exercises using paper and pencil (Lorusso et al., 2006; Lorusso et al., 2011). During the database searches no Brazilian studies were found describing systematic NR programs for DD.

Based on these results, Lima et al. (2014) proposed a neuropsychological rehabilitation program focused on students with DD with the objective of stimulating the EF through learning strategies. The clinical rationale for such interventions includes the involvement of EFs on the supervision and top-down control of information processing; with higher reading processes (i.e., comprehension); with school performance; and their role as indicators of psychological development.

Psychoeducation Sessions that provide information and educate about DD and the NR program: overall process, session models, equipment and accessories used.	Orientation Meetings with parents and teachers during the rehabilitation process that have as objectives answering questions, monitoring the use of strategies, establishing rewards, and agreeing to changes in the patient's environment.
Executive functions applied to study competencies Sessions with the patient that have as objectives learning EF strategies concerning time management, learning how to finish homework, how to take notes and how to study for exams.	Executive functions applied to reading Sessions with the patient that have as objectives learning EF strategies for text comprehension.

Figure 3. Modules of the neuropsychological rehabilitation program for the EF.

Program elaboration consisted of four stages including development of a theoretical basis, structural organization, analysis by independent expert judges, revision and elaboration of final version. In its final form the NR program comprised 30 sessions divided into four modules (Figure 3).

The NR session structure was based on models of self-regulated learning (Zimmerman, 1986; Pintrich, 2000; Rosário, 2004) and on the Self-Regulated Strategy Development – SRSD (Graham and Harris, 1996; Harris et al., 2012). Self-regulated learning, from a motivational, metacognitive and behavioral perspective, gives the student a high degree of independence in fulfilling educational demands (Zimmerman et al., 2002). Overall, self-regulated learning includes processes such as goal setting, following rules, using adequate cognitive and metacognitive strategies, organizing the study space, efficacious use of resources, monitoring one's own performance, time management, seeking help when needed, maintaining positive belief in self-efficacy; perceiving value in learning, identifying factors that affect learning, anticipating results of actions and experiencing satisfaction with one's own efforts (Schunk and Ertner, 2000).

The SRSD has been applied towards the development of reading and writing abilities among young students (Graham and Harris, 1996) and different studies have shown its efficacy (García-Sánchez and Fidalgo-Redondo, 2006; Schünemann et al., 2013). It represents an instructional approach that combines explicit strategy teaching with self-regulation. It is a model that helps teachers with reading and writing assignments by stimulating self-regulation and EF components. The SRSD strategic instruction includes six stages that, although chronologically organized, can be re-combined or re-applied depending on student needs: (1) Developing and activating prior knowledge; (2) Discussing the strategy; (3) Modeling the strategy; (4) Memorizing the strategy; (5) Lending support to the strategy; (6) Independent practice (Mason et al., 2012; Harris et al., 2012).

The efficacy of the NR program was evaluated by two empirical studies. The first included six students with DD diagnosis, and an average age of 14.67 years (±1.03), who were compared to a control sample of seven students with no learning difficulties using different neuropsychological and ecological instruments to probe EF and reading. The inter- and intragroup analyses before and after tests, indicated an improvement among students with DD in attention, memory, inhibition control, flexibility, verbal fluency, use of learning strategies, and reading comprehension. There was also a decrease in the number of teacher complaints regarding EF problems. The second study followed a single-case experimental design, and was conducted with a 13-year old boy, with DD, in the seventh grade who was evaluated before and after rehabilitation with EF and reading instruments. The individual's performance was compared to those of six control students with no learning difficulties. The NR had positive effects on inhibition control, working memory, planning, on the use of learning and comprehension strategies and on reading comprehension. Altogether, the results from both studies suggest that the NR program efficiently reduced the deficits of students with DD, and has clinical relevance for interdisciplinary treatment (Lima, 2015).

Thus, clinical intervention aimed at EF components and the way they are organized to accomplish goals, can improve the performance of individuals with DD in school activities and reading. The methods and techniques should not only provide stimuli for dysfunctional abilities, but they also should have general effects on other cognitive functions under distinct contexts.

Acknowledgments

The first author received funding of the Coordination for the Improvement of Higher Education Personnel (Capes, Brazil) as part of his doctorate degree.

References

Abrisqueta-Gomez, J. (2012). Reabilitação cognitiva baseada em evidências científicas: recomentações para a prática clínica (Cognitive rehabilitation based on scientific evidence: reccomendations for clinical practice). In: Abrisqueta-Gomez J. *Reabilitação neuropsicológica: abordagem interdisciplinar e modelos conceituais na prática clínica.* Porto Alegre: Artmed.

American Psychiatric Association - APA (2014). *DSM-5: Manual Diagnóstico e Estatístico de Transtornos Mentais* (DSM-5: Diagnostic and Statistical Manual of Mental Disorders). 5 ed. rev. Porto Alegre: Artes Médicas.

Badian, N. A. (1997). Dyslexia and the double deficit hypothesis. *Annals of Dyslexia*, 47, 69-87.

Barnett, S. M., and Ceci, S.J. (2002). When and where do we apply what we learn? A taxonomy for far transfer. *Psychological Bulletin* 128, 612-637.

Bakker, D. J (1990). Neuropsychological treatment of dyslexia. New York, NY: Oxford University Press.

Bakker, D. J., Licht, R., and Kappers, E.J. (1995). Hemisphere specific treatment of dyslexia. In: G. Tramontana, and S. R. Hooper (Eds.), *Advances in child neuropsychology* (Vol. 3, pp. 144-177). New York/Berlin: Springer-Verlag.

Brosnan, M., Demetre, J., Hamill, S., Robson, K., Shepherd, H., and Cody, G. (2002). Executive functioning in adults and children with developmental dyslexia. *Neuropsychologia*, 40, 2144-2155.

Ciasca, S. M., Rodrigues, S.D., Salgado-Azoni, C.A., and Lima, R.L. (2015). *Transtornos de aprendizagem: neurociência e interdisciplinaridade* (Learning disorders: neuroscience and interdisciplinarity). São Paulo: Book Toy.

Ciccerone, K. D., Dahlberg, C., Kalmar, K., Langenbahn, D.M., Malec, J.F. et al. (2000). Evidence-based cognitive rehabilitation: recommendations for clinical practice. *Archives of Physical Medicine and Rehabilitation*, 81, 1596-1615.

Diamond, A. (2013). Executive functions. *Annual Review of Psychology*, 64, 135-168.

Facoetti, A., Trussardi, A. N., Ruffino, M., Lorusso, M. L., Cattaneo, C., Molteni, M., and Zorzi, M. (2010). Multisensory spatial attention deficits are predictive of phonological decoding skills in developmental dyslexia. *Journal of Cognitive Neuroscience*, 22, 1011-1025.

Facoetti, A., Lorusso, M. L., Paganoni, P., Cattaneo, C., Galli, R., and Mascetti, G. G. (2003). The time course of attentional focusing in dyslexic and normally reading children. *Brain and Cognition*, 53, 181-118.

Fawcett, A. J. (2011). Balance and reading are separate symptoms of dyslexia. *Developmental Medicine and Child Neurology*, 53, 292-297.

Galuschka, K., Ise, E., Krick, K., and Schulte-Körne, G. (2014). Effectiveness of treatment approaches for children and adolescents with reading disabilities: a meta-analysis of randomized controlled trials. *Plos One*, 9, 1-12.

García-Sánchez, J. N., and Fidalgo-Redondo, R. (2006). Effects of two types of self-regulatory instruction programs on students with learning disabilities in writing products, processes, and self-efficacy. *Learning Disability Quarterly* 2006, 29, 181-211.

Ginarte-Arias, Y. (2002). Rehabilitación cognitiva (cognitive rehabilitation). Aspectos teóricos y metodológicos (theoretical and methodological aspects). *Revista de Neurología*, 35, 870-876.

Gori, S., Cecchini, P., Bigoni, A., Molteni, M., Facoetti A. (2014). Magnocellular-dorsal pathway and sub-lexical route in developmental dyslexia. *Frontiers in Human Neuroscience*, 8, 1-11.

Graham, S., Harris, K.R. (1996). Addressing problems in attention, memory, and executive functioning: an example from Self-Regulated Strategy Development. In: Lyon R, Krasnegor N (Eds.) *Attention, memory, and executive function*. Baltimore: Brookes.

Gindri, G., Frison, T. B., Oliveira, C., Zimmermann, N., Netto, T. M., Landeira-Fernandez, J. et al. (2012). Métodos em reabilitação neuropsicológica (Methods in neuropsychological rehabilitation). In: Landeira-Fernandez J, Fukusima S (orgs.). *Métodos em neurociência*. São Paulo: Manole.

Harris, K. R., Graham, S., Mason, L. H., and Friedlander, B. (2012). *Powerful writing strategies for all students*. Baltimore: Paul H Brooks.

Heim, S., Tschierse, J., Amunts, K., Wilms, M., Vossel, S., Willmes, K. et al. (2008). Cognitive subtypes of dyslexia. *Acta Neuroliologiae Experimentalis*, 68, 73-82.

Helland, T., and Asbjørnsen, A. (2000). Executive functions in dyslexia. *Child Neuropsychology*, 6, 37-48.

Kluwe-Schiavon, B., Viola, T.W., Grassi-Oliveira, R. (2012). Modelos teóricos sobre construto único ou múltiplos processos das funções executivas (Theoretical models of single construct or multiple processes of executive functions). *Revista Neuropsicología Latinoamericana*, 4, 29-34.

Lima, R. F. (2015). *Neuropsychological rehabilitation program in executive functions for students with developmental dyslexia: elaboration and efficacy*. State University of Campinas; Campinas/SP, Brazil.

Lima, R. F., Salgado-Azoni, C. A., and Ciasca, S. M. (2013a). Attentional and executive deficits in Brazilian children with developmental dyslexia. *Psychology* 4, 1-6.

Lima, R. F., Salgado-Azoni, C. A., and Ciasca, S. M. (2013b). Atenção e funções executivas em crianças com dislexia do desenvolvimento (Attention and executive functions in children with developmental dyslexia). *Psicologia em Pesquisa*, 7, 208-19.

Lima, R. F.; Salgado-Azoni, C. A.; and Ciasca, S. M. (2013c). Reabilitação neuropsicológica na dislexia do desenvolvimento: revisão integrativa da literatura (Neuropsychological rehabilitation in developmental dyslexia: integrative literature review). *Anais do XXII Congresso Brasileiro e II Congresso Internacional da ABENEPI*. Belo Horizonte, Minas Gerais. p. 140.

Lima, R. F.; Alves, R. J. R.; Salgado-Azoni, C. A.; and Ciasca, S. M. (2014). Neuropsychological rehabilitation for promoting executive functioning in students with developmental dyslexia. *Annals of II World Dyslexia Forum*. Belo Horizonte, Minas Gerais, p. 29.

Loschiavo-Alvares, F.Q., Sediyama, C.Y.N., Rivero, T.S., Nicolato, R., Neves, F. et al. (2011). Tools for efficacy's assessment of neuropsychological rehabilitation programs: a systematic review. *Child Neuropsychiatry*, 8, 1-11.

López-Luengo, B. (2001). Orientaciones en rehabilitación cognitiva (Guidance on cognitive rehabilitation). *Revista de Neurología*, 33, 383-387.

Lorusso, M. L., Facoetti, A., Paganoni, P., Pezzani, M., and Molteni, M. (2006). Effects of visual hemisphere-specific stimulation versus reading-focused training in dyslexic children. *Neuropsychological Rehabilitation*, 16, 194-212.

Lorusso, M. L., Facoetti, A., and Bakker, D. J. (2011). Neuropsychological treatment of dyslexia: does type of treatment matter? *Journal of Learning Disabilities*, 44, 136-149.

Lyon, G. R., Shaywitz, S. E., and Shaywitz, B. A. (2003). Defining Dyslexia, comorbidity, teachers' knowledge of language and reading: a definition of dyslexia. *Annals of Dyslexia*, 53, 1-14.

Mason, L. H., Reid, R., and Hanagan, J. L. (2012). *Building comprehension in adolescents*. Baltimore: Paul H Brooks.

Menghini, D., Finzi, A., Benassi, M., Bolzani, R., Facoetti, A., Giovagnoli, S. et al. (2010). Different underlying neurocognitive deficits in developmental dyslexia: A comparative study. *Neuropsychologia*, 48, 863-72.

Miotto, E. C. (2015). Conceitos fundamentais, história, modelos teóricos em reabilitação neuropsicológica e planejamento de metas (Fundamental concepts, history, theoretical models in neuropsychological rehabilitation and planning goals). In: Miotto E. C. (org). *Reabilitação neuropsicológica e intervenções comportamentais*. Rio de Janeiro: Rocca.

Miyake, A., Friedman, N. P., Emerson, M. J., Witzki, H., and Howerter, A. (2000). The unity and diversity of executive functions and their contributions to complex "frontal lobe" tasks: a latent variable analysis. *Cognitive Psychology*, 41, 49-100.

Moura, O., Simões, M. R., and Pereira, M. (2015). Executive functioning in children with developmental dyslexia. *The Clinical Neuropsychologist*, 28(Suppl. 1), S20-41.

Nikaedo, C. C. (2015). Funções executivas na infância: conceitos da avaliação dinâmica aplicados à intervenção (Executive functions in children: dynamic evaluation of concepts applied to the intervention). In: Miotto EC (org.). *Reabilitação neuropsicológica e intervenções comportamentais*. Rio de Janeiro: Rocca.

Pintrich, P. R. (2000). The role of goal orientation in self-regulated learning. In: Boekaerts M; Pintrich PR, Zeidner M. (eds.) *Handbook of self-regulation*. Academic Press.

Reiter, A., Tucha, O., Lange, K.W. (2005). Executive functions in children with dyslexia. *Dyslexia*, 11, 116-31.

Rosário, P. S. L. (2004). *Estudar o Estudar: As (Des)venturas do Testas* (Study the study: The (Un) venturas the Brows). Porto, Porto Editora.

Sánchez-Carpintero, R., and Narbona, J. (2004). El sistema ejecutivo y las lesiones frontales en el niño (The executive system and frontal lesions in children). *Revista de Neurología*, 39, 188-91.

Schünemann, N., Spörer, N., Brunstein, J.C. (2013). Integrating self-regulation in whole-class reciprocal teaching: A moderator–mediator analysis of incremental effects on fifth graders' reading comprehension. *Contemporary Educational Psychology*, 38, 289-305.

Schunk, D. H., Ertmer, P. A. (2000). Self-regulation and academic learning: Self-efficacy enhancing interventions. In: Boekaerts M, Pintrich PR, Zeidner M. (eds.) *Handbook of self-regulation*. Academic Press.

Sesma, H. W., Mahone, E. M., Levine, T., Eason, S. H., and Cutting L. E. (2009). The contribution of executive skills to reading comprehension. *Child Neuropsychology*, 15, 232-246.

Soriano-Ferrer, M. (2004). Implicaciones educativas del déficit cognitivo de la dislexia evolutiva. *Revista de Neurología*, 38(Supl. 1), S47-52.

Stein, J. (2001). The magnocellular theory of developmental dyslexia. *Dsylexia*, 7, 12-36.

Tirapu-Ustárroz, J., García-Molina, A., Luna-Lario, P., Roig-Rovira, T., Pelegrín-Valero, C. (2008). Modelos de funciones y control ejecutivo (I) (Models of executive control and functions (I)). *Revista de Neurología*, 46, 684-92.

Tucha, O., Tucha, L., Kaumann, G., König, S., Lange, K. M., Stasik, D., Streather, Z., Engelschalk, T., and Lange, K. W. (2011). Training of attention functions in children with attention deficit hyperactivity disorder. *Attention Deficit and Hyperactivity Disorders*, 3, 271-283.

Varvara, P., Varuzza, C., Sorrentino, A. C. P., Vicari, S., and Menghini, D. (2014). Executive functions in developmental dyslexia. *Frontiers in Human Neuroscience* 2014 8: 1 8.

Wilson, B. (2008). Neuropsychological rehabilitation. *Annual Review in Clinical Psychology*, 4, 141-116.

Wilson, B.A. (2013). Neuropsychological rehabilitation: State of the science. *South African Journal of Psychology*, 43, 267-277.

Wolf, M., and Bowers, P. G. (1999). The double-deficit hypothesis for the developmental dyslexias. *Journal of Educational Psychology*, 91, 415-438.

World Health Organization – WHO (2008). *The ICD-10 Classification of Mental and Behavioural Disorders descriptions and diagnostic guidelines*. Geneva: World Health Organization.

World Health Organization – WHO (2001). *International Classification of Functioning, Disability and Health: ICF*. Geneva.

Yelín, B. (1996). Rehabilitación cognitiva en el traumatismo craneal cerrado em niños (Cognitive rehabilitation in children em closed head injury). *Revista de Neurología*, 24, 1393-1397.

Zimmerman, B. J. (1986). Development of self-regulated learning: which are the key subprocesses? *Contemporary Educational Psychology*, 11, 307-313.

Zimmerman, B. J., Bonner, S., and Kovach, R. (2002). Understanding the principles of self-regulated learning. In: Zimmerman, B. J., Bonner, S., and Kovach, R. *Developing self-regulated learners: beyond achievement to self-efficacy.* Washington, American Psychological Association.

BIOGRAPHICAL SKETCH

Dr. Ricardo Franco de Lima is a clinical psychologist, with specializations degree in child neurology and neuropsychology. He has master and doctorate degree in medical sciences (Faculty of Medical Sciences, State University of Campinas – UNICAMP, Brazil). He is currently a member of the "Laboratory of Learning Disabilities and Attention Disorders" (DISAPRE - UNICAMP), and coordinates the "Research Center of Attention and Learning" (CIAPRE). His research focuses on: developmental dyslexia, neuropsychological rehabilitation and executive functions. E-mail: ricardolima01@yahoo.com.br. Web-site: http://disapre.wordpress.com

Professor Sylvia Maria Ciasca is a psychologist, with specialization degree in neuropsychology. She has master degree in Neuroscience and Behavior (University of São Paulo – USP, Brazil) and doctorate in medical sciences (State University of Campinas – UNICAMP). Professor Sylvia is currently associate professor at Department of Neurology (UNICAMP), and coordinates the "Laboratory of Learning Disabilities and Attention Disorders" (DISAPRE - UNICAMP). Her research focuses on: learning disabilities, attention disorder, higher cortical functions, and neuropsychology. E-mail: sciasca@mpc.com.br.

In: Dyslexia: Perspectives, Challenges and Treatment Options ISBN: 978-1-63485-328-6
Editor: Marilyn Frazier

Chapter 13

INTEGRATION OF PROPRIOCEPTIVE SIGNALS, POSTURAL CONTROL AND DYSLEXIA

***P. Quercia*[1] *and L. J. Feiss*[2]**
[1]Department of Ophthalmology, University Hospital, Dijon, France
Univ. Bourgogne Franche-Comté, Dijon, France
[2]Office of Ophthalmology, Beaune, France

ABSTRACT

The traditional conception of perception is largely influenced by the idea that sensory organs are passive sensitive surfaces awaiting stimulation, processing sensory information with the goal of constructing representations of the sensory world. A new trend, however, emphasizes the active and predictive nature of perception. It conceptualizes perception as a continuous interaction between sensory variation and the motor properties of the organism. This view considers perception and action as two interlinked and inseparable phenomena which could practically be described as two facets of the same process. Therefore, all the mechanisms involved at the developmental level, including the installation of motor control loops, are likely to intervene in the existence of perceptual developmental disorders. Proprioception, which plays a central role in motor control and in perception of motion, merits examination of its possible role in developmental disorders such as dyslexia.

The study of proprioception in dyslexics is validated by the following elements:

- In the 80s, Henrique Martins da Cunha noted that many patients with proprioceptive dysfunction responsible for muscular pain of postural origin were also dyslexic. It evokes the hypothesis that proprioception may play a role in the reading disorders of these children.
- Recordings on the stabilometric platform confirm the instability of dyslexics in a static position and clinical examination confirms that all dyslexic children show symptoms suggestive of postural deficiency syndrome.
- The correlation index between the ocular signs described in this syndrome and the presence of specific learning disabilities is very high (+0.90).
- Experimental manipulations of proprioception in a population of dyslexic children show that they have difficulty integrating proprioceptive information.

Keywords: dyslexia, proprioception, postural control, attention

INTRODUCTION

The origin of developmental dyslexia remains hypothetical. In addition to some genetic factor, researchers have evoked an ontogenetic dysfunction of a part of the brain or cerebellum, abnormal magnocellular pathways, a temporal deficit in the processing of sounds and, most often, a neurodevelopmental origin with inadequate development of phonological awareness and the subsequent development of phonological difficulties. This could result in a developmental disturbance in the dyslexic which affects the organization of sounds and the use of visual symbols upon which the acquisition of reading skills depends [1].

While visual and auditory functions have been widely studied, a possible role for proprioception which is part of somesthesia aroused little interest. Recent studies on multisensory integration have demonstrated a close relationship, beginning at the level of the primary cortex, between somesthesia, hearing and vision in the creation of a perceptual coherence of the world around us [2]. These interactions are prolonged in the associative cortical areas and even at the level of certain basal ganglia that have a role in integration for these three senses [3].

PROPRIOCEPTION: A VERY SPECIAL SENSE

Unlike other senses proprioception does not reside in a specific organ. It is distributed in all of the body's muscles. It does not work independently, but in connection with other sensory organs whose function is strongly influenced by the brain's constant reception of information on the orientation of sensors in the body.

To date, two essential functions appear to be linked to proprioceptive activity:

1. *Postural control*: the vertical position of the body, unstable when standing still or moving, requires precise regulation of the center of gravity. This accuracy is only possible if the brain constantly receives proprioceptive information on the state of tension in all muscles. It is from these impulses, associated with sensory information from the eyes, inner ear and plantar surface that the brain can send specifically adapted orders to the muscular system to maintain body stability with minimal energy expenditure. The entire unit functions as a self-regulating, self-sufficient sensorimotor system based on a constant interaction of a copy of efferent motor instructions and predictive internal motor models [4]. There is thus a constant coming and going of information, organized around sensorimotor control loops, which in fact makes perception and action two interlinked and inseparable phenomena. Proprioception plays a crucial role when learning the relationships between perception and action since the quality of muscular information feedback must be high. Its role diminishes over time in favor of the establishment of an effective copy of efferent signals. Proprioception retains a role as a detector of errors

between the command center and the execution of the command center's motor instructions [5].

2. *The spatial localization of sensory information*: visually, spatial localization is very dependent on retinal image topography and the copy of efferent signals created during the central instigation of eye movements. Ocular proprioception would again act to detect the frequent motor errors occurring during the acquisition of reading skills [6]. It has been shown that experimental modification of ocular proprioceptive neuromuscular spindle activity by vibration at specific frequencies changes the visual localization of observed objects. This effect has also been shown by vibrating extra-ocular muscles which participate in an ocular function: for example the superior rectus muscle of the eye that allows one to look up and the trapezius muscle that tilts the shoulders back to accompany the movement of the head inherent to looking up. Further research has led to the identification of "informational proprioceptive chains" extending from the eye to the foot and implicating all muscles involved in postural control [7]. Beyond its role in the spatial localization of viewed objects, ocular proprioception integrates visual attention abilities [8].

Auditory spatial localization depends on sound reflection from the curves and folds of the auricle in the vertical plane and the temporal comparison of sound between both ears in the horizontal plane. When several sounds are present, it is possible to discern the location of each source by analyzing certain intrinsic qualities of the overall perceptual stream (different pace, sudden changes of intensity or spectral form, temporal differences in sound wave release...) [9]. However detecting the position of the head with cervical proprioception, itself closely linked to eye and body proprioception, is essential in these complex situations.

Due to its intervention in the maintenance and information transport of our senses in the space around us, muscle proprioception has been described as "the sense that enables us to make sense of the other senses" [10].

A Historical Note

Henrique Martins da Cunha originally suggested the possibility of a relationship between proprioception and development of dyslexia in the 1980's [11]. Specializing in physical rehabilitation, this physician found numerous patients who complained of chronic migrating pain with no plausible explanation provided by radiological assessment. Careful observation of these patients revealed that they had subconsciously adopted poor postures which would explain the pain. He proposed that the cause for this posturing is faulty integration of proprioceptive information that, in association with other signals from the inner ear, retina and plantar surfaces, was already known at the time as the regulator for body posture. The dysfunction of this system causes a set of varied clinical signs called postural deficiency syndrome (PDS). Patients with this syndrome complain of migratory pain, dizziness and attention disorders as well as reading difficulties suggestive of dyslexia.

Diagnosis and Treatment of Proprioceptive Dysfunction

Currently, the clinical analysis of proprioception is based on the detection of the clinical signs of PDS [12]. The examination searches for asymmetry of muscle tone in the muscles involved in maintaining posture. Scoliotic attitude is the primary finding and, based on the predominance of torsion or anterior-posterior torso displacement, several types of PDS have been described. The projection of the head forward is often accompanied by a low position of the tongue with persistence of an infantile swallowing and buccal respiration with the development eventually of dental malocclusion. In these cases, the frequency of hypopnea is high and this may cause attention disorders. Along with the presence of this tonic asymmetry, the examination reveals visual-spatial disorders responsible for micro-vertical heterophorias whose essential feature is lability during stimulation of postural sensors.

Proprioception can be changed through a therapeutic tripod:

- *Very low power prisms* included in spectacle lenses. They will deflect the light reaching the retina and thereby change the perception of visual space as well as cervical proprioception and the underlying proprioceptive chains. They must eliminate the labile micro-heterophoria. They act primarily on the oblique eye muscles whose regulation is related to postural reflexes.
- *Insoles discreetly thickened*, respecting the response threshold and the topography of pressure sensors in plantar skin.
- *Maintenance of postures* respecting postural muscle physiology and exercises of specific muscles in order to eliminate asymmetry in the tonicity of muscles providing stability and countering gravity's call.

In certain frequently appearing cases, adjuvant treatment of the stomatognathic apparatus is required. The trigeminal nerve innervation of both oral sensitivity and ocular proprioception increases the effect of the prisms by modifying stomatognathic information [13].

Postural Deficiency Syndrome and Dyslexia

We examined a group of 60 children with a mean age of 11.8 ± 1.8 years on whom neuropsychological assessment using standardized tests confirmed the diagnosis of dyslexia [12]. Each child was examined for subjective and objective clinical signs of of PDS. The PDS rate found was close to 100%. The study was completed in another center by looking at PDS rates in a group of 100 patients aged 6 to 25 years seen successively by a family physician for problems other than learning difficulties. The examiner found 13 children with PDS among whom four new cases of a specific learning disorder were diagnosed while 7 others had previous diagnoses (of learning disorders) according to the criteria proposed by the DSM5. The correlation index between the presence of proprioceptive dysfunction and a specific learning disorder in this study is +0.90. The strongly positive predictive value 0.84 and the negative predictive value of 1 suggest that the diagnosis of specific learning disorders can be questioned in the absence of PDS [14].

POSTURAL CONTROL AND DYSLEXIA

Postural stability can be studied using a force platform ((TechnoConcept®France) [15]. The device measures the position of the center of pressure at a frequency of 40Hz. It consists of a rigid surface on which three force sensors are placed in the form of an equilateral triangle. The center of pressure is associated with the projection of the center of gravity of the examined subject. Its variations are visible on a graded scale. Measurements of the oscillations of the body define the characteristics of the postural system of the observed subject. Measuring deviations from the average position gives a reflection of the accuracy and efficiency of the system that a subject uses to maintain stability. The variations in and of themselves give an idea of the tactics that the subject employs to maintain stability.

To evaluate the hypothesis of a relationship between proprioceptive disorders and dyslexia, we conducted a study with the force platform on a group of 50 dyslexic children (mean age 11.5 +/- 1.8 years) and on a group of normal-readers including 40 children (mean age 12.4 +/- 1.7 years) [16]. The children were only evaluated for 25.6 seconds in the bipedal position since it soon became clear that the dyslexic group had significant difficulties trying to remain stable for the usual adult test duration of 51.2 seconds. In the mono-pedal position, the evaluations lasted only 12.8 seconds for the same reasons. The recordings were made with eyes both open and closed, in the bipedal position and finally on just the right or the left foot. The analysis of the results was based on:

- The length of the statokinesigram, which corresponds to the path made by the center of pressure during measurement,
- The standard deviation (SD) of the center of pressure displacement (CoP) on the lateral and anterior-posterior axis,
- The weighted average of the frequency spectrum (Mean Power Frequency - MPF) calculated for the lateral axis and for the anterior-posterior axis.

The Kolmonorov-Smirnoff and Cochran tests were used to verify the normalcy of the data distribution and the homogeneity of their variance. The threshold value was 5%. For statistical validation we used analysis of variance of two factors (dyslexic group + controls) and visual condition (eyes open + eyes closed) with several measurements made in the bipedal position and then in the mono-pedal mode on the right and then the left foot. Since a significant proportion of children had great difficulty standing on one foot during the test, we only used data from (we were only able to calculate the proportion of) the children who managed to stay completely mono-pedal during the acquisition period. To identify dyslexic subjects with abnormal postural performance, we have applied the procedure for evaluation of deviance from the norm as a complement to the bipedal study. This procedure sets a threshold for n SD as the mean of the control group for each parameter. Since control subjects may also occasionally have abnormal postural performance, we calculated the mean and standard deviation of the control group for each parameter of the measurements made in the resting position. As a result, three control subjects who had abnormal performance based on the deviance value (+/- 1.65 SD) were excluded. The mean and SD of each parameter in the control group were recalculated and the dyslexics were identified by their deviation from the mean.

In the bipedal mode, with eyes open or closed, the dyslexic group showed abnormal postural performances except with regard to the CoP on the displacement in the lateral axis. Postural performances of both groups are altered when tested with eyes closed. If we look at the proportion of dyslexic children as a function of the number of postural parameters deviating significantly from the mean, more than half appear to have abnormal postural performance, except for the MPF of the lateral axis.

In the mono-pedal mode, 25% of control subjects showed difficulties in maintaining posture while on the left foot and could not be recorded during the entire data acquisition period, while they had no difficulty maintaining posture when tested standing on the right foot. For the remaining 75%, the performances were impaired on the left foot test when compared to the right foot test results, especially with eyes closed. Dyslexics showed significant difficulty maintaining mono-pedal posture, right or left, especially with eyes closed (80% right foot and 60% left foot test failures).

This effect was not correlated with their reading discrepancies.

This study thus reveals different postural constants in dyslexics and normal readers that could be evidence of a different proprioceptive function for each group.

POSTURAL CONTROL IN SIBLINGS OF DYSLEXICS

Siblings of dyslexic children may be normal readers even though dyslexia has a partially genetic origin. This is why it seemed interesting to look for any similarities or differences in the examination results on the force platform between a group of dyslexic children, a group of supposedly normal reader siblings of dyslexics and a group of children with no notion of dyslexia in their family (unpublished). The 3 groups had a total of 68 children: 22 dyslexics with 13 boys and 9 girls, 19 siblings of dyslexics with 12 boys and 7 girls and 27 normal readers with 8 boys and 19 girls (mean ages respectively of 10 years 9 months, 11 years 4 months and 10 years 9 months). The average reading delay for the dyslexics was 36.5 months (minimum -19 months, maximum - 80 months) while the normal readers showed an average advance of 21 months (min 0 months, max +68 months). The results for the 19 brothers and sisters of dyslexics split them into 2 subgroups with 8 normal readers (42%) showing an average advance of 13.8 months (min 5 months max 30 months) and 11 children (58%) demonstrating a 12.5 month delay in comparison to the statistical norm for the age (minimum -4 months; maximum -27 months).

The test was conducted first with fixation on a vertical line at 40 cm, then with eyes closed. Each test lasted 30 seconds. The data retained were: the ellipse of the surface of confidence (surface determined by removing 10% of the most erratic results), the average speed of displacement, the average displacement on the X and on the Y axis, the standard deviation of X and the standard deviation of Y.

The analysis of the data showed that during the recordings with eyes open, the postural stability of dyslexics was disrupted with a significant difference for the surface ($p = 0.002$), trace length on the y-axis (p = 0.01) the standard deviation for the y-axis (p = 0.0002) and average speed (p = 0.017). This difference in stability was also found with eyes closed in 3 of the measurements: surface (p = 0.003), y-axis trace length (p = 0.017) and y-axis standard deviation (p = 0.003). A comparison of the dyslexics' siblings with the normal readers group shows that none of the criteria used in the analysis of balance on the platform had any significant difference, with eyes either open or closed. Within the group of siblings of dyslexics, the comparison between normal readers and delayed readers shows that with open eyes, only the average speed is different (p = 0.047) whereas with closed eyes there is a significant difference with regard to the length in the x-axis (p = 0.014), the length in the y-axis (p = 0.027) and the average speed (p = 0.018).

In this study, the group of dyslexic children shows greater volatility than the group of siblings of dyslexics, whether with eyes open or closed. That balance is more difficult and that the standard deviations are different suggest more frequent and chaotic maneuvers to maintain position. Within the dyslexics' siblings, instability was also demonstrated among those who have a reading delay. The speed of movement of the center of pressure is altered with eyes open or closed. However it is more difficult to be categorical due to the limited number of children in these two subgroups.

POSTURAL CONTROL, DYSLEXIA AND QUALITY OF ATTENTION

The possible presence of a modified postural control mechanism in dyslexics made it important to try to understand what relationship could exist between these postural abnormalities and reading difficulties. Rather than directly testing such a complicated cognitive mechanism as decoding a text, we gave a much simpler task involving attention to dyslexic children and sought the presence of any correlation with postural disorders [17].

Three groups participated in this protocol: 12 untreated dyslexic children (mean age 11.6 +/- 2.1), 15 dyslexic children with a previous treatment (mean age = 12.5 +/- 1.5) and 12 normal reader children as controls (mean age 10.6 +/- 1.7). Eligibility for the dyslexic treatment group was based on the use of glasses with postural prisms, postural insoles as well as postural reprogramming exercises for at least 3 months.

Center of pressure displacements (CoP) were recorded for 30 seconds on a force platform operating at 40 Hz. The child was asked to remain as calm as possible during two specific test conditions. In the control condition, the child was asked to fixate on a point 40 cm distant. The second condition, required horizontal fixation on a black paper sheet (European A4 format) containing a modified Stroop test consisting of 50 cells (10 rows and 5 columns) also placed at a distance of 40 cm. Each box contained a word defining a color but written in a different color (for example the word "green" written in red). All boxes formed an array 23.2 cm long by 8.5 cm high. The child was asked to find how many times two words (e.g., "red" and "green") were written on the table. Four different names of colors (blue, red, green, yellow) were possible. The number of words was different for each color. The choice of colors was selected in randomized fashion for each child. The purpose of this test was not to evaluate the number of right answers but to increase the cognitive demand while standardizing the oculomotor strategy. Both conditions (simple fixation and pseudo-Stroop) were performed in random order. To obtain groups operating under the most similar conditions possible, the group of treated dyslexic children was tested even though the children had removed the prismatic glasses and the insoles a few minutes prior to testing ([2, 5] min). We wanted to know if the potential effects of a treatment modifying postural control were directly related to this treatment or rather to some cerebral reprogramation possessing an after-effect of a certain duration. All variables (ellipse surface confidence to 90%, average velocity and variance along the X axis and the Y axis) were treated with a 2-factor ANOVA: 3 Groups (dyslexics, treated dyslexics and controls) and 2 conditions (simple fixation and pseudo-Stroop).

The pseudo-Stroop task only disrupted postural stability in the dyslexic group. The results showed a main effect group ($F(2,36) = 3.36$, $p = 0.046$) and an interaction X Conditions Group ($F(2,36) = 4.06$, $p = 0.026$). A breakdown of this interaction revealed that the average speed of the CoP is greater for the dyslexic group when they perform the pseudo-Stroop task when compared with values observed for the control and treated dyslexic groups. This is true for both the pseudo-Stroop and simple fixation tasks ($p < 0.046$). Within the same dyslexic group, the average speed of CoP displacement is more important for the pseudo-Stroop task than for simple fixation ($p < 0.098$). The differences in the other parameters (area of the ellipse and the movement along axes X and Y) were not significant.

In the treated group, 13 of the 15 children studied show a clear reduction of the average speed of the CoP displacement for the pseudo-Stroop task in comparison to simple fixation. This result is highly significant (t-test in pairs, $t(14) = 5.64$ $p << 0.001$). A positive treatment effect is also visible on the 90% confidence ellipse for displacement of the CoP (t-test paired $t(14) = 2.54$ $p = 0.023$). This improvement is present in 12 out of 15 children. It is not correlated with the decrease in the average speed of movement of the CoP ($r = 0.45$). The treatment seems to improve postural stability when children are subjected to a cognitive task. This would appear to support a persistent cerebral after-effect since the children had removed the various elements of the treatment a few minutes before the test.

DIAGNOSIS INTEGRATION OF PROPRIOCEPTIVE SIGNALS, POSTURAL CONTROL AND DYSLEXIA

We then investigated whether the integration of proprioceptive signals during maintenance of equilibrium on the platform while performing a task requiring attention was different in dyslexic children compared to children who are normal readers [18]. For this study we compared the stability while on a stabilometric platform of 30 untreated dyslexics (mean age = 11 ± 2.1), 51 dyslexics who received a proprioceptive treatment over 3 months (mean age = 11 ± 1.5) and 42 normal readers (mean age = 11.6 ± 2.1). The integration of proprioceptive information was modified in each of these groups with the classic technique of applying the co-vibrations of 85 Hz on the tendons of the muscles of the ankles. At the same time, the children were asked either to fix a point 50 cm distant at eye level or to count stars on an A4 sheet with 2 different sizes in a set of 80 stars.

The 2 attentions x 2 vibrations conditions were performed in a random order. The attention task was thus performed two times for each child. Basic parameters of the CoP displacement were analyzed: surface of the 90% confidence ellipse, mean velocity, and standard deviations along the medial-lateral and anterior-posterior axes. All postural dependent variables were thus submitted to 3 x 2 x 2 ANOVAs with group (dyslexic without treatment, treated dyslexic and control), vibration (no-vibration and 85Hz vibration) and tasks (fixation vs. attention) with repeated measures of these three factors. Post hoc comparisons were performed using the Fisher least significant differences test.

For the surface of the 90% confidence ellipse of the CoP displacement, results of the ANOVA showed a significant main effect of group ($F(2,107) = 3.5$, $p = 0.03$), a significant main effect of vibration ($F(1, 107) = 99.3$, $p << 0.01$), no significant group x vibration interaction ($F(2,107) = 0.6$, $p = 0.54$), no significant effect of the attention task but rather a tendency ($F(1,107) = 3.2$, $p = 0.07$), no group x attention interaction ($F(2,107) = 1.2$, $p = 0.29$), a significant vibration x attention interaction ($F(1,107) = 7.1$, $p << 0.01$) and finally no significant interaction between group, vibration and attention ($F(2,107) = 0.2$, $p = 0.84$).

After analysis of the mean velocity of the CoP displacement, results of the ANOVA showed a significant main effect of group ($F(2,107) = 3.1$, $p = 0.05$), a significant main effect of vibration ($F(1, 107) = 764$, $p << 0.01$), a significant group x vibration interaction ($F(2,107) = 3.4$, $p = 0.04$), a significant effect of the attention task ($F(1,107) = 29$, $p << 0.01$), no group x attention interaction ($F(2,107) = 0.6$, $p = 0.5$), a significant vibration x attention interaction ($F(1,107) = 15.8$, $p << 0.01$) and finally no significant interaction between group, vibration and attention ($F(2,107) = 0.1$, $p = 0.9$). The mean velocity of the CoP displacement was smaller for the control group under the 85Hz-vibrations in comparison to the dyslexic and treated dyslexic groups ($p = 0.046$ and $p = 0.002$ respectively) for both attention tasks. There was no significant difference between the dyslexic and the treated dyslexic group ($p = 0.4$).

Concerning the x-std and y-std, the ANOVA showed no significant main effect of group ($F(1,107) = 1.97$, $p = 0.14$), a significant main effect of vibration ($F(1, 107) = 81.9$, $p << 0.01$), no significant group x vibration interaction ($F(2,107) = 0.21$, $p = 0.80$), no significant effect on the attention task ($F(1,107) = 1.1$, $p = 0.3$), no group x attention interaction ($F(2,107) = 1.7$, $p = 0.18$), a significant vibration x attention interaction ($F(1,107) = 15.6$, $p << 0.01$) and finally no significant interaction between group, vibration and attention ($F(2,107) = 0.02$, $p = 0.98$).

Concerning the y-std, results of the ANOVA showed a significant main effect of group ($F(2,107) = 3.7$, $p = 0.03$), a significant main effect of vibration ($F(1,107) = 65.5$, $p << 0.01$), no significant group x vibration interaction ($F(2,107) = 0.4$, $p = 0.68$), a significant main effect of the attention task ($F(1,107) = 9.1$, $p << 0.01$), no group x attention interaction ($F(2,107) = 0.9$, $p = 0.39$), no significant vibration x attention interaction ($F(1,107) = 0.05$, $p = 0.81$) and finally no significant interaction between group, vibration and attention ($F(2,107) = 0.15$, $p = 0.86$).

Examining the results of a one-way ANOVA for counting the stars shows more errors in untreated dyslexics compared to the treated and control groups ($F(2,108) = 4.12$, $p = 0.019$) with no difference between the latter two groups ($p > 0.05$). Note that the attention performance is not correlated with data obtained on the platform ($|rs| < 0.12$).

This effect was not correlated with their reading discrepancies.

Taken together the results show that during the modification of the proprioceptive information the mean velocity of the center of pressure displacement increased significantly more in the dyslexic and the treated dyslexic groups than in the control group, irrespective of the attention task. Attention performance of treated children is similar to that of control children when vibration is not applied. The lack of correlation between the data on the stabilometric force platform and attention performance suggests that treatment modifying postural regulation acts at another level rather than just on its own regulation. That this study shows, however, that the integration of proprioceptive information is different in dyslexics indicates that it may be interesting to study the role of proprioception in the multisensory integration of dyslexics.

Discussion

Through three successive protocols, study on a force platform of a large number of dyslexic children (130) in the same age group shows that these children have deteriorated postural stability compared to that of normal reader controls. These results exceed those given by other studies that show abnormalities of balance and posture in approximately 50% of dyslexics but not more. It is possible that this difference is related to the fact that we used more sensitive and better-adapted criteria for the study of postural disorders, while others have used instruments such as the accelerometer or the technique of motion capture [19, 20]. However, the use of a stabilometric platform has also given divergent results. Poblano found no significant difference between the groups of dyslexics and non-dyslexics using essentially the X-mode [21]. Ramus proposed a similar conclusion to that of Poblano by testing a population of dyslexics having made it into a university which is not representative, however, of the general dyslexic population. The proprioceptive maturity of an adult is indeed not comparable to that of children whose average age is 11.5 years [22]. Another study by Kapoula confirmed that postural control of dyslexic children, required in this study to perform an attention task, is less altered when the usual age for learning to read has passed [23] For Rochelle, postural abnormalities were primarily related to the presence of attention disorders in dyslexia [24]. These disorders were not assessed in our study. For Barela, motor coordination and postural control disorders present in dyslexics are evidence of a disturbance in ambulatory automatisms [25]. For Viholainen, the relationship between postural disorders and dyslexia could correspond to a co-occurrence through a shared genetic mechanism but no causal relationship [26].

To date, the presence of postural control difficulties in dyslexic children has found no certain explanation and our studies suggest 5 non-exclusive possibilities often intertwined:

1. *An altered relationship between attention and balance.* Indeed degradation of postural control already exists in our studies even when cognitive demand is low. However, the difference between the postural performances of the two populations increases if we add a visual attention task more complex than simply fixation of a point. Conversely, a lack of automation of postural control is known to impair cognitive performance when the dyslexic is asked to perform a task requiring attention.
2. *Disruption of the narrow links between vision, eye movement and the cerebellum.* The imbalance may indeed vary according to whether the visual information is of central or peripheral origin, moving or stationary, but also according to whether the eye movements are imposed, especially if they are needed for convergence. A therapeutic modification of vision, combined with action on other postural sensors, seems capable of reconstructing static balance in the dyslexic that is equivalent to

that found in normal readers. The visual sensor input is modified using oblique prisms of very low power (2-3 diopters) normalizing low level vertical heterophorias, of which the essential feature is lability during stimulation of postural sensors [27]. They are constantly found in children with dyslexia when the examination is carried out in accordance with a highly specific protocol [27]. They reflect a disorder of the stability of binocular torsion, which depends on the oblique eye muscles whose action is closely linked to postural reflexes. This is not surprising since this type of vertical heterophoria is known to alter balance in young, healthy, non- dyslexic adults and that the same alterations can be obtained in this population using vertical prisms of very low power [28, 29]. In our study, treatment also improves attention abilities and this suggests that it may recalibrate the relationship between cognitive demand and postural control. Note that the protocols used did not distinguish whether treatment improves attention capabilities or acts directly on postural control, giving the child the ability to focus on another task. The effect must also be analyzed taking into account that this was not a double-blind study. The effect of treatment may correspond to a reprogramming of the CNS since it persists when prisms and insoles are removed for several minutes. The overall results suggest that balance control and cognitive demand are linked and could interact in developmental dyslexia. They are in agreement with the Nicolson and Fawcett studies on dyslexic motor disorders that are the origin of the cerebellar theory of dyslexia [30].

3. *The Stein proposal for disruption of the magnocellular system in dyslexia* [31]. The retinal-colliculus pathway, representing approximately 10% of retinal axons, couples with the oculomotor nuclei to control the direction of gaze. These neurons are part of the magnocellular system that handles visual information necessary for postural regulation. This sensorimotor organization, highly optimized in humans, would be highly dependent on learning. It allows for gaze to be directed very precisely to particularly informative points. Gradually it would allow the construction of the visual exploration strategies that can be considered as genuine perceptual automatisms. Experience would suffice for the expert to construct complete information from partial signs. Reading requires such skills due to the need to fall on the center of gravity of words to develop an automated decoding system [32].
4. *The fact that the disturbances recorded on the stabilometric platform do not correlate directly to the reading level deficit suggests that there is no direct relationship between the dyslexic disorder and postural control.* Postural disturbances are present in both the untreated and treated groups even when attention capacity improves in the latter reaching that of normal readers. This reinforces the idea of a co-occurrence. Like reading, maintaining body stability involves multiple sensory skills. Thus disruption of postural control could simply reflect a dysfunction appearing once the brain has the need to activate a multimodal system to perform a given function [33].
5. *The co-vibration effect that changes proprioception in a region important for balance and equilibrium, results in a greater alteration of stability in dyslexic children*. This effect suggests that integration of proprioceptive information is significantly altered in these patients. Contrary to vision and hearing, proprioception is a sense that is rarely mentioned in studies on dyslexia, especially when discussing the movement disorders that may accompany dyslexia. Its intervention is however

particularly important during acquisition of motor capabilities that requires a proprioceptive feed back before the motor skills are able to be managed by higher level internal motor models. Remember that proprioception is at the heart of postural control as a consequence of its role in the spatial localization of sensory information [7]. Its status is the result of posture and it is the essential means of postural control. The regulation of automated proprioception occurs in the cerebellum and its role is central at this level for learning automated motor tasks, particularly in the eye. While it is certain that postural control is subject to several sensors and feed-forward phenomena drawn from internal motor models, the idea of a special role for proprioception in the dyslexic child is new. Proprioception merits study in developmental disorders such as dyslexia, notably concerning disturbances in visual attention since ocular proprioception, whose function is closely linked to general proprioception, is known to have the ability to modulate visual attention.

Conclusion

The hypothesis of a disturbance altering proprioceptive postural control in dyslexics opens a new horizon on the relationship between cognition, motor skills and sensory perception in this population. Until recently, the traditional concept of perception has been largely influenced by the idea that the sensory organs are sensitive surfaces in passive expectation of stimulation and that the resulting treatment of sensory information leads to the construction of representations of the material world. A written text is only one specific aspect of these representations. Going beyond this concept, a new trend emphasizes the active and predictive nature of perception. It is based on the notion of a continuous interaction between sensory and motor changes in the properties of the organism. As proof of an actual motor cognition, this view sees perception and action as two interlinked and inseparable phenomena that are in fact two facets of the same process [34]. Thus, all human activity is a mix of sensorimotor activity and perception with obvious consequences for cognition, particularly regarding the representation of sounds and images. The latter may thus no longer be studied without regard to its underlying motor activity. Therefore, all mechanisms involved at the developmental level and during implementation of motor control loops have possible roles in the origin of perceptual developmental disorders.

References

[1] Peterson RL, Pennington BF. Developmental dyslexia. *Annu Rev Clin Psychol.* 2015;11:283-307.

[2] Cappe C, Thut G, Romei V, Murray MM. Auditory-visual multisensory interactions in humans: timing, topography, directionality, and sources. *J Neurosci.* 2010 Sep 22;30(38):12572-80.

[3] Cappe C, Rouiller EM, Barone P. (2012)Cortical and Thalamic Pathways for Multisensory and Sensorimotor Interplay. In: Murray MM, Wallace MT, Editors. *The*

Neural Bases of Multisensory Processes. (Chapter 2). Boca Raton (FL): CRC Press/Taylor and Francis;

[4] Allum JH, Bloem BR, Carpenter MG, Hulliger M, Hadders-Algra M. Proprioceptive control of posture: a review of new concepts. *Gait Posture*. 1998 Dec 1;8(3):214-242.

[5] Proske U, Gandevia SC. The proprioceptive senses: their roles in signaling body shape, body position and movement, and muscle force. *Physiol Rev*. 2012 Oct;92(4):1651-97.

[6] Weir CR. Proprioception in extraocular muscles. *J Neuroophthalmol*. 2006 Jun;26(2):123-7.

[7] Roll R, Velay JL, Roll JP. Eye and neck proprioceptive messages contribute to the spatial coding of retinal input in visually oriented activities. *Exp Brain Res*. 1991;85(2):423-31.

[8] Odoj B, Balslev D. Role of Oculoproprioception in Coding the Locus of Attention. *J Cogn Neurosci*. 2016 Mar;28(3):517-28.

[9] Middlebrooks JC, Green DM. Sound localization by human listeners. *Annu Rev Psychol*. 1991;42:135-59.

[10] Roll JP, Albert F, Ribot-Ciscar E, Bergenheim M. "Proprioceptive signature" of cursive writing in humans: a multi-population coding. *Exp Brain Res*. 2004 Aug;157(3):359-68.

[11] Martins da Cunhà H, Alves da Silva O. Postural Deficiency Syndrome. J Fr Ophtalmol, 1986;9:747-755. 3.

[12] Quercia P, Seigneuric A, Chariot S, Vernet P, Pozzo T, Bron A, Creuzot-Garcher C, Robichon F. Ocular proprioception and developmental dyslexia. Sixty clinical observations. *J Fr Ophtalmol*. 2005 Sep;28(7):713-23.

[13] Quercia P, Feiss L, Michel C. Developmental dyslexia and vision. *Clin Ophthalmol*. 2013;7:869-81.

[14] Virlet L. Specific learning disorders and proprioceptive deficiency syndrome: frequency, correlation and the value of detection testing. 2014-5-2. 2nd Day scientific session SOFTAL Available from: http://www.softal.fr/IMG/pdf/softa-poster-7_avril_14_-virlet-.pdf.

[15] G. Bizzo, N. Guillet, A. Patat, P. M. Gagey, Specifications for building a vertical force platform designed for clinical stabilometry. *Med. Biol. Eng. Comput*. 23 (1985) 474–476.

[16] Pozzo T, Vernet P, Creuzot-Garcher C, Robichon F, Bron A, Quercia P. Static postural control in children with developmental dyslexia. *Neurosci Lett*. 2006 Aug 7;403(3):211-5.

[17] Vieira S, Quercia P, Michel C, Pozzo T, Bonnetblanc F. Cognitive demands impair postural control in developmental dyslexia: a negative effect that can be compensated. *Neurosci Lett*. 2009 Sep 22;462(2):125-9.

[18] Quercia P, Demougeot L, Dos Santos M, Bonnetblanc F. Integration of proprioceptive signals and attentional capacity during postural control are impaired but subject to improvement in dyslexic children. *Exp Brain Res*. 2011 Apr;209(4):599-608.

[19] Moe-Nilssen R, Helbostad JL, Talcott JB, Toennessen FE. Balance and gait in children with dyslexia. *Exp Brain Res*. 2003 May;150(2):237-44.

[20] Stoodley CJ, Fawcett AJ, Nicolson RI, Stein JF. Impaired balancing ability in dyslexic children. *Exp Brain Res*. 2005 Dec;167(3):370-80.

[21] Poblano A, Ishiwara K, de Lourdes Arias M, García-Pedroza F, Marín H, Trujillo M. Motor control alteration in posturography in learning-disabled children. *Arch Med Res.* 2002 Sep-Oct;33(5):485-8.

[22] Ramus F. Developmental dyslexia: specific phonological deficit or general sensorimotor dysfunction? *Curr Opin Neurobiol.* 2003 Apr;13(2):212-8.

[23] Kapoula Z, Bucci MP. Postural control in dyslexic and non-dyslexic children. *J Neurol.* 2007;254(9):1174–1183.

[24] Rochelle KS, Talcott JB. Impaired balance in developmental dyslexia? A meta-analysis of the contending evidence. *J Child Psychol Psychiatry.* 2006 Nov;47(11):1159-66.

[25] Barela JA, Dias JL, Godoi D, Viana AR, de Freitas PB. Postural control and automaticity in dyslexic children: the relationship between visual information and body sway. *Res Dev Disabil.* 2011;32(5):1814–1821.

[26] Viholainen H, Aro M, Ahonen T, Crawford S, Cantell M, Kooistra L. Are balance problems connected to reading speed or the familial risk of dyslexia? *Dev Med Child Neurol.* 2011;53(4):350–353.

[27] Quercia P, Quercia M, Feiss LJ, Allaert F. The distinctive vertical heterophoria of dyslexics. *Clin Ophthalmol.* 2015 Sep 25;9:1785-97.

[28] Matheron E, Kapoula Z. Vertical phoria and postural control in upright stance in healthy young subjects. *Clin Neurophysiol.* 2008;119 (10):2314–2320.

[29] Matheron E, Lê TT, Yang Q, Kapoula Z. Effects of a two-diopter vertical prism on posture. *Neurosci Lett.* 2007;423(3):236–240.

[30] Nicolson RI, Fawcett AJ. Developmental dyslexia, learning and the cerebellum. *J Neural Transm Suppl.* 2005;(69):19-36.

[31] Stein J. The magnocellular theory of developmental dyslexia. *Dyslexia.* 2001 Jan-Mar;7(1):12-36.

[32] Beauvillain C, Dore K, Baudouin V. The 'center of gravity' of words: evidence for an effect of the word-initial letters. *Vision Res.* 1996 Feb;36(4):589-603.

[33] Harrar V, Tammam J, Pérez-Bellido A, Pitt A, Stein J, Spence C. Multisensory integration and attention in developmental dyslexia. *Curr Biol.* 2014 Mar 3;24(5):531-5.

[34] Jeannerod M, Jacob P. Visual cognition: a new look at the two-visual systems model. *Neuropsychologia.* 2005;43(2):301-12.

In: Dyslexia: Perspectives, Challenges and Treatment Options ISBN: 978-1-63485-328-6
Editor: Marilyn Frazier

Chapter 14

A FEW REMARKS ON MAGNOCELLULAR RESPONSES AND BRIEF STIMULI

Bernt Christian Skottun*
Ullevaalsalleen, Oslo, Norway

Abstract

A number of authors have proposed that dyslexia is linked to a deficiency in the magnocellular system. Contrast sensitivity is likely to be the most direct and reliable psychophysical test on magnocellular integrity. However, contrast sensitivity has provided little support for a magnocellular deficiency in dyslexia. That the lack of support is not simply the result of reduced test sensitivity is indicated by the fact that a number of studies have found positive evidence for deficits of a nature incompatible with a magnocellular deficiency. One of these studies found deficits to briefly presented stimuli of high spatial frequency. Since brief stimuli in relative terms have larger amplitudes at higher temporal frequencies and since magnocellular cells tend to give larger responses than do parvocellular cells at high temporal frequencies it has been suggested that brief stimuli predominantly activate the magnocellular system and that deficits which manifest themselves with brief stimuli may be attributed to this system. In the present report the temporal amplitude spectra of rectangular pulses have been calculated. It is found that although brief stimuli, in relative terms, have higher amplitudes than longer stimuli at higher temporal frequencies, all rectangular pulses have their largest amplitudes at the lowest temporal frequencies. This makes it difficult to draw any conclusions about the involvement of the magno- versus the parvocellular systems on the basis of stimulus duration. Furthermore, the fact that deficits observed with brief stimuli have been found only, or predominantly, at high spatial frequencies is irreconcilable with a magnocellular deficiency irrespective of the temporal aspect of the stimuli. Thus, it is possible for there to be contrast sensitivity deficits linked to brief stimuli which are not of magnocellular origin. Consequently, one cannot rely upon brief stimuli to assess the integrity of the magnocellular system.

Keywords: dyslexia, temporal frequency, spatial frequency, Fourier Transform, schizophrenia

*E-mail address: berntchrskottun@gmail.com

It has been proposed that dyslexia is the result of a deficiency in the magnocellular portion of the visual system (see e.g., Stein, 2014). Because all studies that have examined contrast sensitivity in monkeys following the placing of lesions in the magno- or parvocellular layers of their Lateral Geniculate Nuclei (LGNs) have found magnocellular lesions to cause reduced sensitivity at low ($<$ 1.5 cycles/degree approximately) spatial frequencies while parvocellular lesions cause deficits at medium and high frequencies (for references see Skottun, 2000) contrast sensitivity is likely to be the most reliable and direct psychophysical test of magnocellular integrity. This is also supported by human psychophysics which has found contrast detection at low and high spatial frequency to be mediated by mechanisms having different temporal characteristics (Tolhurst, 1975; Legge, 1978).

Studies of contrast sensitivity in dyslexic readers have generally found little evidence for deficiencies at low spatial frequencies (Skottun, 2000, 2015). That this is not merely the result of a lack of test sensitivity is demonstrated by the fact that a number of studies have obtained evidence for differences between dyslexic readers and controls of kinds which are incompatible with a magnocellular deficiency (Skottun, 2000). An example of this is the study of Gross-Glenn et al. (1995) which found contrast sensitivity deficiencies that were most pronounced at high spatial frequencies (i.e. at 12.0 cycles/degree). (Recently, also Chicchini et al., 2015, have found contrast sensitivity deficits in dyslexia linked predominantly to medium and high spatial frequencies. In this case the deficits were linked to motion stimuli which entails there can be deficient motion perception which is not the result of a magnocellular abnormality.)

Because the contrast sensitivity deficits found by Gross-Glenn et al. (1995) were obtained only, or predominantly, with brief stimuli, it has been suggested that these results could be consistent with a magnocellular deficiency (Stein et al., 2000; Stein, 2014). (That brief stimuli should favor the magnocellular system has also been suggested, or implied, in connection with schizophrenia, Green et al., 2009; Calderone et al., 2013; Kelemen et al., 2013, and in other contexts, Medina et al., 2016.) The present report examines the notion that brief stimuli may be used to selectively, or predominantly, activate the magnocellular system.

Figure 1A shows the temporal profiles of two rectangular pulses, one of 10 ms duration the other 100 ms long. In Figure 1B are shown the normalized amplitude spectra of the two pulses. As is apparent, the shorter pulse (the one of 10 ms duration) has substantially larger normalized amplitudes at higher frequencies than does the longer pulse. This may suggest that brief stimuli may be detected by the magnocellular sytem since this system tends to respond to somewhat higher temporal frequencies than does the parvocellular system. (For a brief discussion of temporal frequency tuning in magno- and parvocellular cells see Skottun & Skoyles, 2008.) However, Figure 1B also makes it clear that in the case of both stimuli the largest amplitudes are found at very low temporal frequencies. Of particular relevance is the fact that the dc component (or 0 Hz component) has the largest amplitudes in both cases. Since the zero harmonic is the sum of the signal and since both the magno- and parvocellular systems integrate stimulation over time-windows up to approximately 100 ms (Legge, 1978) it is difficult to draw any conclusions about the magno- and parvocellular systems based on the temporal frequency spectra of these stimuli.

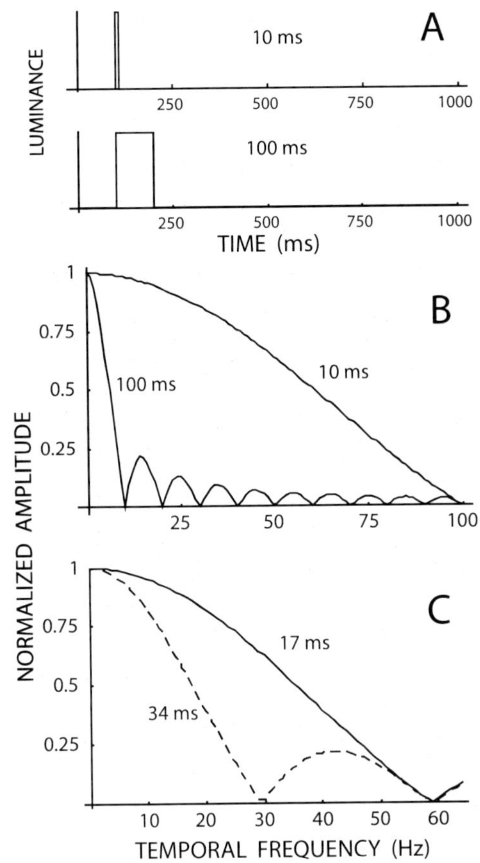

Figure 1. (A) Temporal profiles of rectangular luminance pulses of 10 ms and 100 ms duration. In all the present analyses the Fourier Transform covered a 1.0 s period sampled at 1 ms intervals. (B) Normalized temporal amplitude spectra of the pulses in A. Only amplitudes for frequencies up to 100 Hz are shown. As can be seen, the spectrum of the shorter pulse has a much shallower fall-off with increasing temporal frequency than does the spectrum of the longer pulse. However, both pulses have their largest amplitudes at the lowest temporal frequencies. (C) Normalized amplitude spectra of rectangular pulses of 17 ms (solid line) and 34 ms (dashed line) duration. As can be seen, the largest amplitudes in both spectra are found at 0 Hz. Also apparent are the facts that the spectrum of the 34 ms stimulus has a trough at 29 Hz (as well as at 59 Hz) and the 17 ms stimulus has a trough at 59 Hz. Thus, contrary to what has been alleged these stimuli. for all practical purposes, are not in positions to stimulate the magnocellular system (or any other system for that matter) at these temporal frequencies. (The spectra were generated using *Mathematica* from *Wolfram Research*.

In regard to the study of Gross-Glenn et al. (1995) it has been proposed specifically that the stimuli of 17 ms and 34 ms duration, at which deficits for dyslexic readers were found, should have amplitudes at 59 Hz and 29 Hz, respectively, and that these should have activated the magnocellular system (Stein, 2014). In Figure 1C are shown the amplitude spectra of pulses of 17 and 34 ms duration. As can be seen, consistent with the results in Figure 1B, both pulses have their largest amplitudes at the very lowest temporal frequencies. From 0 Hz both spectra show gradual decline with increasing temporal frequency. The decline is more rapid in the case of the 34 ms stimulus (dashed line). This spectrum reaches a minimum at 29 Hz. Thus, in direct contradiction to what has been proposed the frequency component which should characterize the 34 ms stimulus has essentially zero amplitude. (To be precise, it has less than 1.5 % of the amplitude of the 0 Hz component.) Above 29 Hz the amplitude of this stimulus increases to a secondary peak near 42 Hz after which it declines to a second minimum at 59 Hz.

In the case of the 17 ms pulse the amplitude spectrum shows a monotonic and gradual decline up to 59 Hz where the amplitude is essentially zero. At frequencies above 59 Hz the amplitude increases with frequency. Thus, the 17 ms stimulus has essentially zero amplitude at 59 Hz. Therefore, contrary to what has been proposed, the 34 ms stimulus is not in a position to stimulate anything at 29 Hz and the 17 ms stimulus is not in a position stimulate anything at 59 Hz.

That rectangular pulses of 17 ms and 34 ms duration have zero, or near zero, amplitudes at, respectively, 59 Hz and 29 Hz can be deduced directly from the equation for the Fourier Transform: $F(\omega) = \int f(t)\, e^{i\omega t} dt$, where t is time, $f(t)$ is the signal to be Fourier-analyzed, ω is the temporal frequency and i is $\sqrt{-1}$. Since $e^{i\omega t} = cos(\omega\, t) + i\; sin(\omega\, t)$ this entails that $F(\omega) = \int(f(t)\; cos(\omega\, t))\; dt + \int(f(t)\; i\; sin(\omega\, t))\; dt$.

The integral of both a sine function and of a cosine function over one period is zero (i.e., $\int_0^{2\pi} sin(t)\; dt = \int_0^{2\pi} cos(t)\; dt = 0$). Thus, if $f(t)$ is a rectangular pulse which is non-zero and constant over the duration of one period of a sine function, (i.e., is non-zero and constant over a duration of $1/\omega$) and zero elsewhere then both $\int(f(t)\; cos(\omega\, t))\; dt$ and $\int(f(t)\; i\; sin(\omega\, t))\; dt$ become zero. In the case of a rectangular pulse of 17 ms duration this would occur at 58.82 Hz and in the case of a 34 ms pulse this would take place for a 29.41 Hz stimulus. Since 29 Hz and 59 Hz are the frequencies closest to 29.41 Hz and 58,82 Hz, respectively, the troughs in the amplitude spectrum of the discrete Fourier Transform, in which amplitudes are given only at integer frequency values, are found at these frequencies. (It should also be pointed out that troughs are also found when the duration of the pulse is an integer multiple of the period, i.e. $\int_0^{j2\pi} sin(t)\; dt = \int_0^{j2\pi} cos(t)\; dt = 0$ when j is an integer. This is why the amplitude spectrum of the 34 ms stimulus has a secondary through near 59 Hz.)

As was pointed out above, what makes the findings of Gross-Glenn et al. (1995) irreconcilable with a magnocellular deficiency is the relationship to spatial frequency. Gross-Glenn et al. (1995) found deficits at a spatial frequency of 12.0 cycles/degree but little evidence for deficits at 0.6 cycles/degrees. This is the opposite of what one would expect for a magnocellular deficiency and is irreconcilable with such a deficiency irrespective of the temporal frequency spectra of the stimuli. (For a discussion of contrast sensitivity in relation to dyslexia see Skottun, 2000, 2015.) Further, the fact that Gross-Glenn et al. (1995) found positive evidence for deficits of a nature irreconcilable with a magnocellular deficiency means that these results cannot be made compatible with a magnocellular deficit by assuming insufficient test sensitivity. In addition, the fact that the deficits were found for brief stimuli means that it is possible for there to be deficits unrelated to the magnocellular system which manifest themselves only, or mainly, when tested with briefly presented stimuli. This entails, therefore, that brief stimuli cannot be relied upon to assess the integrity of the magnocellular system.

References

Calderone, D. J., Martinez, A., Zemon, V., Hoptman, M. J., Hu, G., Watkins, J. E., Javitt, D. C., & Butler, P. D. (2013) Comparison of psychophysical, electrophysiological, and fMRI assessment of visual contrast responses in patients with schizophrenia. *NeuroImage*, 67, 153-162.

Cicchini, G. M., Marino, C., Maschetti, S., Perani, D., & Morrone, M. C. (2015) Strong motion deficits in dyslexia associated with DCDC2 gene alteration. *The Journal of Neuroscience*, 35, 8059-8064.

Green, M. F., Butler, P. D., Chen, Y., Geyer, M.A., Silverstein, S., Wynn, J. K., Yoon, J. H., & Zemon, V. (2009). Perception measurement in clinical trials of schizophrenia: Promising paradigms from CNTRICS. *Schizophrenia Bulletin*, 35, 163-181.

Gross-Glenn, K., Skottun, B. C., Glenn, W., Kushch, A., Lingua, R., Dunbar, M., Jallad, B., Lubs, H. A., Levin, B., Rabin, M., Parke, L. A., & Duara, R. (1995) Contrast sensitivity in dyslexia. *Visual Neuroscience*, 12, 153-163.

Kelemen, O., Kiss, I., Benedek, G., & Keri, S., (2013) Perceptual and cognitive effects of antipsychotics in rst-episode schizophrenia:The potential impact of GABA concentration in the visual cortex. *Progress in Neuro-Psychopharmacology & Biological Psychiatry*, 47, 13-19.

Legge, G. E. (1978) Sustained and transient mechanisms in human vision: Temporal and spatial properties. *Vision Research*, 18, 69-81.

Medina, J., Drebing, D. E., Hamilton, R. H., & Coslett, H. B. (2016) Phantoms on the hands: Influence of the body on brief synchric visual percepts. *Neuropsychologia*, In Press. doi: 10.1016/j.neuropsychologia.2016.01.016

Skottun, B. C. (2000) The magnocellular deficit theory of dyslexia: The evidence from contrast sensitivity. *Vision Research*, 40, 111-127.

Skottun, B. C. (2015) The need to differentiate the magnocellular system from the dorsal stream in connection with dyslexia. *Brain and Cognition*, 95, 62-66.

Skottun, B. C., & Skoyles, J. R. (2008) Temporal frequency and the magnocellular and parvocellular systems. *Neuro-Ophthalmology*, 32, 43-48.

Stein, J., Talcott, J., & Walsh, V. (2000) Controversy about the visual magnocellular deficit in developmental dyslexics. *Trends in Cognitive Sciences*, 4, 209-211.

Stein, J. (2014) Dyslexia: the role of vision and visual attention. *Current Developmental Disorders Reports*, 1, 267-280.

Tolhurst, D. J. (1975) Reaction times in the detection of gratings by human observers: A probabilistic mechanism. *Vision Research*, 15, 1143-1149.

In: Dyslexia: Perspectives, Challenges and Treatment Options ISBN: 978-1-63485-328-6
Editor: Marilyn Frazier

Chapter 15

Expert Commentary: Dyslexia in Adulthood - Socio-Emotional Challenges and the Importance of Resilience

Melody M. Terras*[*], *CPsychol. AFBPsS
School of Media, Culture and Society,
University of the West of Scotland, Paisley, UK

Abstract

This commentary provides a synthesis of research concerning the socio-emotional dimension of Dyslexia in adulthood. Lower levels of self-esteem and poorer socio-emotional functioning such as anxiety, depression and behavioural adjustment are documented. Although negative consequences should be considered, it is important to remember that many individuals live and cope with their reading difficulties and experience no significant long term psycho-social problems. Therefore this commentary examines the adaptive coping strategies that may be used and considers the insights that may be derived by adopting a resilience perspective to interpret existing findings and situate future research. The chapter concludes with suggestions for ways in which research concerning the socio-emotional dimension of dyslexia may progress in the future: research must be robust enough, not only to descriptively examine but also to, generate explanatory causal accounts of the complex relationships between external and internal risk and protective factors that operate across the lifespan. It should therefore be longitudinal nature; ambitious, inclusive and integrative in the type and range of methodological techniques used, and be informed by the experiences of individuals with dyslexia.

The advancement of the field and increased linkage between research and practice is essential to the development of evidence-based interventions that have the potential to make a real difference to the lives of individuals with dyslexia.

Keywords: Dyslexia, Adulthood, Socio-emotional functioning, Coping, Resilience

[*] E-mail: melody.terras@uws.ac.uk.

Introduction

The importance of understanding the socio-emotional impact of living with Dyslexia across the life span is being increasingly recognised; with existing research documenting lower levels of self-esteem and poorer socio-emotional functioning. Although negative consequences should be considered, it is important to remember that many individuals with dyslexia interpret, manage and cope in a positive way; and experience no significant long term psycho-social problems; often becoming very successful in life.

The increasing amount of qualitative research exploring the lived experience of dyslexia is extending our understanding of the influence of dyslexia across the lifespan, enriching our appreciation of the challenges and informing interventions about they can managed. In particular this research has highlighted the importance of recognising individual differences in coping and adjustment, and how further research is required to identify the factors that promote and hinder successful psycho-social adjustment (Terras 2012; 2016). To facilitate and inform this process, this expert commentary provides an overview of the socio-emotional challenges that adults with dyslexia may encounter; how they cope; considers the insights that may be derived by adopting a resilience perspective to interpret existing findings and situate future research, and concludes with suggestions for ways in which research concerning the socio-emotional dimension of dyslexia may progress in the future.

Dyslexia: The Socio-Emotional Dimension

Since the reading and spelling difficulties associated with dyslexia persist into adulthood, the emotional and behavioural functioning of adults with dyslexia is an important issue to be addressed (Boetsch, Green and Pennington 1996). Poor socio-emotional functioning is frequently documented in children with dyslexia: children with reading difficulties are almost five times more likely to exhibit anti-social behaviour than children without reading difficulties (Rutter and Yule 1970). Externalising problems such as disruptive behaviour disorders and Attention Deficit Hyperactivity Disorder (ADHD), and Internalising difficulties such as anxiety are well documented in both epidemiological and clinical samples (Willcut and Pennington, 2000) and there is an independent relationship between reading difficulties and behavioural problems after controlling for co-morbidities such as ADHD (Arnold et al. 2005).

In addition to these externalising behaviour problems, individuals with dyslexia often exhibit more frequent emotional and internalising difficulties such as anxiety and depression than those without reading problems (Maughan and Carroll 2006). Insight into the nature of the relationship between dyslexia and internalising difficulties can be derived from recent longitudinal studies of children At-risk from dyslexia (Snowling et al. 2007) which shows that children (12-13 yrs) with a family history of dyslexia who report difficulties with reading exhibited significantly more emotional symptoms than both the control group and those with a family history of dyslexia who showed no reading difficulties. Such findings suggest a strong and possible direct link between anxiety and literacy difficulties (Snowling et al. 2007).

Given the scope and scale of the socio-emotional difficulties experienced in childhood and the educational, occupational and personal challenges that the continuation of reading difficulties bring, it is not unexpected that socio-emotional difficulties persist into adulthood. A recent meta-analysis supports the continuation of internalising problems into adulthood (Klassen et al. 2013); with research indicating poorer socio-emotional function in teenagers with dyslexia in comparison to peers, and an increased risk of anxiety, depression and self-harm in adults (Alexander-Passe 2006, 2015; Riddock, Sterling, Farmer and Morgan 1999; Maughan and Hagell, 1996). Recent evidence also indicates potential increased drug dependence (Yates 2013) and homelessness (McDonald and Deacon 2015) in addition to the well documented high incidence of literacy difficulties in the prison population internationally (Snowling et al. 2000; Gonzalez et al. 2015).

Obviously it is essential to understand the negative consequences of dyslexia in adulthood; however, it is equally, or possibly even more important to recognise that many individuals adapt and cope with their reading difficulties (Boetsch, Green, and Pennington 1996; Maughan and Hagell 1996). Understanding the process of coping and adaptation is key to informing future interventions that have the potential to make a real differences to the lives of adults with dyslexia (Terras 2012; Terras 2016). If this aspiration is to become a reality, then we must (1) establish how and why negative consequences persist; (2) Understand how individuals adapt and cope, and (3) evaluate and develop evidence based interventions. These multiple objectives may best be realised by viewing the psycho-social dimension through a Resilience lens (Terras 2016).

THE IMPORTANCE OF RESILIENCE

There is increasing interest in the concept of resilience as it promotes understanding of how people cope and supports a move away from a deficit approach by promoting the understanding of factors associated with success as well as failure. The concept of resilience is widely applied in the field of mental health (Rutter 2000; Mikami and Hinshaw 2006), so it prudent to use a resilience approach to promote understanding of the socio-emotional functioning of individuals with dyslexia (Terras et al. 2009).

Resilience is "a dynamic process encompassing positive adaptation within the context of adversity" (Luthar, Cicchetti and Becker 2000; pg 543). A resilience perspective aims to understand how individuals cope, or fail to cope with stress and adverse circumstances. It also provides a means to capture individual variation: why are some individuals more vulnerable to risk? What factors, both internal and external, may help or hinder the process of coping and adaptation?

The key elements of a Resilience approach are the identification of Risk and Protective factors and the concept of Cumulative risk. A risk factor can be defined as an aspect of an individual and/or the environment that renders an individual more likely to develop problems. On the other hand, Protective Factors can be defined as factors that act to protect an individual from developing problems in the face of adversity. Because a resilience framework considers both internal and external factors, it acknowledges the social context in which an individual functions, and how their functioning may change over time and therefore considers the influence of Cumulative risk. Cumulative risk captures the fact that individuals may experience more than one risk factor: either externally from the environment, internally, or a combination of both internal and external factors. A resilience framework aims to specify the factors that may put an individual at risk, and the factors that may help or protect an individual against risk and thereby support positive adaptation. However, it is important to remember that a risk factor only increases the likelihood of adverse outcomes, it does not necessarily entail poor outcomes (Margalit 2004).

RISK AND PROTECTIVE FACTORS

Dyslexia as a Risk Factor

From a Resilience perspective, Dyslexia may be regarded as a risk factor that increases the likelihood of adverse outcomes rather than necessarily entailing a negative outcome. The dyslexia risk factor may exerts its influence by interacting with personal characteristics of an individual (e.g., self-esteem, motivation, personality) and their environment (e.g., family and peer relations; levels of educational support) and it is these factors and their interactions, rather the presence of Dyslexia itself, that determine successful psycho-social functioning (Terras 2012, Terras 2016). Applying a Resilience perspective to the psycho-social dimension of dyslexia serves a two-fold function: (1) it facilitates understanding and synthesis of existing and often conflicting research findings concerning psycho-social functioning, and (2) provides a framework within which to situate future research and practice (Terras et al. 2009; Terras 2016). It is to a detailed consideration of these two functions that we now turn.

The identification of risk and protective factors is key to informing interventions which may help minimise risk and maximise protective factors that nurture resilience and promote psycho-social well-being. Protective factors identified in the general literature include supportive relationships, access to good education facilities, participation in sports, small family size and, personal attributes such as good health, even temperament, positive self-esteem, intelligence or good social skills (Rutter and Smith 1995; Rutter 2000). Therefore, such factors should be considered with respect to adults with dyslexia. It is essential to recognise that the existing research data considered below only illustrates the correlates of possible risk and protective factors, as the actual direction of the relationship between many of the variables still needs to be established as much of the existing nature is correlational in nature. However, the consideration of the risk or protective role these factors may play is informative to consider as it can serves as a useful starting point to stimulate future research and discussion.

The Importance of Adaptive Coping

A potentially important protective factor to positive psycho-social adjustment is successful coping (Folkman et al. 1986). Research evidence from both quantitative and especially qualitative methods exploring the lived experience of dyslexia offers insight into how individuals learn to live with dyslexia by developing effective coping strategies e.g., compensating for reading/spelling difficulties by using practical and social skills. One adult who participated in a focus group exploring the day-to-day challenges they experienced (Terras et al. 2009) expressed the following sentiment:

> "You never get rid of it. You get tools to work with it, you get round it, you never get rid of it. You get a better idea how to cope with it"

Coping is how we deal with stress and can formally be defined as "constantly changing cognitive and behavioural efforts to manage specific external and/or internal demands that are appraised as taxing or exceeding the resources of the person" (Lazarus and Folkman 1984; pg 141). The coping strategies that individuals use vary depending on the nature of the stressor; whether it is perceived as a threat, a loss, or a challenge, and the individual characteristics of the person. One of the most influential approaches to characterising coping is that of Endler and Parker (1999) who identified three different categories of coping responses: (1) Task-orientated coping which focuses on prioritizing information and recalling previous attempts to improve current efforts in dealing with a stressful situation; (2) Emotion-orientated coping which focuses on internalizing and externalizing factors that may be used to deal with a particular situation. Internalizing factors include drug and alcohol abuse, and externalizing problems include acting out against friends and family; and (3) Avoidance-orientated coping which can be divided into two sub-categories: distraction and social diversion. Avoidance-orientated coping involves undertaking other tasks to avoid dealing with the stressful one. Examples of avoidance strategies include watching television or going to a party. Distraction strategies focus on doing other things in order to be distracted from the stressful situation. Social diversion strategies include avoiding situations and people where literacy abilities may be tested.

Existing research examining how individuals with dyslexia cope illustrates how a range of different strategies are used, and more importantly highlights which strategies are most adaptive and may therefore function as protective factors. A highly adaptive type of coping is task-focused coping, and this strategy was the dominant one reported by students with dyslexia in a higher education setting (Terras, Ramsay and McMaster 2010) and offers insight into how coping strategies may develop and also how they are related to other important internal variables such as self-esteem which may operate as risk factors. The findings indicate that self-esteem was positively correlated with task-based coping but negatively correlated with emotion-based coping, suggesting that Task-based coping may be used by those with higher self-esteem, whereas Emotion-based coping is used by those with lower self-esteem. There was also a significant negative relationship between Task-based coping and Emotion-based coping suggesting that the use of Emotion-based coping may decrease with the use of Task-based coping.

The adaptive and positive benefits of task-based coping is consistent with the findings of across the age range: Alexander-Passe (2006) who examined the coping strategies used by teenagers with dyslexia and also the work of Maughan et al. (2009) who explored how middle-aged adults with poor reading skills sought assistance to help them cope with their functional literacy impairments. However, it is important to remember that dyslexia brings both practical and emotional challenges and individuals must cope with these emotional challenges on a daily basis.

Emotional Difficulties, Self-Esteem and Stigma

The relationship between coping and emotional wellbeing is complex, and this complexity and interconnectedness may be amplified in individuals with dyslexia who encounter literacy-related stressors on a daily basis and may experience a range of socio-emotional sequela. Therefore the development and use of adaptive coping strategies may help promote resilience and therefore function as an important protective factor for the psycho-social adjustment of individuals with dyslexia.

Insight into potential risk and protective factors can be derived from research examining the risk factors for internalising difficulties in children with dyslexia which include severity of dyslexia, co-morbidity with attention deficit disorder/hyperactivity disorder, amount of perceived social support and being female; protective factors include feeling in tune with the school environment and the family, especially the mother (Muganni et al. 2009) These proposals are consistent with the research discussed earlier illustrating the high rate of internalising problems in children and adults (Terras et al. 2012) and it is reasonable to assume that given the continuation of internalising problems into adulthood that these risk and protective factors will remain applicable. The existing evidence indicates that they do. For example, evidence from both research and practice indicates that dyslexia impacts negatively upon on self-esteem. However the findings are mixed and it is not always lower (Burden 2008) and any deficits that do exist may be limited to academic domains (Terras, Ramsay and McMaster 2010; Snowling et al. 2007). As noted earlier, there is a complex relationship with self-esteem and negative emotions, some if which may be explained by understanding how individuals cope and understand their dyslexia. Research suggests that understanding the circumscribed nature of reading and spelling difficulties is associated with successful adult psycho-social functioning (Boetsch et al. 1996; Maughan and Hagell 1996). However, dyslexia is often experienced as stigmatising and embarrassing, and individuals are reluctant to discuss their difficulties and frequently conceal their problems from family members, friends and employers (Gerber 2012; Nalavany, Carawan and Sauber 2015). Such concealment behaviour can have wide spread repercussions as it can negatively influence self-esteem, emotional adjustment, relationships, possibly via misattributions of behaviour, which may further impact on relationships and the availability of social support that is essential to help people cope.

The Importance of Support

Support is an important protective factor. However, relationships are frequently strained as a result of poor understanding of the impact of dyslexia and how to cope by both the individual themselves and by others. Strain is often apparent from an early age in terms of peer and family relationships in terms of parental stress, differences in parenting style and sibling relationships (Terras et al. 2009; Bonifacci, et al. 2014). This strain may continue into adulthood in terms of personal relationships and even the relationship with their own children (Alexander-Passe 2013). The protective function of perceived support in adulthood is further demonstrated by research evidence indicating that successful intervention and support were often associated with positive feelings of increased confidence and self-esteem (Terras et al. 2004).

Individuals with dyslexia may be doubly disadvantaged in terms of support: not only are family/personal relationships strained, educational experiences are often negative which further limits opportunities for support, from teachers and peers, thereby reducing its protective influence. Coping with reading and spelling difficulties, especially in the context of school, is frequently reported as stressful, anxiety provoking and damaging to self-esteem and can have a compelling impact on the emotional health and self-esteem of adults with dyslexia (Terras et al. 2004; Nalavany, Carawan and Brown 2011).

To summarise, when the existing evidence base concerning the psych-social functioning of adults with dyslexia is viewed through a resilience lens it offers interesting insights into potential risk and protective factors. The presence of Dyslexia alone may be a specific risk factor for increased internalising, anxious and depressive symptomatology. Thankfully dyslexia is only a risk factor and it does not necessarily entail a negative outcome (Terras 2012), as this potential negative influence may be tempered by a range of protective influences such as adaptive coping strategies, good self-esteem and understanding of the nature of their reading and associated difficulties, positive educational experiences, and good family and social support.

THE WAY FORWARD: INTEGRATION AND METHODOLOGY

The utility of a resilience perspective lies in its integrative, explanatory and research value. It provides a framework not only to integrate existing research findings but also a means to situate and stimulate future research which will progress our understanding of the psycho-social dimension of dyslexia. Applying a Resilience perspective supports a move away from a focus on deficits and help promote an understanding of the factors associated with successful functioning and adjustment as well as failure (Terras et al. 2009; Terras 2016).

As noted earlier, many interesting insights have been offered from qualitative research and much of the existing evidence base concerning socio-emotional functioning is often cross-sectional and largely correlational in nature, and only allows the identification of potential risk and protective factors. Therefore future research should adopt a longitudinal approach to obtain a more detailed understanding of the nature of the relationship between dyslexia and socio-emotional and behavioural difficulties across the lifespan. Longitudinal studies are being increasingly used to establish the developmental trajectory, aetiology and cognitive aspects of reading difficulties (Dilnit et al. 2016; Xia et al. 2016; Snowling and Melby-Lervåg 2016).

Future longitudinal research aimed at deepening and progressing our understanding of the socio-emotional dimension of dyslexia would benefit from adopting a mixed-methodology which includes both qualitative and qualitative approaches. Quantitative measures with a sufficiently large sample size will support the application of computational and statistical modelling techniques such as structural equation modelling to detect causal relationships (Zevin and Miller 2016) and assist with greater robustness and generalisation of findings and aid the identification of risk and protective factors. The use of qualitative methodologies which allow exploration of the lived experience within the same study will add greater depth and aid a more nuanced interpretation of the quantitative findings.

It is therefore encouraging to note that recent longitudinal studies within the cognitive domain are adopting a resilience-based approach. Studies examining children at familial risk of Dyslexia have identified protective factors that modify the expression of a dyslexic predisposition with results indicating that children at familial risk of dyslexia who have good oral language skills may be able to compensate for reading failure by drawing upon their semantic skill to offset the impact of weaker phonological decoding abilities when reading. Suggesting that good verbal skills may be a protective factor in enabling early compensation for children at risk of dyslexia. Other protective factors identified include the timing and quality of the intervention, attentional ability, and an environment that fosters high levels of print exposure (Mutter and Snowling 2009). A number of predictors of poor outcome i.e., risk factors are also identified such as: severity, co-occurrence of attentional problems, maths problems, poor fine motor skills and spoken language impairments.

The adoption of a longitudinal lifespan approach is essential as the socio-emotional functioning of adults with dyslexia cannot be understood in isolation; emotional adjustment must be viewed in context generally, and in a developmental context in particular. We need to understand if and how difficulties develop, evolve and/or dissipate across the lifespan; how the socio-emotional and cognitive facets of dyslexia interact in order to identify the developmental trajectory of associated risk and protective factors. Interestingly, Mutter and Snowling (2009) also situate their research more widely by considering the influence of psycho-social influences by recommending that children are encouraged to engage in non-academic activities to help promote their more general self-esteem in the context of potentially poor academic achievement. Furthermore they also highlight the influence of environmental factors such as failure to recognise a reading difficulty; poor teaching, lack of learning support resources, low level of home support and poor family relations. It is interesting to note that many of these environmental factors, especially self-esteem, quality of educational support and family support are consistent with those identified as playing a role in psycho-social outcomes. Therefore a resilience perspective may not only help promote and consolidate research on psycho-social functioning but may also help to integrate research on the cognitive and psycho-social dimensions and thereby provide us a more global understanding of dyslexia (Terras 2012).

Despite the potential usefulness of viewing dyslexia through a resilience lens, it is necessary to recognise deficiencies within existing resilience research: The two most notable are: (1) the multi-dimensional nature of resilience, and (2) the need to move from a descriptive to an explanatory level (Luthar, Cicchetti and Becker 2000). The complex and multi-dimensional nature of resilience is actually a strength when considering the functioning of individuals with dyslexia. The finding that resilience may not apply across all domains nicely captures the individual differences in psycho-social functioning that are documented in both the research literature and encountered in practice. It is important to note that there is variability not only between individuals, but also within individuals across different domains of psycho-social functioning and over time. The second criticism is more serious and the inherent danger of applying a purely descriptive framework should be noted and addressed. If our understanding is to progress then we must not only identify risk and protective factors to the socio-emotional well-being of individuals with dyslexia, we must explore and understand how they operate at an explanatory level i.e., develop an understanding of the actual processes that underlie the operation of risk and protective factors. As noted previously, this may be best be achieved by adopting a more rigorous approach to the research methodologies used to ensure that robust statistical techniques that support the identification of causal linkages as opposed to simple associative relationships can be applied.

To conclude, the adoption of a resilience approach to help interpret current findings and situate future research offers an exciting way forward. Future research is required to develop our understanding of the risk and protective factors that influence the socio-emotional functioning of individuals with dyslexia. Future research must be robust enough, not only to descriptively examine but also to, generate explanatory causal accounts of the complex relationships between external and internal risk and protective factors that operate across the lifespan. It should therefore be longitudinal in nature; be ambitious, inclusive and integrative in the type and range of methodological techniques used, and be informed by the experiences of individuals with dyslexia. Such information may be derived not only from methodologies that allow examination of the lived experience across the lifespan. but also from practice. It may be informative to develop the scope of the relationship between research and practice; clearly the need for evidence-based practice remains paramount but it is also important to develop the two-way interactive relationship between and practice and research, with practice-derived insights functioning as a stimulus to future research and systematic evaluations. Our awareness of the socio-emotional aspects of living with Dyslexia on a daily basis has been raised by research examining how individuals cope and adapt with the functional and emotional sequela of dyslexia (Terras et al. 2012) and if this understanding is to be developed in the future then greater integration of the cognitive and psych-social dimensions of dyslexia is required; a resilience-based approach is well-placed to support this.

REFERENCES

Alexander-Passe, N. (2015). Dyslexia: Investigating Self-Harm and Suicidal Thoughts/Attempts as a Coping Strategy. *J. Psychol. Psychother.*, *5*(224), 2161-0487.

Alexander-Passe, N. (2013). Dyslexia, Dating, Marriage and Parenthood. NY: Nova Science/.

Alexander-Passe, N. (2006). How dyslexic teenagers cope: An investigation of self-esteem, coping and depression. *Dyslexia*, 12, 256–275.

Burden, R. (2008), Is dyslexia necessarily associated with negative feelings of self-worth? A review and implications for future research. Dyslexia, 14: 188–196.

Budren, R., and Burdett, J. (2005). Factors associated with successful learning in pupils with dyslexia: A motivational analysis. *British Journal of Special Education*, 32(2), 100–104.

Dilnot, J., Hamilton, L., Maughan, B., and Snowling, M. J. (2016). Child and environmental risk factors predicting readiness for learning in children at high risk of dyslexia. *Development and psychopathology*, 1-10.

Endler, N. S., and Parker, J. D. A. (1999). Coping Inventory for Stressful Situations: CISS Manual (2nd ed.). New York: Multi-Health Systems.

Folkman, S., Lazarus, R. S., Gruen, R. J., and DeLongis, A. (1986). Appraisal, coping, health status, and psychological symptoms. *Journal of personality and social psychology*, *50*(3), 571.

Gerber, P. J., and Price, L. A. (2012). Self-disclosure in adults with learning disabilities and dyslexia. Supporting Dyslexic Adults in Higher Education and the Workplace, 136.

Gonzalez, J. M. R., Cannell, M. B., Jetelina, K. K., and Froehlich-Grobe, K. (2015). Disproportionate Prevalence Rate of Prisoners With Disabilities Evidence From a Nationally Representative Sample. *Journal of Disability Policy Studies*, 1044207315616809.

Humphrey, N. (2002). Teacher and pupil ratings of self-esteem in developmental dyslexia. *British Journal of special education*, *29*(1), 29-36.

Klassen, R. M., Tze, V. M., and Hannok, W. (2013). Internalizing Problems of Adults with Learning Disabilities A Meta-Analysis. *Journal of learning disabilities*, *46*(4), 317-327.

Lazarus, R. S. and Folkman, S. (1984). Stress, Appraisal and Coping. New York: Springer.

Luthar, S. S., Cicchetti, D., and Becker, B. (2000). The construction of resilience: A critical evaluation and guidelines for future work. *Child Development*, 71(5), 543–562.

Macdonald, S. J., and Deacon, L. (2015). 'No sanctuary': Missed opportunities in health and social services for homeless people with dyslexia? *Social Work and Social Sciences Review*, *17*(3), 78-93.

Margalit, M. (2004). Second-generation research on resilience: Social-emotional aspects of children with learning disabilities. *Learning Disabilities Research and Practice*, 19(1), 45–48.

Maughan, B., and Hagell, A. (1996). Poor readers in adulthood: Psycho-social functioning. *Development and Psychopathology*, 8, 457-476

Maughan, B., and Carroll, J. (2006). Literacy and mental disorders. *Current Opinion in Psychiatry*, 19, 350–354.

Maughan, B., Messer, J., Collishaw, S., Pickles, A., Snowling, M., Yule, W., and Rutter, M. (2009). Persistence of literacy problems: spelling in adolescence and at mid-life. *Journal of Child Psychology and Psychiatry*, *50*(8), 893-901.

Mikami, A. Y., and Hinshaw, S. F. (2006). Resilient adolescent adjustment among girls: Buffers of childhood peer rejection and attention-deficit/hyperactivity disorder. *Journal of Abnormal Child Psychology*, 34(6), 823–837.

Mugnaini, D., Lassi, S.,Giampaolo M., and Albertini., G. (2009). Internalizing correlates of Dyslexia. *World Journal of Pediatrics*, 5(4), 255-264.

Nalavany, B. A., Carawan, L. W. and Brown, L. J. (2011), Considering the role of traditional and specialist schools: do school experiences impact the emotional well-being and self-esteem of adults with dyslexia? *British Journal of Special Education*, 38: 191–200.

Nalavany, B. A., Carawan, L. W., and Sauber, S. (2015). Adults with dyslexia, an invisible disability: the mediational role of concealment on perceived family support and self-esteem. *British Journal of Social Work*, *45*(2), 568-586.

Ozernov-Palchik, O., and Gaab, N. (2016). Tackling the 'dyslexia paradox': reading brain and behavior for early markers of developmental dyslexia. *Wiley Interdisciplinary Reviews: Cognitive Science*, *7*(2), 156-176.

Riddock, B., Sterling, C., Farmer, M., and Morgan, S. (1999). Self-esteem and anxiety in the educational histories of adult dyslexic students. *Dyslexia*, 5, 227–248.

Snowling, M. J., and Melby-Lervåg, M. (2016). Oral Language Deficits in Familial Dyslexia: A Meta-Analysis and Review. Psychological Bulletin.

Snowling, M. J., Muter, V., and Carrol, J. (2007). Children at family risk of dyslexia: A followup in early adolescence. *Journal of Child Psychology and Psychiatry*, 48(6), 609–618.

Rutter, M. (2000). Psychosocial influences: Critiques, findings, and research needs. *Development and Psychopathology*, 12, 375–405.

Terras M. M. (2016). Dyslexia in Adulthood: Experiences, Coping and the Importance of Resilience. Proceedings of the British Dyslexia Association 10th International Conference, 10-12 March 2016, Oxford.

Terras, M. M. (2012). Dyslexia and Psycho-social Adjustment: A Resilience Perspective, In Alexander-Passe, N. (Ed) Dyslexia and Mental Health: An investigation from differing perspectives. NY: Nova Science Publishers. Inc.

Terras M. M., Ramsay, J. and McMaster, L. (2010). Dyslexia in Adulthood: Experiential impact, Coping strategies and technology use. Proceedings of the British Psychological Society Annual Conference, 14-16 April, Stratford-upon-Avon.

Terras M. M., Thompson L. C., and Minnis, H. (2009). Dyslexia and Psycho-social Functioning: An exploratorystudy of the role of self-esteem and understanding. *Dyslexia*, 15(4), 304-327.

Terras, M. M., MacKenzie E., Thompson L., Minnis, H., (2004). I feel very, very small: Reflections on living with dyslexia. Proceedings of the 6th British Dyslexia Association International Conference, University of Warwick, 27th-30 March 2004.

Willcutt, E. G., and Pennington, B. F. (2000). Psychiatric comorbidity in children and adolescents with reading disability. *Journal of Child Psychology and Psychiatry*, 41(8), 1039–1048.

Xia, Z., Hoeft, F., Zhang, L., and Shu, H. (2016). Neuroanatomical anomalies of dyslexia: Disambiguating the effects of disorder, performance, and maturation. *Neuropsychologia*, *81*, 68-78.

Yates, R. (2013). Bad mouthing, bad habits and bad, bad, boys: an exploration of the relationship between dyslexia and drug dependence. *Mental health and substance use*, *6*(3), 184-202.

Zevin, J. D., and Miller, B. (2016). Introduction to the special issue. Advancing the state-of-the-science in reading research through modelling. *Scientific Studies of Reading*, *20*(1), 1-5.

RELATED NOVA PUBLICATIONS

DYSLEXIA AND DEPRESSION: THE HIDDEN SORROW

Author: Neil Alexander-Passe (London South Bank University, London, UK)

ISBN: 978-1-60876-118-0 Publication Date: 2010

This book is the culmination of fifteen years of the author's research into dyslexia. As a dyslexic himself, the author grew up with many difficulties in dealing with both family and school life. As an adult he wanted to understand more about dyslexia, how it affects individuals and be better prepared if dyslexia affected his own children. So he began an academic study of the emotional effects, rather than educational interventions, based on the collection of the neurological deficit symptoms defined as dyslexia.

The book begins by reviewing the cause and effects of depression, starting from anxiety and leading through defensive mechanisms to depression. Parallels were made to other learning disability groups who also suffer from depression, suggesting that groups that experience exclusion from mainstream society are at higher risk of depression.

The book also investigates dyslexia, by reviewing past empirical research into its symptoms and diagnosis, into how it affects individuals at school, at home and lastly in the workplace. Such a review was felt to be needed to enlighten the reader to the historical aspect of dyslexia, which many believe to be 'medical in cause, but educational in treatment'. Whilst dyslexia may have been recognised by many medical minds for over a century, it has only been fully recognised by educationalists for less than a decade, thus the study of secondary manifestations due to a lack of recognition by teachers is the basis for this book. A review is also given of several of the authors own published works, of which two form pilot studies for this book.

The main study of N=29 adult dyslexics used both qualitative (Interpretative Phenomenological Analysis-IPA) and quantitative methodologies. IPA was found to be beneficial in understanding the life experiences and secondary manifestations in participants.

The majority of participants were only diagnosed as dyslexic after leaving school and this the author finds typical of the many dyslexics he has encountered. Whilst the study set out to investigate depression as a sub-factor, it turned out to be the main focus of the study, as the majority of those who took part were depressed at some points in their child and/or adult lives. Gender also turned out to be an important variable in understanding how male and female dyslexics cope with the educational experiences they encountered.

In the discussion chapter, three hypothetical models of how dyslexics cope are suggested based on parenting type and style, through an investigation of cause and effect, leading to proposed interventions to tackle helplessness developing from mainstream education.

This book is a suitable reference book for a range of individuals, beginning with researchers in the field; to educationalists looking to understand the secondary and long-term effects of the condition; to parents of dyslexics looking to understand their children; and finally to dyslexics themselves, who are looking to understand their condition better. It is hoped that dyslexics who read this book will realise that their feelings of being an outsider are typical of those living with a 'hidden' disability or disorder that touches every part of their lives.

This book has been an emotional journey for both the author and those who took part in the study. Many participants noted that they knew very few, if any, dyslexics and their interview was the first time they had taken time to understand and discuss their dyslexia and how the effects of their childhood and school experiences had manifested themselves into lifelong secondary psychological and emotional affects.

Dyslexia and Creativity: Investigations from Differing Perspectives

Editors: Neil Alexander-Passe (London, UK)

ISBN: 978-1-61668-552-2 Publication Date: 2010

'Dyslexia and Creativity: An Academic Perspective' is the first in a series to investigate under-researched areas of dyslexia. It has come from a need to investigate a much quoted but little researched and substantiated area of dyslexia, namely positive attributes or talents that have come out of having a learning disability. Whilst traditional understanding of creativity is solely concerned with the arts, wider investigation suggests it includes many other careers, from cooking to sport, business to politics. Thus creativity can be seen is all areas of society.

As dyslexia is traditionally perceived to be a disability affecting reading and writing, many imagine that dyslexics are unable to attain in our word-based society. However many have, and these include world leaders and celebrities, in a range of areas. Those believed to be dyslexic, include:

- Inventors (Leonardo da Vinci, Albert Einstein, Thomas Edison and Michael Faraday),
- Artists (Leonardo da Vinci, David Bailey, Pablo Picasso, Andy Warhol, Auguste Rodin),
- Actors (Tom Cruise, Robin Williams, Kiera Knightly, Keanu Reeves, Whoppi Goldberg),
- Sports people (Mohammed Ali, Sir Steven Redgrave, Magic Johnson, Bruce Jenner, Nolan Ryan, Sir Jackie Stewart),
- Political leaders (Winston Churchill, John F Kennedy, George Washington), and
- Business people (Sir Richard Branson, Henry Ford, William Hewlett, Charles Schwab, Ted Turner)

So how can they be dyslexic and attain to such high standards? What is that they have, in addition to their difficulties that allow them to reach international success?

One explanation is that dyslexics develop compensation skills as a reaction to their difficulties; another suggests that the dyslexic brain is neurologically different, and a third sees dyslexics as part of the next stage in human evolution, with superior abilities for our modern age.

However research to date has been unable to support the claim that dyslexics are creative or have visual-spatial talents in excess of the normal population. Thus this book aims to shed light on the issue, through three types of perspectives: (1) Academic Perspectives; (2) Personal Perspectives; and (3) Alternative Perspectives.

'Dyslexia and Creativity: An Academic Perspective' is the collection of sixteen perspectives, from authors and artists from the US, UK, Sweden and Australia, which aim to enlighten the reader to new academic research, personal views of dyslexic artists, and an investigative interview study challenging dyslexic artists to 'what makes the dyslexic artist unique'.

'Dyslexia and Creativity: An Academic Perspective' is an ideal reference book for researchers, educators, artists, and dyslexics who seek understanding of their creative abilities.

Dyslexia and Mental Health: Investigations from Differing Perspectives

Editor: Neil Alexander-Passe (Middlesex University, London, UK)

ISBN: 978-1-62100-432-5 Publication Date: 2012

This is the second book of this series, the first being 'Dyslexia and Creativity'. This format has been found to be advantageous to inform readers that looking at issues from a singular angle can cause distortion, so several points of reference are used to better understand complex problems. Enclosed you will find the work of nine professors and other researchers in the field, some taking highly academic perspectives, whilst others prefer a more down-to-earth style. Chapters are also included from neurologists, educational psychologists and employment specialists, who give alternative ways to understand the topic. No one continent has the whole picture, thus a worldwide span is required to do the subject justice, with the authors reflecting this concept. (Imprint: Nova)

Dyslexia: A Visual Approach

Author: Carlo Aleci (Department of Ophthalmology, The Gradenigo Hospital, Turin, Italy)

ISBN: 978-1-62618-534-0 Publication Date: 2013

Even if the ophthalmological aspects of developmental dyslexia are generally considered negligible in comparison to the cognitive and phonological ones, a growing body of evidence suggests in many patients the presence of deficiencies related to a neuronal subpopulation along the visual pathway. Still, even in the limited area of neuro-ophtalmological research, there is no general agreement on the mechanisms underlying reading impairment and on how the aetiological element determines the phenotype, that is to say the typical symptomatology. Nevertheless, the spatial and temporal vision in dyslexics seem to be defective.

The purpose of this work is to report in a critical way the state of the art visual research in developmental dyslexia, without considering the aspects that go beyond our competence. In the second part of the treatise, the personal approach to the visuoperceptive impairment in this clinical condition is phenomenological rather than aetiological: it investigates the problem from the perceptive symptoms and signs rather than from the causal hypothesis and from the anatomofunctional demonstration.

Without claiming to exhaust the subject, we have pursued a triple aim: trying to shed light on one of the most debated and controversial questions, providing a rigorous and comprehensive overview on the current acquisitions, and, why not, offering some cues to those who intend to contribute to solve this problem.

Leaders, Visionaries and Dreamers: Extraordinary People with Dyslexia and Other Learning Disabilities

Authors: Paul J. Gerber (School of Education, Virginia Commonwealth University, Richmond, VA, USA)

and Marshall H. Raskind (Bainbridge Island, WA, USA)

ISBN: 978-1-62808-873-1 Publication Date: 2013

This book is an in-depth look at 12 incredible people with LD and dyslexia whose lives are characterized by major accomplishments and contributions that they have made in their respective fields as well as on the contemporary American scene. These men and women are from a variety of fields – arts and literature, science, politics and sports. Included are individuals such as Gavin Newsom, Lieutenant Governor of California; Gaston Caperton, former governor of West Virginia and President of the College Board; MacArthur Fellowship "Genius Award"-winning paleontologist, Jack Horner; one of America's pre-eminent visual artists, Chuck Close; actor Henry Winkler and financier Charles Schwab.

The book is not framed as a "feature piece" but one that develops the trials, tribulations and triumphs in unique ways, befitting those who have become extraordinarily successful despite the odds. The writing is constructed to explore a myriad of underlying dynamics of accomplishment to give the reader a thematic view of LD and dyslexia by hearing the voices of those included in the book. The content for the book was derived from extensive interviews and is presented in a reader-friendly format from what has been gleaned from research and the prevailing wisdom in this area over the last 25 years.

INDEX

E

H

I

L

M

N

P

R

S

T

W